Depression and Personality

Series Editors

Mariane Krause
Millennium Institute for Research in Depression and Personality;
School of Psychology
Pontificia Universidad Católica de Chile, Santiago
RM-Santiago, Chile

Guillermo de la Parra
Millennium Institute for Research in Depression and Personality;
Department of Psychiatry
Pontifical Catholic University of Chile
Santiago, RM - Santiago, Chile

Alemka Tomicic
Millennium Institute for Research in Depression and Personality;
Faculty of Psychology
Universidad Diego Portales
Santiago, RM - Santiago, Chile

The Depression and Personality book series presents cutting edge knowledge regarding the causes, treatment, and prevention of depression from a perspective that takes into account the interaction between depression and personality and the influences of multiple dimensions that contribute to the development, maintenance, and exacerbation of depression in different populations. The series is published in collaboration with the Millennium Institute for Research in Depression and Personality (MIDAP), a scientific center of excellence in Chile made up of psychologists, psychiatrists and professionals from various areas of social sciences and health, who seek to generate knowledge based on a multidimensional understanding of depression.
MIDAP's characteristic multidimensional and multidisciplinary approach implies the development of an empirically-based model that takes into account the etiology, prevention, intervention, and rehabilitation of depression. This multidimensional and multidisciplinary model is evidenced in the titles of the series, which cover, individually or in combination, the following topics:

1. Basic bio-psycho-social structures and processes involved in depression and its interaction with the personality.
2. Health promotion and psychosocial intervention strategies that would prevent early conditions associated with the development of depression and personality dysfunction.
3. Psychotherapeutic interventions and mechanisms involved in symptomatic relief and change processes in diverse types of depressive patients.
4. Rehabilitation and reintegration interventions oriented to reduce the chronicity of depression and to maintain gains after treatment, as well as, topics regarding early-life maltreatment and co-morbid personality dysfunction as risk factors of chronic or recurrent courses of depression.

More information about this series at http://www.springer.com/series/16388

Guillermo de la Parra • Paula Dagnino
Alex Behn
Editors

Depression and Personality Dysfunction

An Integrative Functional Domains Perspective

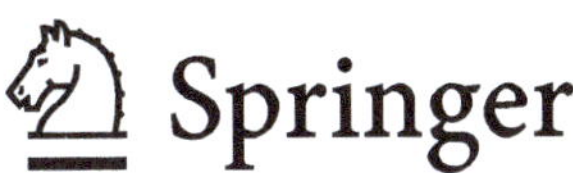

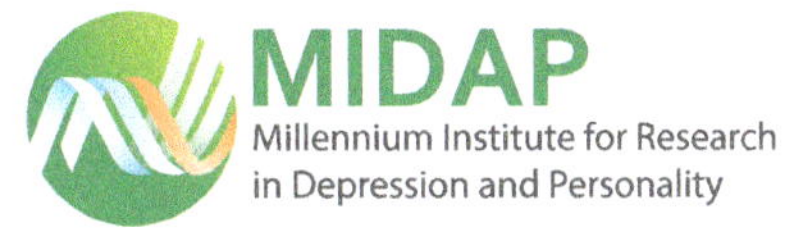

Editors
Guillermo de la Parra
Millennium Institute for Research in
Depression and Personality;
Department of Psychiatry
Pontificia Universidad Católica de Chile
Santiago, RM - Santiago, Chile

Paula Dagnino
Millennium Institute for Research
in Depression and Personality;
Faculty of Psychology
Universidad Alberto Hurtado
Santiago, RM - Santiago, Chile

Alex Behn
Millennium Institute for Research
in Depression and Personality;
School of Psychology
Pontificia Universidad Católica de Chile
Santiago, RM - Santiago, Chile

ISSN 2662-3587 ISSN 2662-3595 (electronic)
Depression and Personality
ISBN 978-3-030-70698-2 ISBN 978-3-030-70699-9 (eBook)
https://doi.org/10.1007/978-3-030-70699-9

This Springer imprint is published by the registered company Springer Nature Switzerland AG
The registered company address is: Gewerbestrasse 11, 6330 Cham, Switzerland

About the Series Editors

Mariane Krause Mariane Krause is a professor at Pontificia Universidad Católica de Chile's School of Psychology. She obtained her doctoral degree at Freie Universität Berlin (Germany). Her areas of research are change processes in psychotherapy, depression, and the interaction between sociocultural and mental health conditions. She has led several research projects in these areas, with funding from the Millennium Scientific Initiative of the Ministry of Economy, Development, and Tourism (ICM-Chile), the National Committee of Scientific and Technological Research (CONICYT-Chile), and the United Nations Development Program. Currently, she is the principal investigator at the Millennium Institute for Research in Depression and Personality (MIDAP), a Chilean center of excellence in research, which received funding for 10 years starting in 2015. Since 2017, she is the principal investigator of the Latin American Network in Psychotherapy Process Research, funded by the National Committee of Scientific and Technological Research (CONICYT-Chile). Between 2013 and 2016, she was president of the Latin American Chapter of the Society for Psychotherapy Research. In 2016, she received the National Award of the Chilean Society for Clinical Psychology. Currently she is president of the Society for Psychotherapy Research.

Guillermo de la Parra Guillermo de la Parra, M.D., Ph.D., is full professor of psychiatry in the Department of Psychiatry at Pontificia Universidad Católica de Chile. He received his Ph.D. from the Ulm University, Germany. He has developed three interest areas: First, he has been interested in offering therapeutic services to socioeconomically vulnerable patients. For this reason, he has founded psychotherapy units in public institutions and the University Outpatient Clinic, as a space for care, research, and teaching. Second, as former president of the International Society for Psychotherapy Research, he has been interested in bridging the gap between cultures and also between research and clinical practice, applying and assessing evidence-based models in Psychotherapy Units. Third, his research in the frame of the Millennium Institute for Research in Depression and Personality (MIDAP), in a country where depressive illness is relevant, has been devoted to the depressive patient, his/her personality style, and personality structure in its relation to depression. In recent times, he has developed models of psychotherapeutic competencies for the treatment of complex depression in primary healthcare, based on the MIDAP model.

Alemka Tomicic Alemka Tomicic, Ph.D., is associated researcher at the Center of Studies in Clinical Psychology and Psychotherapy and director of the School of Psychology both in the Faculty of Psychology at Universidad Diego Portales. She obtained her doctoral degree from the Pontificia Universidad Católica de Chile. Dr. Tomicic has done studies in three areas of research. In the first one, research in psychotherapeutic process and patient-therapist interaction, she has focused on the interactive phenomena that underlie the process of change of psychotherapy patients. For its part, in the second area, namely studies on the subjective construction of mental health problems, she has centered on first- and second-person experiences relating to mental health problems and/or psychological treatment and psychotherapy, as well as on the subjective meanings attributed to these experiences. Finally, in the third research area, regarding mental health and psychotherapy in the context of sexual and gender diversity, Dr. Tomicic has focused on the clinical and psychotherapeutic skills needed to carry out sensitive and well-informed psychological interventions on the social determinants of mental health affecting LGBTI+ patients. Also, these three topics of her concern have found a place in the Millennium Institute for Research in Depression and Personality (MIDAP), in which she is part as associated researcher.

Series Editors' Preface: Depression and Personality: A Multidimensional Perspective

The aim of this book series on depression and personality is to provide their readers cutting-edge knowledge regarding the causes, treatment, and prevention of depression from a perspective that takes into account the interaction between depression and personality and the influences of multiple dimensions that contribute to the development, maintenance, and exacerbation of depression in different populations. This series arises as a collaboration between the Millennium Institute for Research in Depression and Personality (MIDAP) and Springer.

MIDAP is a research center made up of psychologists, psychiatrists, and professionals from various areas of social sciences and health who seek to generate knowledge based on a multidimensional understanding of depression in interaction with personality, with the objective of maximizing the effectiveness of interventions by identifying the agents and mechanisms of change involved in prevention, psychotherapy, and rehabilitation.

Around 200 researchers and students make up MIDAP's scientific team, coming mainly from its 6 host institutions: Pontificia Universidad Católica de Chile, Universidad de Chile, Universidad del Desarrollo, Universidad de La Frontera, Universidad de Valparaíso, and Universidad Diego Portales. MIDAP is part of several international scientific networks that include researchers from most Latin American countries, the USA, Canada, Germany, Switzerland, the UK, Italy, Spain, and Portugal.

In the year 2015, MIDAP developed due to two historical research initiatives: the Chilean "Psychotherapy and Change Research Group," which now includes researchers from nine Latin American countries, and the Millennium Nucleus "Psychological Intervention and Change in Depression," a Chilean state-funded research center. In the framework of these scientific initiatives, a combination of psychological, psychosocial, and psychophysiological approaches to depression were examined and tested. This multidimensional approach to the study of depression was continued by MIDAP, including, at the same time, a differentiated analysis of personality and all the relevant dimensions involved in depression and personality disorders.

MIDAP's research activities follow four lines of research:

1. Basic bio-psycho-social structures and processes involved in depression and its interaction with the personality
2. Health promotion and psychosocial intervention strategies that intend to prevent early life conditions associated with the development of depression and personality dysfunction
3. Psychotherapeutic interventions and mechanisms involved in symptomatic relief and change processes in diverse types of depressive patients
4. Rehabilitation and reintegration interventions oriented to reduce the chronicity of depression and to maintain its benefits gained through treatment, as well as to address topics regarding childhood adversity and co-morbid personality dysfunction as risk factors of chronic or recurrent courses of depression

MIDAP's multidimensional and multidisciplinary approach aims to construct an empirical model that takes into account the etiology, prevention, intervention, and rehabilitation of depression. This approach addresses the relationship between depression and personality, along with the multiple dimensions of human functioning that have been empirically linked to this disorder. Thus, MIDAP developed systematic research on each of these dimensions, which include developmental, cognitive, emotional, and behavioral variables, as well as others of a psychophysiological and genetic nature. MIDAP pursues this multidimensional scientific agenda using a variety of methods and multiple research designs and analytic strategies, including cross-sectional, longitudinal, experimental, and naturalistic designs; process-and outcome-oriented studies; as well as action/applied research and quantitative and qualitative data-analyses strategies.

So far, knowledge on depression and personality developed by MIDAP, together with current findings from other research initiatives in each of the aforementioned dimensions, can be organized in two main categories leading to two different (but related) perspectives in the understanding of mental disorders. The first is an individual's life path, which begins before birth and continues to influence contemporaries and descendants after death. Life paths are influenced by – placed in a continuum – biogenetic determinants at one end and social determinants at the other end, which, in turn, influence each other. The second category comprises current contextual determinants of human well-being, including biological as well as sociocultural conditions involved in the onset and maintenance of disorders and their treatments.

As an example of the precedent, initial results of a longitudinal study, developed by MIDAP in collaboration with other Chilean centers and institutes, show the high prevalence of depressive symptomatology in women from disadvantaged socioeconomic sectors (Hojman et al., 2018). From the life path perspective, poverty could be seen as a causal determinant of depression through its relation with childhood adversity (e.g., Ridley et al., 2020), shaping the biopsychosocial development of a person. From the perspective of current contextual determinants, it can be both a triggering factor or a chronic stressor in daily life of people, thus making the initial causal conditions of depression more acute (Krause et al., 2018). Furthermore, this example includes the gender dimension, which can also be read from the perspective of social determinant factors, as life-span conditions or as current contextual socio-cultural determinant, manifested in both cases through inequality, discrimination, and violence against women.

These two perspectives are relevant when researchers focus on the conditions for the occurrence of depression or personality disorders, or when trying to determine the best interventions to prevent or heal people with these disorders. For example, from the life path perspective, studies on depression, epigenetics, and psychotherapy show that genetic sensitivity is involved in the fact that some individuals develop depression whereas others under the same conditions do not, and that, paradoxically, the higher genetic sensitivity relates positively to a greater benefit from psychotherapeutic intervention (e.g., Jimenez et al., 2018). From the perspective of current social and cultural determinants, findings range from the interaction of daily life stressors and social support with depressive disorders (Dagnino et al., 2017) to the identification of barriers for accessing competent and high-quality health services, including psychotherapy (Krause et al., 2018).

These are examples of how the multidimensional and multidisciplinary approach has implied the development and empirical testing of a model that takes into account the etiology, prevention, intervention, and rehabilitation of depression and personality. This model is evidenced in the titles of the series that range from the relationship between depression and personality dysfunction through the etiology of depression (including fundamental topics like suicide, treatment, child development, and psychotherapeutic process research) to the development and evaluation of intervention strategies, namely prevention and psychotherapy.

Specifically, the book series intends to cover, individually or combined, the following topics: depression and personality dysfunction, etiopathogenic theories and models in depression, prevention and management of depression, early socio-emotional development and depression, and psychotherapy process research in depression and personality disorders.

The first book of the series (*Depression and Personality Dysfunction: An integrative functional domains perspective*; editors: Guillermo de la Parra, Paula Dagnino, Alex Behn) presents an authoritative and up-to-date review of the clinical interaction between depression and personality dysfunction. The book covers this issue from the perspective of problems in domains of personality dysfunction that drive complex depressive presentations. First, a state of the art is presented, followed by contributions about domains of personality dysfunction thought to participate in complex depression. Finally, integrative models to think about complex depression – diagnostically and clinically – are presented. The book is thus meant to be a scientific and clinical guide for understanding and treating patients with complex depression. For a comprehensive description of this book, see "about the first book" in the section below.

The second book, entitled *Etiopathogenic Theories and Models in Depression* (editors: Juan Pablo Jiménez, Alberto Botto, Peter Fonagy) addresses depression as a complex psychopathological construct of high phenotypic heterogeneity. This book seeks to review different theories and models about depression, which belong to different etiopathogenic levels (from the molecular to the socio-cultural) understanding depression as a complex phenomenon in which the different explanatory levels interact with each other. The book examines conditions where the integrated consideration of different explanatory levels illuminates how depression originates and is maintained. The increasing knowledge about the interaction of these etiopathogenic levels is relevant when it comes to making therapeutic decisions with depressed patients or groups of patients. Such an integrated perspective is of high translational value for clinical practice.

The third book is devoted to new perspectives in the prevention and management of depression (editors: Vania Martínez Nahuel, Claudia Miranda-Castillo). This book presents current evidence on prevention, and the timely and appropriate management of depression in people of different ages. It includes a review of: innovation in global prevention and treatment, interventions based on mindfulness and contemplative practices, interventions in primary healthcare centers for adolescents and adults, the challenges in the management of depression and self-harm in mental health services for adolescents, a dimensional approach to management based on the description of mood disorders as a spectrum, and interventions for the elderly and their caregivers.

In a fourth book (editors: María Pía Santelices, Claudia Capella), the theme is how to promote child socioemotional development and thus prevent depression in the present and future. The book addresses different prevention and intervention strategies that favor children's socio-emotional development or prevent depressive illness and/or personality dysfunctions, which concerns researchers as well as professionals who work with children.

A further book of this series addresses suicide and suicide risk in different populations (editors: Susana Morales Silva, Jorge Barros Beck, Orietta Echávarri Vesperinas) with the purpose of offering effective tools (based on clinical experience and research findings) to health professionals that work with people at risk for suicide.

The series also includes a book that updates the empirical knowledge about the psychotherapeutic process in depression and personality disorders (editors: Mariane Krause, Daniel Espinosa, Olga Fernández). This book covers the evolution of psychotherapeutic change, significant episodes, and different change mechanisms, including patients' characteristics, and therapeutic activities involved in change processes.

The books that comprise this series are meant to be read by professionals working in the field of mental health (psychologists, psychiatrists, psychotherapists, primary care physicians, etc.), as well as by undergraduate and graduate students interested in acquiring a deeper knowledge of a multidimensional comprehension of depression and personality and tools for its prevention and intervention. Other targeted readers are researchers and academics, as some of the books in the series provide information on operational aspects for teaching and studying depression, personality, and its associated health problems.

Acknowledgments

The production of this book and its publication has been only possible thanks to our committed contributors, all of them notable scientists and clinicians who believed in this project and worked diligently on their chapters. They have all made important contributions to the field, and now important contributions to this book. We are truly and profoundly impressed and grateful for their work.

The ideas that led to the development of this book emerged in the setting of a rich and productive environment of scientific exchange and openness to new frontiers of academic and clinical work in the areas of depression and personality dysfunction. This environment is the Millennium Institute for Research in Depression and Personality (MIDAP) which has produced 6 years of dedicated, rigorous, and broad scientific work in this area. To this extent, we are immensely grateful to Mariane Krause who inspired and led so much of the way in the development of MIDAP and to Juan Pablo Jimenez who has led this endeavor during the past years, further consolidating MIDAP´s work in Chile, Latin America, and the world. The international nature of contributions for this book documents the international scope of the institute´s work and highlights the fundamental idea that research in mental health is a global endeavor.

MIDAP is a government-funded research institute, and the book project as well as many of its chapters were reliant on work funded by the Agencia Nacional de Investigación y Desarrollo (ANID) and the Millennium Science Initiative. We are grateful for the existence of this agency and the remarkable work conducted in supporting local scientific initiatives.

MIDAP´s capacity to sustain a remarkable and productive research agenda in the areas of depression and personality dysfunction is also due to its host institutions; thus, we are grateful to the Pontificia Universidad Católica de Chile, the Universidad de Chile, the Universidad de la Frontra, the Universidad del Desarrollo, the Universidad de Valparaiso, and the Universidad Diego Portales for supporting the work of the Institute.

We are appreciative of the dedicated assistance of Alexandra Epstein during all phases of editorial preparation of the book.

About This Book

This book is consistent with MIDAP's perspective of understanding depression as a complex multicausal and multilevel phenomenon and personality disorders from a dimensional view, where it is preferred to talk about personality dysfunction rather than disorder. In that sense, the authors were put on a "forced foot": their contributions, product of their researches, revisions, and studies had to follow the perspective of functional domains. This challenge was met with enthusiasm by the various authors of the chapters and the result, as the reader will see, was successful.

The first chapter, "Depression and Personality Dysfunction: Towards the Understanding of Complex Depression," by Mariane Krause and Alex Behn, presents an integrative and dense synthesis of the state of the art regarding the relationship between depression and personality, a relationship that leads "to common or overlapping intermediate phenotypes."

The next 10 chapters are arranged in three parts: Part I: Domains of Personality Dysfunction Complicating the Presentation and Treatment of Depression; Part II: Integrative Models of Depression and Personality Dysfunction: Implications for Diagnosis and Treatment; and Part III: Concluding Remarks.

Part I includes Chap. 2, "The Functional Domain of Identity" by Klaus Schmeck, Susanne Schlüter-Müller, and Nelson Valdés-Sanchez in which they emphasize how the therapeutic approach of the depressed adolescent should take into account the bidirectional influence between identity formation and depression. In Chap. 3, "The Functional Domain of Affect Regulation," Carolina Altimir, Cecilia de la Cerda, and Paula Dagnino make an exhaustive review of the subject, understanding affect regulation from "a developmental perspective based on attachment theory and developmental research, including emotion processing models derived from psychological and neuroscientific research." In Chap. 4, "The Functional Domain of Self-Other Regulation," Nicolás Lorenzini, Peter Fonagy, and Patrick Luyten, after presenting an updated literature review including their own studies, propose a model for understanding the relationship between depression and personality dysfunction "based on three of the main component systems of the functional domains perspective of the Research Domain Criteria Initiative: stress regulation (negative valence and arousal/regulatory systems), reward (positive valence systems), and mentalizing (system for social processes or social cognition) systems", this, from a "developmental psychopathology perspective." In Chap. 5 "The Domain of Social Dysfunction in Complex Depressive Disorders," Devika Duggal, Eric Fertuck, and Steven Huprich directly focus on the five functional domains that can make depression complex: "occupational functioning, romantic and sexual relationships, leisure activities, affiliation and attachment, and social support networks." Chapter 6, "Neurobiological Findings Underlying Personality Dysfunction in Depression: From Vulnerability to Differential Susceptibility," by Alberto Botto and Caroline Leighton reviews, at the level of neurobiological evidence and the gene-environment relationship, the interaction between depression and personality, focusing on "differential sensitivity to environmental stimuli," which has consequences for both, susceptibility to depression and its psychotherapeutic treatment. This first part ends with Chap. 7, "The Functional Domain of Self-Criticism," in which Ulrike Dinger-Ehrenthal, Christina Löw, and Johannes Ehrenthal discuss the impact of personality dysfunction according to the "Structural Integration Axis of the Operationalized Psychodynamic Diagnosis System (OPD-2)" and how this dysfunction in its interaction with self-criticism affects depressive manifestations and their response to treatment.

Part II begins with Chap. 8, "Complex Depression and Early Adverse Stress: A Domain-Based Diagnostic Approach," written by Paul Vöhringer, Pablo Martinez, and Sergio Gloger. The authors present here a model of complex depression determined by childhood adversity, whose clinical manifestations would allow it to be differentiated from non-complex depression. In Chap. 9, "Complex Depression in High-Pressure Care Settings: Strategies and Therapeutic Competences," Guillermo de la Parra, Ana Karina Zúñiga, Paula Dagnino, and Elyna Gómez-Barris expand the term of complex depression not only to the aspects of personality (traits and dysfunctions) or the evolution and comorbidity of the illness but to the social context which surrounds the patient. Furthermore, the authors discuss how the characteristics of institutions, where public mental health professionals intervene, are an additional factor that contributes to the complexity of depression. They conclude by providing guidelines for the treatment of these complex patients in high-pressure care settings. Part II ends with Chap. 10, "Modular Treatment for Complex Depression According to Metacognitive Interpersonal Therapy," by Antonella Centonze, Paolo Ottavi, Angus MacBeth, Raffaele Popolo, and Giancarlo Dimaggio, in which they propose the detail of specific treatment strategies for specific dysfunctions, consistent with the general perspective of this book.

Part III ends the book with Chap. 11, "Where do we come from? Where are we moving to? Towards the development of precision psychotherapy," by Guillermo de la Parra, Alex Behn, and Paula Dagnino. After reviewing and comparing the different chapters, the authors wonder if, within the framework of the functional domain's perspective, we are in a position to speak of precision psychotherapy, paraphrasing the term *precision medicine* that comes from oncology.

In short, we think that the reader has in his/her hands a stimulating piece, completely in tune with the results of contemporary research and in line with the paradigm shift and the epistemological changes of the current *Zeitgeist* of an interrelated, complex reality, far from narrow categories.

Mariane Krause
Guillermo de la Parra
Alemka Tomicic

References

Dagnino, P., Pérez, C., Gómez, A., Gloger, S., & Krause, M. (2017). Depression and attachment: how do personality styles and social support influence this relation? *Research in Psychotherapy: Psychopathology, Process and Outcome, 20(1),* 53–62. https://doi.org/10.4081/ripppo.2017.237

Hojman, D., Krause, M., Llaupi, M., Rojas, G., & Verges, A. (2018). Salud Mental en el Chile de hoy. *Notas Centro de Estudios de Conflicto y Cohesión Social [COES], 15.* http://www.elsoc.cl/publicaciones-elsoc/informes

Jiménez, J., Botto, A., Herrera, L., Leighton, C., Rossi, J., Quevedo, Y., Silva, J., Martinez, F., Assar, R., Salazar, L., Ortiz, M. Ríos, U., Barros, P., Jaramillo, K, & Luyten, P. (2018). Psychotherapy and Genetic Neuroscience: An Emerging Dialog. *Frontiers in Genetic, 257*(9). https://doi.org/10.3389/fgene.2018.00257

Krause, M., Espinosa, H. D., Tomicic, A., Córdoba, A. C., & Vásquez, D. (2018). Psychotherapy for depression from the point of view of economically disadvantaged individuals in Chile and Colombia. *Counselling and Psychotherapy Research 18(2):*178–189. https://doi.org/10.1002/capr.12171

Ridley, M., Rao, G., Schilbach, F., & Patel, V. (2020). Poverty, depression, and anxiety: Causal evidence and mechanisms. *Science, 370*(6522). https://doi.org/10.1126/science.aay0214

Contents

Contributors

Carolina Altimir Facultad de Psicología, Universidad Alberto Hurtado, Santiago, Chile

Millennium Institute for Research in Depression and Personality (MIDAP), Santiago, Chile

Alex Behn Escuela de Psicología, Pontificia Universidad Católica de Chile, Santiago, Chile

Millennium Institute for Research in Depression and Personality (MIDAP), Santiago, Chile

Alberto Botto Departamento de Psiquiatría y Salud Mental Campus Oriente, Facultad de Medicina, Universidad de Chile, Santiago, Chile

Millennium Institute for Research in Depression and Personality (MIDAP), Santiago, Chile

Antonella Centonze Centro di Terapia Metacognitiva Interpersonale, Rome, Italy

Paula Dagnino Facultad de Psicología, Universidad Alberto Hurtado, Santiago, Chile

Millennium Institute for Research in Depression and Personality (MIDAP), Santiago, Chile

Cecilia de la Cerda Departamento Disciplinario de Psicología, Facultad de Ciencias Sociales, Universidad de Playa Ancha, Valparaiso, Chile

Millennium Institute for Research in Depression and Personality (MIDAP), Santiago, Chile

Guillermo de la Parra Departamento de Psiquiatría, Escuela de Medicina, Pontificia Universidad Católica de Chile, Santiago, Chile

Millennium Institute for Research in Depression and Personality (MIDAP), Santiago, Chile

Giancarlo Dimaggio Centro di Terapia Metacognitiva Interpersonale, Rome, Italy

Ulrike Dinger-Ehrenthal Klinik für Allgemeine Innere Medizin und Psychosomatik, Universitätsklinikum Heidelberg, Universität Heidelberg, Heidelberg, Germany

Devika Duggal City College and Graduate Center, City University of New York, New York, NY, USA

Johannes C. Ehrenthal Department Psycholgie, Universität zu Köln, Köln, Germany

Eric A. Fertuck City College and Graduate Center, City University of New York, New York, NY, USA

Peter Fonagy Research Department of Clinical, Educational and Health Psychology, University College London, London, UK

Millennium Institute for Research in Depression and Personality (MIDAP), Santiago, Chile

Sergio Gloger Psicomédica Clinical & Research Group, Santiago, Chile

Departamento de Psiquiatría y Salud Mental Este, Facultad de Medicina, Universidad de Chile, Santiago, Chile

Elyna Gómez-Barris Departamento de Psiquiatría, Escuela de Medicina, Pontificia Universidad Católica de Chile, Santiago, Chile

Millennium Institute for Research in Depression and Personality (MIDAP), Santiago, Chile

Steven Huprich Michigan State University College of Human Medicine, East Lansing, MI, USA

University of Detroit Mercy, Detroit, MI, USA

Mariane Krause Escuela de Psicología, Pontificia Universidad Católica de Chile, Santiago, Chile

Millennium Institute for Research in Depression and Personality (MIDAP), Santiago, Chile

Caroline Leighton Departamento de Psiquiatría y Salud Mental Campus Oriente, Facultad de Medicina, Universidad de Chile, Santiago, Chile

Millennium Institute for Research in Depression and Personality (MIDAP), Santiago, Chile

Nicolás Lorenzini Research Department of Clinical, Educational and Health Psychology, University College London, London, UK

Christina A. Löw Klinik für Allgemeine Innere Medizin und Psychosomatik, Universitätsklinikum Heidelberg, Universität Heidelberg, Heidelberg, Germany

Psychologisches Institut, Universität Heidelberg, Heidelberg, Germany

Patrick Luyten Faculty of Psychology and Educational Sciences, KU Leuven (University of Leuven), Leuven, Belgium

Research Department of Clinical, Educational and Health Psychology, University College London, London, UK

Millennium Institute for Research in Depression and Personality (MIDAP), Santiago, Chile

Angus MacBeth Department of Clinical and Health Psychology, School of Health in Social Science, University of Edinburgh, Edinburgh, Scotland

Pablo Martinez Hospital Clínico de la Universidad de Chile, Universidad de Chile, Santiago, Chile

Millennium Institute for Research in Depression and Personality (MIDAP), Santiago, Chile

Paolo Ottavi Centro di Terapia Metacognitiva Interpersonale, Rome, Italy

Raffaele Popolo Centro di Terapia Metacognitiva Interpersonale, Rome, Italy

Susanne Schlüter-Müller Department of Child and Adolescent Psychiatric Research, Psychiatric University Hospitals, University of Basel, Basel, Switzerland

Millennium Institute for Research in Depression and Personality (MIDAP), Santiago, Chile

Klaus Schmeck Department of Child and Adolescent Psychiatric Research, Psychiatric University Hospitals, University of Basel, Basel, Switzerland

Millennium Institute for Research in Depression and Personality (MIDAP), Santiago, Chile

Nelson Valdés-Sánchez Psychology Department, Universidad Santo Tomás, Santiago, Chile

Millennium Institute for Research in Depression and Personality (MIDAP), Santiago, Chile

Paul A. Vöhringer Universidad de Chile, Santiago, Chile

Tufts University, Boston, MA, USA

Millennium Institute for Research in Depression and Personality (MIDAP), Santiago, Chile

Ana Karina Zúñiga Programa de Doctorado en Psicoterapia, Pontificia Universidad Católica de Chile y Universidad de Chile, Santiago, Chile

Millennium Institute for Research in Depression and Personality (MIDAP), Santiago, Chile

Chapter 1
Depression and Personality Dysfunction: Towards the Understanding of Complex Depression

Mariane Krause and Alex Behn

Abstract This introductory chapter presents a focused survey of the literature on the interaction between depression and personality, which represents one of the approaches to the issue of *complex depression*, which is treated from different perspectives throughout this book. Patients who, in addition to a depression, present with personality dysfunction are more than twice as likely to be nonresponders to treatment compared to patients with common, stand-alone depression. Furthermore, personality styles and the level of structural integration of personality are, as well, related to severity and to the response to treatment. For this reason, in order to assess *complex depression* and to improve treatment, it is important to deepen our understanding of the interaction of depression and personality. We examine this issue from the perspective of functional domains that are differentially affected in depression concurrent with personality dysfunction and specific personality styles, as well as how the co-occurrence of both impacts on the severity of the condition. The chapter outlines the complex and multimodal relationships between depression and personality dysfunction, discussing specific models for the interaction between depression and borderline personality disorder, on one hand, and personality styles and structural personality integration, on the other hand.

Keywords Depression · Personality disorders · Personality dysfunction · Intermediate phenotypes · Personality styles · Complex depression

---

M. Krause (✉) · A. Behn
Escuela de Psicología, Pontificia Universidad Católica de Chile, Santiago, Chile

Millennium Institute for Research in Depression and Personality (MIDAP), Santiago, Chile
e-mail: albehn@uc.cl

G. de la Parra et al. (eds.), *Depression and Personality Dysfunction*, Depression and Personality, https://doi.org/10.1007/978-3-030-70699-9_1

1.1 Introduction

Due to its high lifetime prevalence worldwide (10–15% of the population; Lépine & Briley, 2011) and high subjective and societal costs, major depressive disorders (MDD) need to be better understood. When depression is severe and long-lasting, it results in intense suffering for affected individuals, and also for their loved ones, leading as well to a significant decline in social and vocational functioning. Depression increases the risk for suicidality, comorbidity with other mental health conditions, and chronic physical illness and impairs physical and psychosocial functioning (Spijker, van Straten, Bockting, Meeuwissen, & van Balkom, 2013). Additionally, depression is a recurrent illness (DeRubeis, Siegle, & Hollon, 2008), with 50–60% of patients experiencing a second episode, 70% of these a third one, and 90% of these a fourth episode (Hart, Craighead, & Craighead, 2001). This means that many patients with this disorder spend up to 21% of their lives clinically depressed (Vos et al., 2004). Treating depression is a worldwide priority, but treatment effectiveness needs to be improved because only 30–40% of patients enrolled in randomized clinical trials (RCTs) show remission of symptoms (Craighead & Dunlop, 2014).

Further research in depression is urgent to improve detection and treatment of those affected. However, depression is a heterogeneous clinical phenomenon (Buch & Liston, 2020), presenting itself very differently across individuals and probably stemming from differential etiopathogenetic mechanisms (Cai, Choi, & Fried, 2020). This heterogeneity may be partially responsible for lack of substantive progress in treatment effectiveness. The interaction between depression and personality dysfunction is one domain suitable to parse out some aspects of the heterogeneity of depression. The term *complex depression* has been proposed by our group to understand depressive presentations that are further complicated by personality dysfunction (Behn, 2019). Nowadays the term has been extended to include other conditions that add severity to the course of the disorder and imply difficulties for its treatment, such as psychosocial stressors, early life maltreatment, risk of suicide, conditions related to the health system, and treatment, which is addressed throughout this book.

In this chapter *complex depression* will be examined through the lens of functional domains related to personality functioning, namely, affect regulation, identity, self and other regulation, socio-cognitive functioning, self-criticism (a form of self-dysregulation particularly important in depression), and neurobiological underpinnings related to depression complicated by personality dysfunction.

Generally speaking, complexity in mental health problems refers to the aggregation of difficulties or affected domains on top of the presenting problem (e.g., depression) and it refers to an intrinsically multidimensional construct, because depression can be complicated by comorbid mental health disorders. For the purposes of this chapter, complexity is restricted to the interaction between depressive symptomatology (i.e., a depressive phenotype) and personality dysfunction, including a dimensional component that admits subthreshold or mild personality dysfunction and a categorical component indicative of the presence of a personality disorder.

Regarding the latter, we will focus on borderline personality disorder (BPD) because this disorder concentrates most of the empirical research on personality pathology, and thus, more robust conclusions can be drawn from the depression and personality disorders literature. We will also examine personality styles as related to specific depressive phenotypes and personality structural integration.

1.2 The Overlap Between Depression and Personality Dysfunction in Classification Systems

The interaction between depression and personality functioning is relevant for the scientific understanding of the heterogeneity and complexity of depression as well as for the improvement of treatment options. Before we delve into co-occurrence or mutual influence models between both disorders, it is useful to discuss the general problem of symptomatic superposition between depression and personality pathology and the diagnostic difficulties that emerge.

The debate regarding a strict separation versus the superposition between depression and personality disorders is not new. In the 1960s Akiskal and McKinney (1973) argued in a widely cited study published in *Science* that depression is a single and stable clinical entity with strong diagnostic borders with other clinical entities. This may be considered a strong positioning regarding the borders with all other diagnostic entities from the mood disorders specialist perspective of the time. On the other hand, Gunderson and Phillips (1991) have argued that BPD, the most prototypical personality disorder, exhibits a weak and nonspecific relationship to depression. Both perspectives, one stemming from the mood disorders field and the other from de BPD field, are examples of the notion that both disorders are quite different clinical entities with robust diagnostic borders. Furthermore, both perspectives assume that depression and personality disorders are distinct clinical entities that can be clearly differentiated at the phenotypic and at the etiological level. Yet, very frequently, both disorders present together. As a way to bridge this gap and achieve common ground, Klein and colleagues (Klein, Kotov, & Bufferd, 2011) proposed that even though different at the level of its manifest clinical presentations (phenotype), both entities may share common causes, that is, common etiological pathways or affected functional domains. These common etiological pathways can also include intermediate phenotypes that mediate between genomic and symptomatic complexity. Indeed, the notion of an intermediate phenotype may be a key component in understanding how depression and personality disorders are deeply intertwined. Above and beyond the discussion regarding diagnostic limits or superposition of diagnostic entities, we make the argument that studying key functional domains related to personality functioning is a useful approach to examine specific intermediate phenotypes involved in depression heterogeneity. These domains refer to psychological mechanisms related to phenotypic complexity. Intermediate phenotypes could be crucial for the understanding of the complex relationship between depression and personality dysfunction because both disorders are "superficially divergent [but] fundamentally overlapping" (Choi-Kain & Gunderson, 2015, p. 257). Mapping intermediate phenotypes related to both depression and personality disorders is also a viable strategy to improve treatment effectiveness.

Following this reasoning, phenotypic variability can be reconducted to common or overlapping intermediate phenotypes, within specific affected functional domains. Functional domains can cover several intermediate phenotypes. In other words, a particular functional domain affected in depression and BPD, for example, emotional regulation, can contain several different intermediate phenotypes, including negative mood bias or amygdala dysfunction. This view does not suppose direct causal influences between depression and personality dysfunction, but rather, common disease mechanisms within functional domains. Patients frequently present both disorders because they have similar causal influences, but a patient's depression is not caused by his or her personality problems (Behn, Herpertz, & Krause, 2018). Following this idea, major depressive disorder and BPD can be understood as two distinct disorders, sharing common affected functional domains, regardless of specific phenotypes (Goodman, Chowdhury, New, & Siever, 2015).

1.3 Depression and Personality Disorders

The comorbidity of depression and personality disorders is a common clinical finding. In a meta-analysis, Friborg et al. (2014) estimated that 45% of patients with major depressive disorder had a concurrent personality disorder, while approximately 60% of patients with a diagnosis of personality disorder also were diagnosed with a depressive disorder. This concurrent presentation has shown to be predictive of more persistent and recurrent depressive episodes (Levenson, Wallace, Fournier, Rucci, & Frank, 2012; Skodol et al., 2011) and related, as well, to an increased probability of psychiatric admissions (Wiegand & Godemann, 2017). Thus, personality dysfunction combined with depressive presentations is not only quite common, but it also results in more complex and severe psychopathology, which obviously has a bearing in prognosis and treatment planning. Additionally, patients with comorbid depressive disorder and personality disorders have typically poorer adherence to treatments and respond worse to antidepressant psychotherapy compared to those patients with a single diagnosis of depression (Newton-Howes et al., 2014). The psychosocial and occupational impairment is also higher for patients with comorbid depression and personality pathology (Markowitz, Skodol, & Bleiberg, 2006) and they have a higher risk of developing additional psychopathology, for example, anxiety (Stein, Hollander, & Skodol, 1993).

For those patients with comorbid depression and BPD, depressive symptomatology is also typically more severe when compared to depressed controls (Köhling et al., 2016). Furthermore, the specificity of concurrent depression and BPD has been explored in depth in a meta-analysis developed by Köhling, Ehrenthal, Levy, Schauenburg, and Dinger (2015). This concurrent presentation is characterized by increased anger and hostility that can be directed also against the self, resulting in increased self-criticism, an aspect previously proposed by Blatt and Zuroff (1992). The functional domain of affect regulation is affected in both, MDD and BPD; however the interaction between this functional domain and the functional domain of social relationships explains some differences between both disorders, where affect dysregulation in BPD with MDD appears to be significantly more reactive to real or perceived interpersonal rejection than in MDD alone (Goodman, New, Triebwasser, Collins, & Siever, 2010). Affected functional domains of impulsivity within depression seem to be mostly indicative of complex depression, including a greater risk for self-injurious behavior and suicidality (Lieb, Zanarini, Schmahl, Linehan, & Bohus, 2004).

The use of Ecological Momentary Assessment (EMA) (Shiffman, Stone, & Hufford, 2008) has been crucial to further understand these intertwined disease mechanisms at the intermediate phenotype level. A study using this methodology found that patients presenting MDD alone compared to those with MDD and BPD did not exhibit differential patterns of affect dysregulation but were indeed distinguished by interpersonal reactivity (Köhling et al., 2016). Even though it is possible that in this specific study EMA calibration was not intense enough to detect differences between both groups in patterns of affect dysregulation, results are still quite interesting and suggestive. In fact, mood disturbances in depression have been largely considered to be episodic, more sustained, and less reactive to environmental interpersonal stressors. Conversely, in BPD, affect dysregulation has been typically considered to be chronic rather than episodic and is characterized by intense fluctuations and extremely high reactivity to interpersonal stressors, most notably to interpersonal rejection and abandonment (Staebler, Helbing, Rosenbach, & Renneberg, 2011). It is only due to the publication of long-term longitudinal studies that these assumptions regarding stark differences can be looked at critically. According to this literature, depression frequently exhibits a recurrent course and inter-episodic maintenance of residual symptoms is quite common (Frodl, Möller, & Meisenzahl, 2008). According to Klein (2010), when depression exhibits an early onset, it is characterized by significant impairment in interpersonal functioning, comparable to BPD, and most likely related to personality dysfunction (Herpertz, Steinmeyer, & Saß, 1998). On the other hand, according to longitudinal studies, some of them spanning decades, BPD patients typically lose their most intense, diagnostic threshold symptomatology with the passage of time (Zanarini, 2018). When remission occurs in BPD, it is very likely to be sustained across measurement waves in longitudinal studies, thus exhibiting even less recurrence than common depression (Paris & Zweig-Frank, 2001).

1.4 Functional Domains Implicated in Depression and Personality Dysfunction

Personality functioning includes multiple psychological and neurobiological domains operating in an integrated way. These systems include cognitive functioning and identity, affect regulation, behavioral control, and interpersonal functioning. Such functional domains may include several intermediate phenotypes and define personality pathology in recent classifications, including DSM-5 Alternative Model and the new ICD-11 classification. In fact, specific phenotypes for personality disorders (e.g., narcissistic, histrionic, schizoid, etc.) are dropped altogether in ICD-11 in favor of a single diagnosis of personality disorder based on deficits in self and interpersonal functioning. Only BPD is retained as a qualifier, likely because of insurance coverage issues (Herpertz et al., 2017). Crucial to these new diagnostic models is the dimensional conceptualization of personality dysfunction in a gradient of severity. Based on the assessment of functional domains, the clinician needs to decide whether or not a personality disorder is present and then estimate the severity. A careful evaluation of the level of the personality dysfunction within a continuum of severity is proposed by current diagnostic guidelines, including the ICD-11 and the DSM-5 Alternative Model. Dimensionality is thus a key component in the functional domains perspective, and even sub-threshold personality vulnerabilities need to be taken into account as they can complicate depression and result in chronicity or recurrence, as well as on early onset and resistance to treatment as usual for common depression (Newton-Howes et al., 2014). Variability in deficits of functional domains implicated in complex depression may result in different phenotypes diagnostically and, clinically, allows to tailor interventions in order to prioritize treatment of most affected functional domains. As an example, a depressed patient with increased behavioral dysregulation possibly related to the functional domain of impulsivity will require treatment alternatives that mainly focus on this domain, for example, skills training in the context of dialectical behavioral therapy (DBT). On the other hand, a patient with no behavioral dysregulation but prominent affectation of the functional domain of identity (e.g., lack of self-concept clarity and self-direction) will likely benefit from treatment alternatives that improve identity functioning, for example, components of transference-focused psychotherapy (TFP). This diverse and patient-centered approach has been advanced, for example, in the setting of integrated modular treatments (Livesley, Dimaggio, & Clarkin, 2015).

Several domains of functioning related to personality dysfunction can further complicate depressive symptomatology and thus benefit from a functional domains perspective for diagnosis and treatment planning. An excellent although not recent review by Hasler, Drevets, Manji, and Charney (2004) presents specific intermediate phenotypes for depression, including mood bias towards negative emotions, impaired reward functioning, impaired learning and memory, and increased stress sensitivity. Goodman et al. (2010) have summarized this literature specifically comparing BPD with MDD and focusing primarily on shared biological endophenotypes. A recent meta-analysis reviews one of the main neurobiological endophenotypes related to BPD, namely, the hypothalamic-pituitary-adrenal axis which may help explain stress-related symptoms. Specific functional domains related to self and other functioning include metacognitive capacities related to the understanding of self-states and empathy (Dimaggio & Brüne, 2016); difficulties related to hypermentalizing, particularly in the context of intimate relationships (Sharp et al., 2016); and insecure attachment styles (Bo & Kongerslev, 2017). From a trait perspective, interpersonal hostility, rejection sensitivity, and low agreeableness have also been identified as components of personality dysfunction implicated in complex depression (Hirsch, Quilty, Bagby, & McMain, 2012; Zufferey, Caspar, & Kramer, 2019). Intense mental pain, although present in BPD and MDD, appears to be particularly reactive to interpersonal rejection in BPD (Fertuck, Karan, & Stanley, 2016). Emotion dysregulation has been prominently related to personality dysfunction, particularly in patients with BPD (Dixon-Gordon, Peters, Fertuck, & Yen, 2017) with relatively well-known neurobiological underpinnings as indicated in a fairly recent meta-analysis (Schulze, Schmahl, & Niedtfeld, 2016). Within the functional domain of affect regulation, specific intermediate phenotypes can be further identified, including difficulties in emotional awareness (De Panfilis, Ossola, Tonna, Catania, & Marchesi, 2015) and emotional expression and modulation (Berenson, Downey, Rafaeli, Coifman, & Paquin, 2011; Mancke, Herpertz, Kleindienst, & Bertsch, 2017). The functional domain of self and cognitive processes has been related to specific biases for negative information processing as well as binary, "black or white" thinking (Kramer, Vaudroz, Ruggeri, & Drapeau, 2013).

1.5 Depression, Personality Styles, and Structural Personality Integration

In 1974 Sydney Blatt proposed that depression may be a by-product of deficits in the structure of object relations, developing the idea of two distinct forms of depression (Blatt, 1974, 2004, 2008). These forms of depression would be anchored in personality styles, implying dysfunction in different dimensions. The different personality styles would emerge from two main developmental tasks: self-definition and relatedness. As a result, depression could be conceptualized as the consequence of disruptions in the course of these developmental tasks, leading to two different forms of depression: introjective and anaclitic. Introjective depression would show deficits in self-integrity and in self-esteem (typically extreme self-criticism; Blatt & Zuroff, 1992), whereas anaclitic depression would be characterized by a disruption of interpersonal relatedness (typically fears of abandonment). The self-critical (introjective) and dependent (anaclitic) types of depression have been measured through the Depressive Experience Questionnaire (DEQ; Blatt, D'Afflitti, & Quinlan, 1976; Blatt, Zohar, Quinlan, Zuroff, & Mongrain, 1995).

These different types of depression have been studied from the perspective of neurophysiological, psychological, and psychosocial variables (de la Parra, Dagnino, Valdés, & Krause, 2017). Silva, Vivanco-Carlevari, Barrientos, Martinez, Salazar and Krause (2017) provided experimental evidence indicating that biological stress reactivity (cortisol in saliva) of individuals is modulated by their positioning within the anaclitic or introjective polarity, with self-critical individuals exhibiting more objective biological stress reactivity compared to dependent individuals, but anaclitics showing higher scores in self-report instruments. Thus, personality predispositions in the anaclitic versus introjective continuum could indicate a specific vulnerability for the development of depression, particularly when an individual is confronted with stressors. Rodríguez et al. (2017) studied the dependent versus self-critical functioning in relation to cognitive tasks and mentalization, finding longer reaction times in cognitive tasks for dependent individuals, and a poorer performance in mentalization for high self-critical individuals.

On the dimension of psychological variables, Dagnino, Pérez, Gómez, Gloger, and Krause (2017) reported differences in attachment between introjective and anaclitic participants. While introjective depressive patients showed higher anxious and avoidant attachment, anaclitic patients only showed anxious attachment. In this study, likewise previously mentioned by Rodríguez et al. (2017), higher levels of self-criticism go along with more depressive symptomatology. In psychotherapy, introjective patients are more likely to drop out from treatment, and those that complete treatment show less improvement in depressive symptoms, compared to anaclitic participants (de la Parra et al., 2017). Similar results have also been observed in psychosocial interventions (Olhaberry et al., 2015), with less improvement of maternal depression and higher avoidant and anxious attachment scores in self-critical participants. On the basis of these findings, it can be stated that the introjective personality style adds severity to depression and complexity for its treatment.

A relevant question is how these personality styles relate to personality structural functioning, as it is understood from the perspective of the Operationalized Psychodynamic Diagnosis System (OPD Task Force, 2008), implying the availability of mental functions for the regulation of the self and its relationships with others. Five levels of structural integration are defined by the degree of availability of these mental functions, within a continuum, including high integration (level 1), moderate integration (level 2), low integration (level 3), and disintegration (level 4) (de la Parra et al., 2017). A self-rating questionnaire was developed to assess these structural levels in research settings (OPD Structure Questionnaire, OPD-SQ, Schauenburg et al., 2012).

Research with the OPD system has shown that lower structural levels in personality functioning go along with higher mental health symptomatology (Zimmermann et al., 2012). Relating structural functioning to personality styles, Dagnino (2015) found that high self-criticism was associated with less integrated structural functioning, measured by the OPD system. Following this line of research, de la Parra et al. (2017) studied structural personality functioning (measured by the OPD) and personality styles (measured by the DEQ) in clinical and nonclinical samples. Their results show, first, that lower structural levels in personality functioning were related to higher levels of depressive symptomatology and, additionally, that the correlation between self-criticism and structural functioning was significantly higher than between dependency and structural functioning.

These studies give support to the hypothesis that personality styles related to depression are not independent from structural personality functioning. Furthermore, they support the idea that both, the self-critical personality style and the lower integration of structural functioning, add complexity to depression. Therefore, both models can be useful to untangle aspects of the heterogeneity of depression that have to be taken into account in research and for treatment efficacy.

1.6 Conclusions

This chapter approached the topic of *complex depression* from the review of the literature regarding the interaction of depression and personality dysfunction with the aim of contributing to a better understanding of the heterogeneity of depression. It is an empirical and clinical fact that depression is a notoriously heterogeneous clinical syndrome, and this heterogeneity can be established at an empirical and conceptual level by taking into consideration personality. We have shown that patients who, in addition to a depression, present personality dysfunction are more than twice as likely to be nonresponsive to treatment compared to patients with common, stand-alone depression. We have advanced the idea that a functional domains perspective provides adequate coverage of personality functioning and can work as a framework for the identification of specific affected intermediate phenotypes that contribute complexity in depression.

Nevertheless, there is an ongoing debate about the symptomatic superposition between depression and personality pathology, which we addressed in the first section of this chapter. The different positions argue in favor of a strict separation versus the superposition between depression and personality disorders. This debate can be addressed with the inclusion of a *common cause* hypothesis at the level of shared affected intermediate phenotypes within functional domains.

In the next section, we reviewed findings about the comorbidity of depression and personality disorders, which lies around between 45% (patients with major depressive disorder diagnosed also with a personality disorder) and 60% (patients with a personality disorder that also were diagnosed with a depressive disorder). Personality dysfunction combined with depression is not only common, but results in more severe psychopathology and poorer adherence to treatments. We have argued that, from a functional domains perspective, comorbidity estimates are highly likely because of shared affected intermediate phenotypes, in particular the functional domain of affect regulation and modulation.

In the third section of this chapter, we proposed that underlying functional domains related to personality functioning would be a useful approach to examine specific intermediate phenotypes involved in depression heterogeneity. These intermediate phenotypes could be crucial for the understanding of the complex relationship between depression and personality dysfunction and also be a viable strategy to improve treatment effectiveness. Symptom heterogeneity can be vast, but vulnerability in relevant functional domains can reduce this heterogeneity and be an important input for treatment design, specifically for the development of differential treatment components for patients that share these affected intermediate phenotypes.

With the idea that even sub-threshold personality vulnerabilities need to be taken into account, as they can complicate depression, we devoted the fourth section of this chapter to two conceptual models of personality functioning, with their corresponding empirical research, including Sydney Blatt's polarity of relatedness and self-definition in personality development, resulting in different personality styles and different types of depression, and the model of levels of structural personality integration, proposed the OPD task group. Interestingly, research findings for both models establish the relationship between personality and severity of depression. In Blatt's model the higher impairment in self-definition adds severity to depression; in the OPD model's case, lower levels of personality integration are related to more complex and severe depressive presentations.

In conclusion, the evidence we presented along this chapter indicates that personality disorders and dysfunctions, personality styles, as well as the level of structural integration of personality, add severity to depression and lead to a poorer response to habitual treatments. For this reason, personality is a crucial dimension for explaining severe depression, and a functional domain perspective is a useful framework to address research, diagnosis, and treatment planning. This understanding is the basis for the development of detection strategies and treatments designed specifically to address personality dysfunctions and styles that are responsible for the poor outcome of standard interventions in cases of *complex depression*.

Acknowledgments This work was funded by the ANID-Millennium Science Initiative/ Millennium Institute for Research on Depression and Personality-MIDAP.

References

Akiskal, H. S., & McKinney, W. T. (1973). Depressive disorders: Toward a unified hypothesis: Clinical, experimental, genetic, biochemical, and neurophysiological data are integrated. *Science, 182*(4107), 20–29.

Behn, A. (2019). Working with clients at the intersection of depression and personality dysfunction: Scientific and clinical findings regarding complex depression. *Journal of Clinical Psychology, 75*(5), 819–823.

Behn, A., Herpertz, S. C., & Krause, M. (2018). The interaction between depression and personality dysfunction: State of the art, current challenges, and future directions. Introduction to the Special Section. *Psykhe, 27*(2), 1–12.

Berenson, K. R., Downey, G., Rafaeli, E., Coifman, K. G., & Paquin, N. L. (2011). The rejection–rage contingency in borderline personality disorder. *Journal of Abnormal Psychology, 120*(3), 681.

Blatt, S. J. (1974). Levels of object representation in anaclitic and introjective depression. *The Psychoanalytic Study of the Child, 29*, 107–157.
Blatt, S. J. (2004). *Experiences of depression: Theoretical, clinical and research perspectives*. Washington, DC: American Psychological Association.
Blatt, S. J. (2008). Two primary configurations of psychopathology. In S. Blatt (Ed.), *Polarities of experiences: Relatedness and self-definition in personality development, psychopathology and the therapeutic process* (pp. 234–245). Washington, DC: American Psychological Association.
Blatt, S. J., D'Afflitti, J. P., & Quinlan, D. M. (1976). Experiences of depression in normal young adults. *Journal of Abnormal Psychology, 85*, 383–389.
Blatt, S. J., & Zuroff, D. C. (1992). Interpersonal relatedness and self-definition: Two prototypes for depression. *Clinical Psychology Review, 12*, 527–562.
Blatt, S. J., Zohar, A. H., Quinlan, D. M., Zuroff, D. C., & Mongrain, M. (1995). Subscales within the dependency factor of the Depressive Experiences Questionnaire. *Journal of Personality Assessment, 64*(2), 319–339.
Bo, S., & Kongerslev, M. (2017). Self-reported patterns of impairments in mentalization, attachment, and psychopathology among clinically referred adolescents with and without borderline personality pathology. *Borderline Personality Disorder and Emotion Dysregulation, 4*(1), 4.
Buch, A. M., & Liston, C. (2020). Dissecting diagnostic heterogeneity in depression by integrating neuroimaging and genetics. *Neuropsychopharmacology, 46*, 1–22.
Cai, N., Choi, K. W., & Fried, E. I. (2020). Reviewing the genetics of heterogeneity in depression: Operationalizations, manifestations, and etiologies. *Human Molecular Genetics*. Ahead of Print. https://doi.org/10.1093/hmg/ddaa115.
Choi-Kain, L. W., & Gunderson, J. G. (2015). Conclusion: Integration and synthesis. In *Borderline personality and mood disorders* (pp. 255–270). New York, NY: Springer.
Craighead, W. E., & Dunlop, B. W. (2014). Combination psychotherapy and antidepressant medication treatment for depression: For whom, when, and how. *Annual Review of Psychology, 65*, 267–300.
Dagnino, P. (2015). Structural vulnerabilities of depression. In *Millennium nucleus research program "psychological intervention and change in depression" meeting*. Santiago, Chile: Universidad de Chile.
Dagnino, P., Pérez, C., Gómez, A., Gloger, S., & Krause, M. (2017). Depression and attachment: How do personality styles and social support influence this relation? *Research in Psychotherapy: Psychopathology, Process and Outcome, 20*, 53–62. https://doi.org/10.4081/ripppo.2017.237
de la Parra, G., Dagnino, P., Valdés, C., & Krause, M. (2017). Beyond self-criticism and dependency: Structural functioning of depressive patients and its treatment. *Research in Psychotherapy: Psychopathology, Process and Outcome, 20*, 43–52. https://doi.org/10.4081/ripppo.2017.236
De Panfilis, C., Ossola, P., Tonna, M., Catania, L., & Marchesi, C. (2015). Finding words for feelings: The relationship between personality disorders and alexithymia. *Personality and Individual Differences, 74*, 285–291.
DeRubeis, R. J., Siegle, G. J., & Hollon, S. D. (2008). Cognitive therapy versus medication for depression: Treatment outcomes and neural mechanisms. *Nature Reviews Neuroscience, 9*(10), 788–796.
Dimaggio, G., & Brüne, M. (2016). Dysfunctional understanding of mental states in personality disorders: What is the evidence? *Comprehensive Psychiatry, 64*, 1–3.
Dixon-Gordon, K. L., Peters, J. R., Fertuck, E. A., & Yen, S. (2017). Emotional processes in borderline personality disorder: An update for clinical practice. *Journal of Psychotherapy Integration, 27*(4), 425.
Fertuck, E. A., Karan, E., & Stanley, B. (2016). The specificity of mental pain in borderline personality disorder compared to depressive disorders and healthy controls. *Borderline Personality Disorder and Emotion Dysregulation, 3*(1), 2.
Friborg, O., Martinsen, E. W., Martinussen, M., Kaiser, S., Øvergård, K. T., & Rosenvinge, J. H. (2014). Comorbidity of personality disorders in mood disorders: A meta-analytic review of 122 studies from 1988 to 2010. *Journal of Affective Disorders, 152*, 1–11.

Frodl, T., Möller, H. J., & Meisenzahl, E. (2008). Neuroimaging genetics: New perspectives in research on major depression? *Acta Psychiatrica Scandinavica, 118*(5), 363–372.

Goodman, M., Chowdhury, S., New, A. S., & Siever, L. J. (2015). Depressive disorders in borderline personality disorder: Phenomenology and biological markers. In *Borderline personality and mood disorders* (pp. 13–37). New York, NY: Springer.

Goodman, M., New, A. S., Triebwasser, J., Collins, K. A., & Siever, L. (2010). Phenotype, endophenotype, and genotype comparisons between borderline personality disorder and major depressive disorder. *Journal of Personality Disorders, 24*(1), 38–59.

Gunderson, J. G., & Phillips, K. A. (1991). A current view of the interface between borderline personality disorder and depression. *The American Journal of Psychiatry, 148*(8), 967–975.

Hart, A. B., Craighead, W. E., & Craighead, L. W. (2001). Predicting recurrence of major depressive disorder in young adults: A prospective study. *Journal of Abnormal Psychology, 110*(4), 633.

Hasler, G., Drevets, W. C., Manji, H. K., & Charney, D. S. (2004). Discovering endophenotypes for major depression. *Neuropsychopharmacology, 29*(10), 1765–1781.

Herpertz, S. C., Huprich, S. K., Bohus, M., Chanen, A., Goodman, M., Mehlum, L., ... & Sharp, C. (2017). The challenge of transforming the diagnostic system of personality disorders. *Journal of personality disorders, 31*(5), 577–589.

Herpertz, S., Steinmeyer, E. M., & Saß, H. (1998). On the conceptualisation of subaffective personality disorders. *European Psychiatry, 13*(1), 9–17.

Hirsch, J. B., Quilty, L. C., Bagby, R. M., & McMain, S. F. (2012). The relationship between agreeableness and the development of the working alliance in patients with borderline personality disorder. *Journal of Personality Disorders, 26*(4), 616–627.

Klein, D. N. (2010). Chronic depression: diagnosis and classification. *Current Directions in Psychological Science, 19*(2), 96–100.

Klein, D. N., Kotov, R., & Bufferd, S. J. (2011). Personality and depression: Explanatory models and review of the evidence. *Annual Review of Clinical Psychology, 7*, 269–295.

Köhling, J., Ehrenthal, J. C., Levy, K. N., Schauenburg, H., & Dinger, U. (2015). Quality and severity of depression in borderline personality disorder: A systematic review and meta-analysis. *Clinical Psychology Review, 37*, 13–25.

Köhling, J., Moessner, M., Ehrenthal, J. C., Bauer, S., Cierpka, M., Kämmerer, A., … Dinger, U. (2016). Affective instability and reactivity in depressed patients with and without borderline pathology. *Journal of Personality Disorders, 30*(6), 776–795.

Kramer, U., Vaudroz, C., Ruggeri, O., & Drapeau, M. (2013). Biased thinking assessed by external observers in borderline personality disorder. *Psychology and Psychotherapy: Theory, Research and Practice, 86*(2), 183–196.

Lépine, J. P., & Briley, M. (2011). The increasing burden of depression. *Neuropsychiatric Disease and Treatment, 7*(Suppl 1), 3.

Levenson, J. C., Wallace, M. L., Fournier, J. C., Rucci, P., & Frank, E. (2012). The role of personality pathology in depression treatment outcome with psychotherapy and pharmacotherapy. *Journal of Consulting and Clinical Psychology, 80*(5), 719–729. https://doi.org/10.1037/a0029396

Lieb, K., Zanarini, M. C., Schmahl, C., Linehan, M. M., & Bohus, M. (2004). Borderline personality disorder. *The Lancet, 364*(9432), 453–461.

Livesley, W. J., Dimaggio, G., & Clarkin, J. F. (Eds.). (2015). *Integrated treatment for personality disorder: A modular approach*. New York, NY: Guilford Publications.

Mancke, F., Herpertz, S. C., Kleindienst, N., & Bertsch, K. (2017). Emotion dysregulation and trait anger sequentially mediate the association between borderline personality disorder and aggression. *Journal of Personality Disorders, 31*(2), 256–272.

Markowitz, J. C., Skodol, A. E., & Bleiberg, K. (2006). Interpersonal psychotherapy for borderline personality disorder: Possible mechanisms of change. *Journal of Clinical Psychology, 62*, 431–444.

Newton-Howes, G., Tyrer, P., Johnson, T., Mulder, R., Kool, S., Dekker, J., & Schoevers, R. (2014). Influence of personality on the outcome of treatment in depression: Systematic review and meta-analysis. *Journal of Personality Disorders, 28*, 577–593.

Olhaberry, M., Mena, C., Zapata, J., Miranda, A., Romero, M., & Sieverson, C. (2015). Terapia de interacción guiada en díadas madre-bebé con sintomatología depresiva materna en el embarazo: un estudio piloto. [Guided interaction therapy in mother-baby dyads with maternal depressive symptomatology in pregnancy: A pilot study]. *Summa Psicológica UST, 12*(2), 63–74.

OPD Task Force (Ed.). (2008). *Operationalized psychodynamic diagnosis OPD-2: Manual of diagnosis and treatment planning*. Cambridge, MA: Hogrefe Publishing.

Paris, J., & Zweig-Frank, H. (2001). The 27-year follow-up of patients with borderline personality disorder. *Comprehensive Psychiatry, 42*(6), 482–487.

Rodríguez, E., Ruiz, J. C., Valdés, C., Reinel, M., Díaz, M., Flores, J., ... Tomicic, A. (2017). Estilos de personalidad dependiente y autocrítico: desempeño cognitivo y sintomatología depresiva [Dependent and self-critical personality styles: Cognitive performance and depressive symptomatology]. *Latinoamericana de Psicología, 49*, 2. https://doi.org/10.1016/j.rlp.2016.09.005

Schauenburg, H., Dinger, U., Komo-Lang, M., Klinkerfuss, M., Horsch, L., Grande, T., & Ehrenthal, J. C. (2012). Der OPD Strukturfragebogen [The OPD structure questionnaire]. In S. Döring & S. Hörz (Eds.), *Handbuch der Strukturdiagnostik* (pp. 284–307). Stuttgart, Germany: Schattauer.

Schulze, L., Schmahl, C., & Niedtfeld, I. (2016). Neural correlates of disturbed emotion processing in borderline personality disorder: A multimodal meta-analysis. *Biological Psychiatry, 79*(2), 97–106.

Sharp, C., Venta, A., Vanwoerden, S., Schramm, A., Ha, C., Newlin, E., ... Fonagy, P. (2016). First empirical evaluation of the link between attachment, social cognition and borderline features in adolescents. *Comprehensive Psychiatry, 64*, 4–11.

Shiffman, S., Stone, A. A., & Hufford, M. R. (2008). Ecological momentary assessment. *Annual Review of Clinical Psychology, 4*, 1–32.

Silva, J. R., Vivanco-Carlevari, A., Barrientos, M., Martínez, C., Salazar, L. A., & Krause, M. (2017). Biological stress reactivity as an index of the two polarities of the experience model. *Psychoneuroendocrinology, 84*, 83–86.

Skodol, A. E., Grilo, C. M., Keyes, K. M., Geier, T., Grant, B. F., & Hasin, D. S. (2011). Relationship of personality disorders to the course of major depressive disorder in a nationally representative sample. *American Journal of Psychiatry, 168*(3), 257–264. https://doi.org/10.1176/appi.ajp.2010.10050695

Spijker, J., van Straten, A., Bockting, C. L., Meeuwissen, J. A., & van Balkom, A. J. (2013). Psychotherapy, antidepressants, and their combination for chronic major depressive disorder: a systematic review. *The Canadian Journal of Psychiatry, 58*(7), 386–392.

Staebler, K., Helbing, E., Rosenbach, C., & Renneberg, B. (2011). Rejection sensitivity and borderline personality disorder. *Clinical Psychology & Psychotherapy, 18*(4), 275–283.

Stein, D. J., Hollander, E., & Skodol, A. E. (1993). Anxiety disorders and personality disorders: A review. *Journal of Personality Disorders, 7*(2), 87–104.

Vos, T., Haby, M. M., Barendregt, J. J., Kruijshaar, M., Corry, J., & Andrews, G. (2004). The burden of major depression avoidable by longer-term treatment strategies. *Archives of General Psychiatry, 61*(11), 1097–1103.

Wiegand, H. F., & Godemann, F. (2017). Increased treatment complexity for major depressive disorder for inpatients with comorbid personality disorder. *Psychiatric Services, 68*(5), 524–527.

Zanarini, M. C. (2018). *In the fullness of time: Recovery from borderline personality disorder*. New York, NY: Oxford University Press.

Zimmermann, J., Ehrenthal, J. C., Cierpka, M., Schauenburg, H., Doering, S., & Benecke, C. (2012). Assessing the level of structural integration using operationalized psychodynamic diagnosis (OPD): Implications for DSM-5. *Journal of Personality Assessment, 94*, 522–532.

Zufferey, P., Caspar, F., & Kramer, U. (2019). The role of interactional agreeableness in responsive treatments for patients with borderline personality disorder. *Journal of Personality Disorders, 33*(5), 691–706.

Part I
Domains of Personality Dysfunction Complicating the Presentation and Treatment of Depression

Chapter 2
The Functional Domain of Identity

Klaus Schmeck, Susanne Schlüter-Müller, and Nelson Valdés-Sánchez

Abstract Establishing a stable identity is one of the main developmental tasks of adolescence. During this vulnerable period of life, many internal and external influences can impair this development, which can result in identity disturbance or diffusion. In the DSM-5 Alternative Model of Personality Disorders, identity disturbance is one of the core aspects of impaired personality functioning, especially in borderline personality disorder. The association between depression and identity disturbance seems to be bidirectional. Severe confusion about oneself can increase the risk of subsequent depression. On the other hand, early starting depression can disturb the process of shaping a stable identity. In empirical studies and clinical practice, there is a frequent comorbidity between personality disorders and depression. Chronic emptiness reflecting a detachment from sense of self is one of the shared symptoms between these two disorders and is linked to identity disturbance. In adolescent patients suffering from depression and personality disorder, identity diffusion, if present, should be a crucial target of psychotherapy.

Keywords Identity disturbance · Personality functioning · Personality disorder · Complex depression · Chronic emptiness

2.1 Introduction

While diagnostical and treatment manuals usually focus on specific disorders, we know from many studies as well as from clinical psychiatric experience that monosymptomatic disorders are rare in mental health (Caspi & Moffitt, 2018; Kessler

K. Schmeck (✉) · S. Schlüter-Müller
Department of Child and Adolescent Psychiatric Research, Psychiatric University Hospitals, University of Basel, Basel, Switzerland

Millennium Institute for Research in Depression and Personality (MIDAP), Santiago, Chile
e-mail: Klaus.Schmeck@upk.ch

N. Valdés-Sánchez
Millennium Institute for Research in Depression and Personality (MIDAP), Santiago, Chile

Psychology Department, Universidad Santo Tomás, Santiago, Chile

G. de la Parra et al. (eds.), *Depression and Personality Dysfunction*, Depression and Personality, https://doi.org/10.1007/978-3-030-70699-9_2

et al., 2005), and if we see a patient suffering from only one mental disorder, then we are, in most cases, faced with the heterogeneity of the disorder. In spite of substantial efforts over the last decades, research on biomarkers, etiology, course of disorders, or treatment approaches with specificity to individual mental disorders have led to frustrating results. Splitting up disorders into distinct diagnoses, the common approach of DSM and ICD, has enhanced the reliability of diagnoses at the expense of their validity. Moreover, psychotherapy research has demonstrated that the use of manualized treatment approaches for single disorder is insufficient for the majority of clinically referred patients who suffer from multiple disorders (Marchette & Weisz, 2017).

As a consequence, several new nosological concepts of mental disorders emerged in the last years. Caspi and Moffitt developed the p-factor model postulating that one general psychopathology factor better explains the structure of psychiatric disorders than the current concepts of distinct categorical conditions used in ICD-10 or DSM-5 (Caspi & Moffitt, 2018). The American National Institute of Mental Health started the RDoC initiative postulating that domains of psychological functioning are more useful to define mental disorders and their neurobiological etiology than the diagnostic concepts of DSM and ICD (Cuthbert, 2014). However, while this new framework stimulated researchers to conceptualize their studies in a different way, the effects on treatment and clinical practice have remained sparse. More promising concepts with a closer connection between classification and treatment emerged with transdiagnostic approaches (Fusar-Poli et al., 2019) or the Hierarchical Taxonomy of Psychopathology (HiTOP) (Kotov et al., 2017) that originates from a sharp critique of the existing classification systems (instability of diagnoses, random boundaries between psychopathology and normality and unclear boundaries between disorders, co-occurrence of disorders, heterogeneity within disorders) and tries to overcome their limitations.

However, all these classification systems, both traditional and new, focus on symptoms, syndromes, disorders, or maladaptive temperamental traits. With the Levels of Personality Functioning Scale (LPFS), the Alternative Model of Personality Disorders (AMPD) of the DSM-5 chapter III (APA, 2013) introduces a fundamentally different aspect, the impairment of self-related and interpersonal personality functioning of an individual in his psychosocial living conditions. This aspect of personality functioning is called "Criterion A" which is used in the AMPD of DSM-5 to determine if a person suffers from a personality disorder, independently from the specific type of the disorder. Identity is one of the four dimensions of the LPFS, and impairment of identity or identity diffusion is one of the core aspects of personality disorders in general and borderline personality disorder (BPD) specifically (Sharp et al., 2015). In this chapter we will delineate the relevance of the concept of identity for the frequent co-occurrence of major depressive disorder (MDD) and borderline personality disorder.

2.2 Personality Functioning

In the dimensional view on personality disorders that has been adopted by DSM-5 and the forthcoming ICD-11, two broad criteria define personality disorders. Five pathological personality traits are used to characterize the temperamental basis of a personality disorder. Temperamental traits are observable already in early stages of development and are widely continuous over the course of development. The second criterion of a disturbed personality is defined as an impairment of self-functioning and interpersonal functioning. In contrast to former conceptualizations of personality disorder, it is not the sum of personality disorder symptoms but instead the maladaptive functioning which constitutes the core of a personality disorder. The four domains of personality functioning are identity, self-directedness, empathy, and intimacy.

The AMPD of DSM-5 integrates many aspects of Kernberg's theory of personality and borderline personality organization. Kernberg defines personality "as an umbrella organization that includes a small number of major component systems: temperament, object relations, character, identity, ethical value systems, and cognitive capability (intelligence)" (Kernberg, 2016, p.147). Temperamental traits are represented in the pathological personality traits of criterion B, identity and character in the criterion A dimensions of identity and self-directedness, and object relations and ethical value systems in the interpersonal dimensions of empathy and intimacy. Kernberg describes internalized affective memory traces as the core of internal representations of relationships with significant others. In contrast to character, that he defines as "the objective, individualized integration of habitual behavior patterns" (2016, p.148), identity shall represent "the subjective correspondent of character in terms of the integration of self-perception and experience and the experience of significant others." (2016, p.148).

2.3 The Functional Domain of Identity

The concept of identity has a long-lasting tradition in Western philosophy, stretching out from Plato and Aristotle to Leibniz, Locke, Kant, and others (Sollberger, 2013). In philosophy, the term "identity" is used as a marker that differentiates one object from another object, thus defining the uniqueness of the target object. The philosopher and early psychologist William James (1890) defined two core domains of identity: the "subjective self" or "I," an intuitive, emotionally experienced vital self-evidence, and the "definitory self" or "ME," the result of a self-reflective process leading to an integrated awareness and knowledge about oneself (Goth et al., 2012). In his anthropology, George Mead (1934) outlined these ideas further.

A milestone in the clinical approach to the concept of identity lies in the contributions of the psychoanalyst Erik H. Erikson, who defines identity as a fundamental organizing principle, which develops throughout life and provides a healthy individual with two major capacities: a sense of continuity within the self and in interaction with others ("self-sameness") and a sense of coherence that enables us to differentiate between self and others ("uniqueness"), a precondition to function autonomously from others (Erikson, 1959). The consolidation of a stable identity can be seen as the main developmental task of an adolescent. Usually, the search for identity is accompanied by phases of identity crises when the rapidly shifting self-experience of the adolescent does no longer correspond to the view of him or her from the perspective of others. The resolution of identity crises strengthens the identity development and leads to a better self-esteem, a more realistic appraisal of self and others, and insight into the effect one has on another (Schmeck et al., 2013). Thus, a stable identity provides predictability and continuity of functioning within a person, across situations, and across time and supports self-reflective functioning, autonomy, and mutually satisfying social exchanges (P. Kernberg et al., 2000).

Another influential theory of identity was developed by Marcia (1966) who differentiates identity formation along the two dimensions of "commitment" and "exploration," The specific combination of high versus low expression on these two dimensions leads to the four states of identity formation "achievement" (high in both exploration and commitment), "foreclosure" (low exploration, high commitment), "moratorium" (high exploration, low commitment), and "diffusion" (high in both exploration and commitment).

2.4 Identity Disturbance

Identity crises, which are part of a normal adolescent development, have to be differentiated from identity diffusion, a pathology of identity that is characteristic for borderline patients and other severe personality disorders (Sharp et al., 2015). According to Kernberg's definition, the lack of integration of the concept of self and of significant others leads to the pathology of identity diffusion, which in combination with the predominant use of immature defenses constitutes borderline personality organization (Kernberg, 1976). Identity diffusion results in a painful sense of incoherence as well as a loss of capacity for self-definition and commitment to values, goals, or relationships. Patients who suffer from identity diffusion appear unreflective or chaotic, give contradictory descriptions about themselves and others, and are unable to perceive contradictions (Clarkin, Yeomans, Kernberg, 1999). An incompletely integrated identity can lead to feelings of chronic emptiness, weak ego-strength indicated by poor anxiety tolerance or impulse control, contrary behavior, and superficiality (Kernberg, 1984). In 2000, Paulina Kernberg presented a concept for understanding identity pathology in children and adolescents and for the differentiation of normal identity crisis from identity diffusion (P. Kernberg et al., 2000). She developed an approach for early interventions in older children and adolescents suffering from identity diffusion to improve their relationships with friends, parents, and teachers, to acquire positive self-esteem and to clarify life goals in order to increase identity integration, adaptive functioning, and adaptive behavior (Foelsch et al., 2014; Kernberg et al., 2000).

2.5 Complex Depression

Depression is a disease that affects millions of people worldwide, characterized by its impact on the mood and affects of individuals, which are usually associated with changes in appetite, fatigue, sleepiness, cognitive difficulties, loss of interest, and enjoyment (Costello et al., 2019). It has become a common mental health problem in adolescents, being a major risk factor for suicide in people aged 15–29 (Global Burden Disease, 2018). More than half of teenagers who commit suicide have often been suffering from a depressive disorder at the time they end their lives. The clinical and diagnostic features of this disorder in adolescents are often similar to those in adults; however, it is more often overlooked in adolescents because there is greater irritability, mood reactivity, and fluctuation of symptoms at this stage of development. It has also been considered an early form (subsyndromal depression) of the diagnosis verified later in adulthood (Birmaher et al., 2004).

There are two diagnoses in the classification systems that include both an impairment and a depressive symptomatology, and these are the adaptation disorder and the dysthymic disorder. The first one is usually brief, has its beginning near the appearance of a stressor, and does not persist beyond 6 months. On the other hand, the second one is characterized by a chronic depressive symptomatology present most of the time in most days and with a minimum duration of 1 year. In addition, two-thirds of adolescents with depression have at least one comorbid psychiatric disorder, and between 10% and 15% usually have two or more comorbidities (Finning et al., 2019). Adolescents with depression are more likely to suffer from anxiety, conduct disorder, substance abuse problems, generalized anxiety disorder, eating disorders, and TDAH (Clarkin, Petrini, & Diamond, 2019; Costello, Foley, & Angold, 2006; Moffitt et al. 2010; Thapar, Collishaw, Pine, & Thapar, 2012). It is precisely for this reason that depression is considered a complex dynamic system that evolves over time, whose relationships between different symptoms can result in episodes that are impossible to predict from a single symptom (Schmittmann, Cramer, Waldorp, Epskamp, Kievit, & Borsboom, 2013). Therefore, the complexity is not determined by whether a patient with depression has responded inadequately to other previous treatments, nor only by its characteristics of being severe, early, recurrent, or chronic (Garland, 2015; Maillard, Pellaton, & Kramer, 2019; Tarrier & Johnson, 2015; Waller & Turner, 2016). Conversely, depression is considered complex when, in addition to the above, it is complicated by psychotic symptoms and/or associated with significant psychiatric comorbidity, resulting from the interactions of biological, psychological, and social factors that hinder treatment (NICE, 2009).

There are some biopsychosocial factors that coexist with depression, complicate the diagnosis, and cause unusual and unpredictable effects. Barton, Armstrong, Wicks, Freeman, and Meyer (2017) have graphed these factors in a diagrammatic map format, which allows a better understanding of how these factors interact with each other, thus facilitating diagnosis and treatment planning. Some of these factors are the following: (a) biological (physical disability, sleep disorder, somatization, chronic fatigue, or stress), (b) psychological (developmental problems, cognitive problems, body/eating disorders, trauma, or anxiety disorders), and (c) social (cultural factors, economic factors, healthcare factors, and work, family, or interpersonal problems). These authors propose four main complications: (a) complexity factors that can create barriers to treatment, (b) complexity factors that delay the patient's preparation for treatment, (c) complexity factors that interfere with the development of the therapeutic alliance, and (d) complexity factors that modify the usual maintenance of a disorder and require a nonstandard process of change. Therefore, depression should be considered as a complex spectrum that encompasses different levels of interaction of factors that end up generating complications and from a network perspective that assumes that the symptoms of one disorder may end up causing symptoms of another disorder. In this way, not only are there symptoms that are not possible to observe directly, and which must be measured indirectly through the presence or absence of other variables that are observable, but also the symptoms do not measure a disorder, but are part of it (Cramer, Waldorp, van der Maas, & Borsboom, 2010; McGrath (2005).

2.6 Relationship Between Identity Disturbance and Complex Depression

Many theories of personality pathology point out that problems in personal and interpersonal functioning during adolescence (Both, Pereira da Cruz, & Goodman, 2019) are considered predictors of personality disorders during adulthood (Clarkin & Huprich, 2011; Feenstra, Busschbach, Verheul, & Hutsebaut, 2011; Hopwood et al., 2011; Kasen et al., 2007). It is for this reason that longitudinal studies have been conducted that have examined the relationship between different phases in identity formation and psychological well-being. There have been studies that have concluded that there are higher levels of depression over time in adolescents who go through the moratorium phase (Luyckx, Goossens, Soenens, Beyers and Vansteenkiste, 2005; Luyckx, Schwartz, Goossens, Soenens, & Beyers, 2008b). These results coincide with those of the cross-sectional studies conducted by Meeus, Van de Schoot, Keijsers, Schwartz, and Branje (2010), who observed that these same adolescents scored higher on several indicators related to problems such as anxiety, depression, negative affect, and the tendency to worry.

This increase in depressive symptoms experienced during adolescence (Meeus, 2016) begins to diminish over time; however, in some cases these symptoms remain even beyond adolescence, reaching subclinical levels that become a diagnosis of depression in adulthood (Dozois & Dobson, 2003; Fischer-Kern et al., 2008; Hankin et al., 2015; Kessler, Berglund, Demler, Jin, Merikangas, & Walters, 2005). These clinical results have motivated more studies that have allowed a deeper understanding of the probable risk factors for the development of depressive symptoms during adolescence, especially considering that one of the basic tasks during this stage of development is precisely the shaping of identity (Erikson, 1968). Therefore, there is always a risk of developing depressive symptoms during this stage because of the permanent uncertainty and instability that adolescents experience as they struggle with the choices and decisions of this stage. This is the case for those adolescents who cannot make and keep firm commitments but remain uncertain about who they are. In this regard, many studies have shown a high significant positive correlation between this feeling of uncertainty and depressive symptoms during adolescence (Klimstra & Denissen, 2017; Luyckx, Klimstra, Duriez, Van Petegem, & Beyers, 2013; Luyckx et al., 2008b; Porfeli, Lee, Vondracek, & Weingold, 2011; Schwartz, Klimstra, Luyckx, Hale, & Meeus, 2012). Ragozini, Sica, and Sestito (2014) observed that a growing reconsideration of engagement and ruminative exploration in adolescents predicted an increase in depressive symptoms (Luyckx et al., 2008a). In this regard, processes of exploring identity formation that are not adapted to reality play a particularly important role in the development of depressive symptoms. However, the directional nature of the association between the two variables remains unclear (Klimstra & Denissen, 2017), as most studies reach conclusions based on the separate analysis of individuals' uncertainty and depression scores in relation to the rest of the sample (Curran & Bauer, 2011).

There are two dominant but opposite perspectives from personality psychology when it comes to explaining the direction of the association between depression and identity development (Becht et al., 2019). However, both theoretical perspectives have received limited support from longitudinal studies. On the one hand, there is the model of vulnerability-predisposition, which suggests that an ineffective treatment for the diffusion of identity could predispose some adolescents to develop depressive symptoms over time (Durbin & Hicks, 2014), specifically those adolescents with low levels of engagement and high levels of identity reconsideration or ruminal exploration (Meeus, van de Schoot, Keijsers, & Branje, 2012; Ritchie et al. (2013). On the other hand, the scar model suggests the opposite, that is, the experience of depressive symptoms influences the capacity of adolescents to form a healthy and integrated identity, characterized by the possibility of establishing strong and stable commitments over time (Durbin & Hicks, 2014; Klimstra & Denissen, 2017). This is because adolescents with depressive symptoms often feel less motivated and uncertain to achieve valuable goals and greater autonomy, these being important skills to develop during adolescence (Becht et al., 2018; Burrow & Hill, 2011; Schwartz et al., 2012).

A major part of BPD patients suffers from comorbid depressive disorders. In these patients, long-term outcome of functioning is predicted primarily by the severity of BPD, while depression is the best predictor of quality of life (Thompson et al., 2019). The presence of a comorbid personality disorder in major depressive disorder (MDD) leads to longer-lasting MDD episodes, an increased risk of recurrence of MDD, a shorter time to recurrence, and higher rates of chronicity (Grilo et al., 2010; Skodol et al., 2011; Bukh, Andersen, & Kessing, 2016), thus demonstrating a negative impact of personality disorders on the long-term outcome of MDD.

Connections can also be found in respect to pathological personality. In the DSM-5-Chap. III algorithm for BPD, depressivity, i.e., a depressive personality style, is among the facets that are defining the disorder. Depressivity is described as "Frequent feelings of being down, miserable, and/or hopeless; difficulty recovering from such moods; pessimism about the future; pervasive shame and/or guilt; feelings of inferior self-worth; thoughts of suicide and suicidal behavior" (American Psychiatric Association, 2013; p.780). Morey et al. (2016) studied the significance of Criterion B domains and facets for all kinds of personality disorders. The facet "depressivity" was significantly correlated with avoidant PD (0.44), depressive PD (0.41), and borderline PD (0.36).

2.7 Chronic Emptiness

Chronic emptiness is one of the symptoms at the interface of depression, BPD, and identity disturbance. While feelings of emptiness, hopelessness, loneliness, or isolation are often part of depressive symptomatology, chronic feelings of emptiness are more closely related to BPD and are one of the nine criteria defining the disorder in DSM-IV and DSM-5. In the alternative diagnostic model for BPD in DSM-5, chronic emptiness is included as one of the symptoms of identity disturbance (APA, 2013). In several studies, chronic emptiness reflecting a detachment from sense of self was linked to identity disturbance (Miller et al., 2020).

Price, Mahler and Hopwood (2019) define chronic emptiness as "a pervasive and visceral sense of detachment spanning intrapersonal, interpersonal, and existential domains of experience as evidenced by a factor structure encompassing feelings of hollowness, absence from one's own life, profound aloneness, disconnection from the world, and chronic unfulfillment" (p. 19).

If compared to other borderline criteria, emptiness was one of the symptoms that remitted most slowly and that was associated with greater impairment across a broad range of psychosocial domains (Ellison, Rosenstein, Chelminski, Dalrymple, & Zimmerman, 2016; Zanarini et al., 2007).

2.8 Case Example

The present complex case focuses on ongoing modifications of the clinical hypotheses and therapeutic approach. This psychotherapeutic process is illustrated through the case of Norah, a 13-year-old adolescent suffering from depressive disorder, suicidal risk, social phobia, and borderline personality disorder.

Norah was referred to psychotherapy by her psychiatrist, whom she had seen for receiving antidepressant medication (fluoxetine) during the last year. Norah was out of school at the beginning of the treatment (finishing 8th grade), with private classes at home and with free exams. She lived with her father, mother, and sister, and there was no family history of mental disorders reported. Two years earlier, Norah and her family moved from her hometown to the capital, which made it very difficult for her to adapt. This case was chosen because it is representative of the therapeutic work done with adolescents diagnosed with identity diffusion.

Norah presented problems in her social relations, specifically, in primary school when she used to be dominant with her schoolmates. Likewise, she presented a relational pattern that led her to idealize her friends, showing herself dependent on them; however, when she became frustrated (e.g., that a friend did not do what she wanted), she ended up devaluing and breaking the bond. According to her parents, since she was a child she showed a high sensitivity to criticism and little tolerance to frustration, which increased with the change of city and the entrance to the new school, where she was a victim of bullying. Her parents decide to change her school again, but she continues to show distrust and fear of experiencing bullying again, responding aggressively to any sign that was interpreted by her in this line. Eventually, she dropped out of school, eliminated all contacts with her friends (Facebook, WhatsApp) and locked herself in her home. Any attempt of approach activated again her distrust ("they do it out of obligation, but they secretly hate me"). She began to be more irritable-aggressive (yelling at both parents and hitting her mother) and disrespectful towards authority, which ended up with parents being overwhelmed (her father used beating to try to calm her down). She lacked a coherent and continuous vision of herself and began to become more dependent on her mother. Norah presented emotional dysregulation, aggression toward her sister, academic problems, distortion of her body image, disturbed interpersonal relationships, many difficulties in establishing commitments, and significant difficulties regarding her roles, values, and choices. She also had marks on both arms due to self-injurious behavior; therefore she always used to wear shirts that covered the cuts. Regarding depressive symptomatology, she showed apathy, lack of motivations, difficulties to concentrate, insomnia, lack of appetite, anhedonia, sadness, and crying most of the time. She also mentioned having had suicidal ideation without attempts. According to the International Neuropsychiatric Interview (MINI-Kid) conducted by the teenage psychiatrist, Norah suffered from a severe major depressive episode (F32.x) (BDI-I = 32) with a mild suicidal risk (F34.1) and social phobia (F40.1). She also fulfilled criteria for a borderline personality disorder according to the Structured Interview for Axis II of the DSM-IV (SCID-II) and identity diffusion according to the Assessment of Identity Development in Adolescence (AIDA; T = 76) (Goth et al., 2012; Valdés, Hernández, Goth, Quevedo, & Borzutzky, 2019).

Norah received a nine-month treatment that included individual sessions (biweekly), family sessions (biweekly), and pharmacological control (biweekly). The interventions were based on the treatment model of Adolescent Identity Treatment (AIT; Foelsch et al., 2014), which adapts the techniques of transference-focused psychotherapy (TFP) for the treatment of adolescents. This model was developed to treat adolescents with severe personality pathology. AIT focuses on improving identity integration, increasing adaptive functioning, increasing productivity toward achieving life goals, and behavior in the areas of self-regulation and interpersonal relationships. A therapeutic contract, psychoeducation, parenting guidelines, and environmental interventions were conducted, with the aim of containing severe self-injurious behaviors and focusing psychotherapy on the experience of the self and the improvement of affective and behavioral regulation.

Norah and her individual therapist (psychologist) were able to bond quickly and set therapeutic goals together. Her low tolerance to frustration was evident from the first sessions on, as was her lack of differentiation from others. Her oscillation between idealization and devaluation, both in extra-transferential relationships (e.g., friends, parents) and with her therapist, was evident at many times when the therapeutic alliance was strained. After the second month of treatment and with a favorable symptomatic evolution, Norah made a two-month cultural exchange trip, which was considered an important milestone within the treatment, since she was able to establish social relationships and achieve a sense of self-efficacy to face different situations. When she returned, she reintegrated into school in a much more adaptive way, but her social relations were still based on mistrust and the projection of her internal conflicts. This was the focus of the individual sessions, in which the psychotherapist clarified, confronted, and interpreted contents, both extra-transferentially and in the therapeutic relationship itself. At the fifth month of treatment, Norah showed substantial improvements in symptomatology (suicidality, self-harm, negative mood, and aggressive behavior), interpersonal relationships, and academic performance (she was regularly attending school and performing at level). There was a decrease in conflicts related to lack of family boundaries, as well as more support from parents to facilitate her separation and individualization. Considering all these achievements, some therapeutic elements were progressively reduced (one session per week). At the end of the treatment, the improvement achieved was maintained, evidencing a more integrated vision of herself and others, as well as a better regulation of her affects and behaviors. Norah was now able to establish and maintain friendly relationships, with further consolidation of identity as a result of greater integration and differentiation of self and other representations, but also in her ability to utilize more mature defense mechanisms and in reduction of immature defenses (e.g., splitting, omnipotent control, denial, projective identification). The pharmacological treatment ended 1 month after the end of the therapy.

2.9 Conclusion

In this chapter we have outlined the close connection between complex depression and personality functioning with a focus on identity integration. A case example of a 13-year-old girl is used to illustrate the association between depressive symptomatology and anguish related to the diffusion of identity. Negative life experiences can influence the onset of depressive symptomatology, as well as difficulties in the development of the individual's identity and subsequent personality (Middledorp, Cath, Beem, Willemsen, & Boomsma, 2008). This difficulty in the formation of identity during adolescence is in itself a generator of stress, reason why the occurrence of a negative vital event would be enough to limit the strategies of confrontation of the individual, and to end up developing a depressive disorder. One hypothesis could be that greater coherence and continuity of identity mediated the effect of the treatment of depression. Therefore, it was not until the identity integration could be improved that the depression improved as well.

This case is an example for the observation that treatment of depression is not successful if there is a comorbid personality pathology that is not addressed. In previous treatments the patient had been treated only for the diagnosis of depression, and her identity diffusion was not addressed. Then the focus of treatment was shifted towards the patient's identity diffusion and the manualized treatment approach AIT (Adolescent Identity Treatment) was used. After 9 months of treatment a maturation of personality functioning occurred, and parallel with this increase in identity integration, the depressive symptomatology decreased.

Gunderson et al. (2004) could demonstrate that improvements in BPD are often followed by improvements in MDD but, in contrast, improvements in MDD are often not followed by improvements in BPD. Thus, comorbid patients do not recover properly if they are treated with a focus on their depressive disorder, and the outcome is better if the focus of treatment lies on the personality disorder (Gunderson et al., 2014). In adolescent patients, whose main developmental task is the establishment of a stable identity, identity diffusion, if present, has to be the crucial target of psychotherapy.

References

American Psychiatric Association. (2013). *Diagnostic and statistical manual of mental disorders* (5th ed.).

Barton, S., Armstrong, P., Wicks, L., Freeman, E., & Meyer, T. D. (2017). Treating complex depression with cognitive behavioural therapy. *The Cognitive Behaviour Therapist, 10*, 1–15. https://doi.org/10.1017/S1754470X17000149

Becht, A. I., Bos, M. G. N., Nelemans, S. A., Peters, S., Vollebergh, W. A. M., Branje, S. J. T., … Crone, E. A. (2018). Goal-directed correlates and neurobiological underpinnings of adolescent identity: A multimethod multisample longitudinal approach. *Child Development, 89*, 823–836. https://doi.org/10.1111/cdev.13048

Becht, A. I., Luyckx, K., Nelemans, S. A., Branje, S. J. T., Vollebergh, W. A. M., & Meeus, W. H. J. (2019). Linking identity and depressive symptoms across adolescence: A multisample longitudinal study testing within-person effects. *Developmental Psychology, 55*, 1733–1742. https://doi.org/10.1037/dev0000742

Birmaher, B., Williamson, D. E., Dahl, R. E., Axelson, D. A., Kaufman, J., Dorn, L. D., & Ryan, N. D. (2004). Clinical presentation and course of depression in youth: Does onset in childhood differ from onset in adolescence? *Journal of the American Academy of Child and Adolescent Psychiatry, 43*, 63–70. https://doi.org/10.1097/00004583-200401000-00015

Both, L. M., Pereira da Cruz, S., & Goodman, G. (2019). Reflective function and identity in adolescents with clinical and nonclinical symptoms. *Trends in Psychiatry and Psychotherapy, 41*, 176–185. https://doi.org/10.1590/2237-6089-2018-0067

Bukh, J. D., Andersen, P. K., & Kessing, L. V. (2016). Personality and the long-term outcome of first-episode depression. *Journal of Clinical Psychiatry*. https://doi.org/10.4088/JCP.15m09823

Burrow, A. L., & Hill, P. L. (2011). Purpose as a form of identity capital for positive youth adjustment. *Developmental Psychology, 47*, 1196–1206. https://doi.org/10.1037/a0023818

Caspi, A., & Moffitt, T. E. (2018). All for one and one for all: Mental disorders in one dimension. *American Journal of Psychiatry, 175*(9), 831–844.
Clarkin, J. F., & Huprich, S. K. (2011). Do DSM-5 personality disorder proposals meet criteria for clinical utility? *Journal of Personality Disorders, 25*, 192–205. https://doi.org/10.1521/pedi.2011.25.2.192
Clarkin, J. F., Petrini, M., & Diamond, D. (2019). Complex depression: The treatment of major depression and severe personality pathology. *Journal of Clinical Psychology, 75*, 824–833. https://doi.org/10.1002/jclp.22758
Clarkin, J. F., Yeomans, F. E., & Kernberg, O. F. (1999). *Psychotherapy for borderline personality*. New York, NY: Wiley.
Costello, E. J., Foley, D. L., & Angold, A. (2006). 10-year research update review: The epidemiology of child and adolescent psychiatric disorders: II. Developmental epidemiology. *Journal of the American Academy of Child & Adolescent Psychiatry, 45*, 8–25. https://doi.org/10.1097/01.chi.0000184929.41423.c0
Costello, L. H., Suh, C., Burnett, B., Kelsay, K., Bunik, M., & Talmi, A. (2019). Addressing adolescent depression in primary care: Building capacity through psychologist and pediatrician partnership. *Journal of Clinical Psychology in Medical Settings*. https://doi.org/10.1007/s10880-019-09680-w
Cramer, A. O. J., Waldorp, L. J., van der Maas, H. L. J., & Borsboom, D. (2010). Comorbidity: A network perspective. *The Behavioral and Brain Sciences, 33*, 137–193.
Curran, P. J., & Bauer, D. J. (2011). The disaggregation of within-person and between-person effects in longitudinal models of change. *Annual Review of Psychology, 62*, 583–619. https://doi.org/10.1146/annurev.psych.093008.100356
Cuthbert, B. N. (2014). The RDoC framework: Facilitating transition from ICD/DSM to dimensional approaches that integrate neuroscience and psychopathology. *World Psychiatry, 13*, 28–35.
Dozois, D. J., & Dobson, K. S. (2003). The structure of the self schema in clinical depression: Differences related to episode recurrence. *Cognition and Emotion, 17*, 933. https://doi.org/10.1080/02699930244000363
Durbin, C. E., & Hicks, B. M. (2014). Personality and psychopathology: A stagnant field in need of development. *European Journal of Personality, 28*, 362–386. https://doi.org/10.1002/per.1962
Ellison, W. D., Rosenstein, L., Chelminski, I., Dalrymple, K., & Zimmerman, M. (2016). The clinical significance of single features of borderline personality disorder: Anger, affective instability, impulsivity, and chronic emptiness in psychiatric outpatients. *Journal of Personality Disorders, 30*(2), 261–270. https://doi.org/10.1521/pedi_2015_29_193
Erikson, E. H. (1959). *Identity and the cycle of life*. New York, NY: Norton & Co..
Erikson, E. H. (1968). *Youth and crisis*. New York, NY: Norton & Co..
Feenstra, D. J., Busschbach, J. J. V., Verheul, R., & Hutsebaut, J. (2011). Prevalence and comorbidity of Axis I and Axis II disorders among treatment refractory adolescents admitted for specialized psychotherapy. *Journal of Personality Disorders, 25*, 842–850. https://doi.org/10.1521/pedi.2011.25.6.842
Finning, K., Ukoumunne, O. C., Ford, T., Danielsson-Waters, E., Shaw, L., Romero De Jager, I., … Moore, D. A. (2019). The association between child and adolescent depression and poor attendance at school: A systematic review and meta-analysis. *Journal of Affective Disorders, 245*, 928–938. https://doi.org/10.1016/j.jad.2018.11.055
Fischer-Kern, M., Tmej, A., Kapusta, N. D., Naderer, A., LeithnerDziubas, K., Löffler-Stastka, H., … Springer-Kremser, M. (2008). The capacity for mentalization in depressive patients: A pilot study. *Psychosomatische Medizin und Psychotherapie, 2008*(54), 368–380. https://doi.org/10.13109/zptm.2008.54.4.368
Foelsch, P. A., Schlüter-Müller, S., Odom, A. E., Arena, H. T., Borzutzky, A., & Schmeck, K. (2014). *Adolescent identity treatment: An integrative approach for personality pathology*. Basel, Switzerland: Springer.

Fusar-Poli, P., Solmi, M., Brondino, N., Davies, C., Chae, C., Politi, P., … McGuire, P. (2019). Transdiagnostic psychiatry: A systematic review. *World Psychiatry, 18*(2), 192–207. https://doi.org/10.1002/wps.20631

Garland, A. (2015). Cognitive behavioural case formulation for complex and recurrent depression. In N. Tarrier & J. Johnson (Eds.), *Case formulation in cognitive behaviour therapy: The treatment of challenging and complex cases*. Routledge.

Global Burden Disease. (2018). Global, regional, and national incidence, prevalence, and years lived with disability for 354 diseases and injuries for 195 countries and territories, 1990–2017: A systematic analysis for the Global Burden of Disease Study 2017. *The Lancet, 392*, 1789–1858. https://doi.org/10.1016/S0140-6736(18)32279-7

Goth, K., Foelsch, P., Schlüter-Müller, S., Birkhölzer, M., Jung, E., Pick, O., & Schmeck, K. (2012). Assessment of identity development and identity diffusion in adolescence – Theoretical basis and psychometric properties of the self-report questionnaire *AIDA. Child and Adolescent Psychiatry and Mental Health, 6*(1), 27.

Grilo, C. M., Stout, R. L., Markowitz, J. C., Sanislow, C. A., Ansell, E. B., Skodol, A. E., … McGlashan, T. H. (2010). Personality disorders predict relapse after remission from an episode of major depressive disorder: A 6-year prospective study. *The Journal of Clinical Psychiatry, 71*(12), 1629–1635. https://doi.org/10.4088/JCP.08m04200gre

Gunderson, J. G., Morey, L. C., Stout, R. L., Skodol, A. E., Shea, M. T., McGlashan, T. H., … Bender, D. S. (2004). Major depressive disorder and borderline personality disorder revisited: Longitudinal interactions. *Journal of Clinical Psychiatry, 65*(8), 1049–1056. https://doi.org/10.4088/jcp.v65n0804

Gunderson, J. G., Stout, R. L., Shea, M. T., Grilo, C. M., Markowitz, J. C., Morey, L. C., … Skodol, A. E. (2014). Interactions of borderline personality disorder and mood disorders over 10 years. *Journal of Clinical Psychiatry, 75*(8), 829–834. https://doi.org/10.4088/JCP.13m08972

Hankin, B. L., Young, J. F., Abela, J. R., Smolen, A., Jenness, J. L., Gulley, L. D., . . . Oppenheimer, C. W. (2015). Depression from childhood into late adolescence: Influence of gender, development, genetic susceptibility, and peer stress. Journal of Abnormal Psychology, 124, 803–816. https://doi.org/10.1037/abn0000089

Hopwood, C. J., Malone, J. C., Ansell, E. B., Sanislow, C. A., Grilo, C. M., McGlashan, T. H., … Morey, L. C. (2011). Personality assessment in DSM-5: Empirical support for rating severity, style, and traits. *Journal of Personality Disorders, 25*, 305–320. https://doi.org/10.1521/pedi.2011.25.3.305

James, W. (1890). *Principles of psychology* (Vol. 1). New York, NY: Henry-Holt & Co..

Kasen, S., Cohen, P., Skodol, A. E., First, M. B., Johnson, J. G., Brook, J. S., … Oldham, J. M. (2007). Comorbid personality disorder and treatment use in a community sample of youths: A 20-year follow up. *Acta Psychiatrica Scandinavica, 115*, 56–65. https://doi.org/10.1111/j.1600-0447.2006.00842.x

Kernberg, O. F. (1976). *Object Relations Theory and Clinical Psychoanalysis*. New York: Jason Aronson.

Kernberg, O. F. (1984). *Severe personality disorders*. New Haven: Yale University Press.

Kernberg, O. F. (2016). What is personality? *Journal of Personality Disorders, 30*(2), 145–156.

Kernberg, P. F., Weiner, A. S., & Bardenstein, K. K. (2000). *Personality disorders in children and adolescents*. New York, NY: Basic Books.

Kessler, R. C., Berglund, P., Demler, O., Jin, R., Merikangas, K. R., & Walters, E. E. (2005). Lifetime prevalence and age-of-onset distributions of DSM–IV disorders in the National Comorbidity Survey Replication. *Archives of General Psychiatry, 62*, 593–602. https://doi.org/10.1001/archpsyc.62.6.593

Klimstra, T. A., & Denissen, J. J. A. (2017). A theoretical framework for the associations between identity and psychopathology. *Developmental Psychology, 53*, 2052–2065. https://doi.org/10.1037/dev0000356

Kotov, R., Krueger, R. F., Watson, D., Achenbach, T. M., Althoff, R. R., Bagby, R. M., … Zimmerman, M. (2017). The Hierarchical Taxonomy of Psychopathology (HiTOP): A dimensional alternative to traditional nosologies. *Journal of Abnormal Psychology, 126*(4), 454–477.

Luyckx, K., Goossens, L., Soenens, B., Beyers, W., & Vansteenkiste, M. (2005). Identity statuses based upon four rather than two identity dimensions: Extending and refining Marcia's paradigm. *Journal of Youth and Adolescence, 34*, 605–618. https://doi.org/10.1007/s10964-005-8949-x

Luyckx, K., Klimstra, T. A., Duriez, B., Van Petegem, S., & Beyers, W. (2013). Personal identity processes from adolescence through the late 20s: Age trends, functionality, and depressive symptoms. *Social Development, 22*, 701–721. https://doi.org/10.1111/sode.12027

Luyckx, K., Schwartz, S., Berzonsky, M., Soenens, B., Vansteenkiste, M., Smits, I., et al. (2008a). Capturing ruminative exploration: Extending the four-dimensional model of identity formation in adolescence. *Journal of Research in Personality, 42*, 58–82. https://doi.org/10.1016/j.jrp.2007.04.004

Luyckx, K., Schwartz, S. J., Goossens, L., Soenens, B., & Beyers, W. (2008b). Developmental typologies of identity formation and adjustment in female emerging adults: A latent class growth analysis approach. *Journal of Research on Adolescence, 18*, 595–619. https://doi.org/10.1111/j.1532-7795.2008.00573.x

Maillard, P., Pellaton, J., & Kramer, U. (2019). Treating comorbid depression and avoidant personality disorder: The case of Andy. *Journal of Clinical Psychology, 75*, 886–897. https://doi.org/10.1002/jclp.22764

Marchette, L. K., & Weisz, J. R. (2017). Practitioner review: Empirical evolution of youth psychotherapy toward transdiagnostic approaches. *Journal of Child Psychology and Psychiatry, 58*, 970–984.

Marcia, J. E. (1966). Development and validation of ego identity status. *Journal of Personality and Social Psychology, 3*, 551–558.

McGrath, R. E. (2005). Conceptual complexity and construct validity. *Journal of Personality Assessment, 85*, 112–124.

Mead, G. H. (1934). *Mind, self, and society*. Chicago, IL: University Press of Chicago.

Meeus, W. (2016). Adolescent psychosocial development: A review of longitudinal models and research. *Developmental Psychology, 52*, 1969–1993. https://doi.org/10.1037/dev0000243

Meeus, W., Van de Schoot, R., Keijsers, L., & Branje, S. (2012). Identity statuses as developmental trajectories: A five-wave longitudinal study in early-to-middle and middle-to-late adolescents. *Journal of Youth and Adolescence, 41*, 1008–1021. https://doi.org/10.1007/s10964-011-9730-y

Meeus, W., Van de Schoot, R., Keijsers, L., Schwartz, S. J., & Branje, S. (2010). On the progression and stability of adolescent identity formation. A five-wave longitudinal study in early-to-middle and middle-to-late adolescence. *Child Development, 81*, 1565–1581. https://doi.org/10.1111/j.1467-8624.2010.01492.x

Middledorp, C. M., Cath, D. C., Beem, A. L., Willemsen, G., & Boomsma, D. I. (2008). Life events, anxious depression and personality: A prospective and genetic study. *Psychological Medicine, 38*, 1557–1565.

Miller, C. E., Townsend, M. L., Day, N., & Grenyer, B. (2020). Measuring the shadows: A systematic review of chronic emptiness in borderline personality disorder. *PLoS One, 15*(7), e0233970. https://doi.org/10.1371/journal.pone.0233970

Moffitt, T. E., Caspi, A., Taylor, A., Kokaua, J., Milne, B. J., Polanczyk, G., … Poulton, R. (2010). How common are common mental disorders? Evidence that lifetime prevalence rates are doubled by prospective versus retrospective ascertainment. *Psychological Medicine, 40*, 899–909. https://doi.org/10.1017/S0033291709991036

Morey, L. C., Benson, K. T., & Skodol, A. E. (2016). Relating DSM-5 section III personality traits to section II personality disorder diagnoses. *Psychological Medicine, 46*(3), 647–655. https://doi.org/10.1017/S0033291715002226

NICE (2009). *Borderline personality disorder: recognition and management*. Clinical guideline. Published: 28 January 2009 https://www.nice.org.uk/guidance/cg78

Porfeli, E. J., Lee, B., Vondracek, F. W., & Weingold, I. K. (2011). A multi-dimensional measure of vocational identity status. *Journal of Adolescence, 34*, 853–871. https://doi.org/10.1016/j.adolescence.2011.02.001

Price, A., Mahler, H., & Hopwood, C. (2019). Subjective emptiness: A clinically significant transdiagnostic psychopathology construct. (pre-print). https://doi.org/10.31235/osf.io/f2x6r
Ragozini, G., Sica, L. S., & Sestito, L. A. (2014). Identity coping in the first years of university: Identity diffusion, adjustment and identity distress. *Journal of Adult Development, 21*, 159–172. https://doi.org/10.1007/s10804-014-9188-8
Ritchie, R. A., Meca, A., Madrazo, V. L., Schwartz, S. J., Hardy, S. A., Zamboanga, B. L., … Ham, L. S. (2013). Identity dimensions and related processes in emerging adulthood: Helpful or harmful? *Journal of Clinical Psychology, 69*, 415–432. https://doi.org/10.1002/jclp.21960
Schmeck, K., Schlüter-Müller, S., Foelsch, P. A., & Doering, S. (2013). The role of identity in the DSM-5 classification of personality disorders. *Child and Adolescent Psychiatry and Mental Health, 7*(1), 27. https://doi.org/10.1186/1753-2000-7-27
Schmittmann, V. D., Cramer, A. O. J., Waldorp, L. J., Epskamp, S., Kievit, R. A., & Borsboom, D. (2013). Deconstructing the construct: A network perspective on psychological phenomena. *New Ideas in Psychology, 31*, 45–53.
Schwartz, S. J., Klimstra, T. A., Luyckx, K., Hale, W. W., III, & Meeus, W. H. (2012). Characterizing the self-system over time in adolescence: Internal structure and associations with internalizing symptoms. *Journal of Youth and Adolescence, 41*, 1208–1225. https://doi.org/10.1007/s10964-012-9751-1
Sharp, C., Wright, A. G., Fowler, J. C., Frueh, B. C., Allen, J. G., Oldham, J., & Clark, L. A. (2015). The structure of personality pathology: Both general ('g') and specific ('s') factors? *Journal of Abnormal Psychology, 124*(2), 387–398.
Skodol, A. E., Grilo, C. M., Keyes, K. M., Geier, T., Grant, B. F., & Hasin, D. S. (2011). Relationship of personality disorders to the course of major depressive disorder in a nationally representative sample. *American Journal of Psychiatry, 168*(3), 257–264. https://doi.org/10.1176/appi.ajp.2010.10050695
Sollberger, D. (2013). On identity: from a philosophical point of view. *Child and Adolescent Psychiatry and Mental Health, 7*(1), 29. https://doi.org/10.1186/1753-2000-7-29
Tarrier, N., & Johnson, J. (2015). *Case formulation in cognitive behaviour therapy: The treatment of challenging and complex cases*. Routledge.
Thapar, A., Collishaw, S., Pine, D. S., & Thapar, A. K. (2012). Depression in adolescence. *Lancet (London, England), 379*(9820), 1056–1067. https://doi.org/10.1016/S0140-6736(11)60871-4
Thompson, K. N., Jackson, H., Cavelti, M., Betts, J., McCutcheon, L., Jovev, M., & Chanen, A. M. (2019). Number of borderline personality disorder criteria and depression predict poor functioning and quality of life in outpatient youth. *Journal of Personality Disorders*, 1–14. https://doi.org/10.1521/pedi_2019_33_411
Valdés, N., Hernández, C., Goth, K., Quevedo, I., & Borzutzky, A. (2019). Adaptación y validación de la versión chilena del Cuestionario para Evaluar el Desarrollo de la Identidad en Adolescentes (AIDA) [Adaptation and validation of the Chilean version of the Questionnaire for Assessing Identity Development in Adolescents (AIDA)]. *Revista Argentina de Clínica Psicológica, XXVIII*(5), 610–623.
Waller, G., & Turner, H. (2016). Therapist drift redux: Why well-meaning clinicians fail to deliver evidence-based therapy, and how to get back on track. *Behaviour Research and Therapy, 77*, 129–137.
Zanarini, M. C., Frankenburg, F. R., Reich, D. B., Silk, K. R., Hudson, J. I., & McSweeney, L. B. (2007). The subsyndromal phenomenology of borderline personality disorder: A 10-year follow-up study. *The American Journal of Psychiatry, 164*(6), 929–935. https://doi.org/10.1176/ajp.2007.164.6.929

Chapter 3
The Functional Domain of Affect Regulation

Carolina Altimir, Cecilia de la Cerda, and Paula Dagnino

Abstract This chapter reviews the concept of affect regulation from the perspective of the functional domain criteria, in an attempt to understand and describe its role for psychopathology, and specifically for depression and personality dysfunction. It incorporates the ongoing discussions within the fields of psychiatry, psychology, and psychopathology research that call for a reformulation of the traditional categorical diagnostic systems that account for both healthy and maladaptive mental functioning. The value of the Research Domain Criteria Initiative (RDoC) for the comprehension as well as the integration of the conceptual diversity of affect regulation is discussed, given its dimensional, transdiagnostic and multilevel perspective for the comprehension of mental functioning. This opens up a window of opportunity for collaboration between different approaches from various disciplines to the understanding of affect regulation, under the spirit of an explanatory pluralism. In this integrative attempt, we have proposed to complement two main approaches to defining and understanding affect regulation: a developmental perspective based on attachment theory and developmental research, and emotion processing models derived from psychological and neuroscientific research. We conclude with a discussion of the contribution of understanding affect regulation in depression and personality disorders based on a dimensional framework for understanding the development of personality and psychopathology. For this purpose, we review two complementary models that focus on relatedness and self-definition as the central coordinates of human mental development and examine the domain of affect regulation along a continuum from normal to abnormal functioning within the levels of operation described in the previous models.

C. Altimir (✉) · P. Dagnino
Facultad de Psicología, Universidad Alberto Hurtado, Santiago, Chile

Millennium Institute for Research in Depression and Personality (MIDAP), Santiago, Chile

C. de la Cerda
Millennium Institute for Research in Depression and Personality (MIDAP), Santiago, Chile

Departamento Disciplinario de Psicología, Facultad de Ciencias Sociales, Universidad de Playa Ancha, Valparaiso, Chile

G. de la Parra et al. (eds.), *Depression and Personality Dysfunction*, Depression and Personality, https://doi.org/10.1007/978-3-030-70699-9_3

Keywords Affect regulation · Personality-depression · Attachment · Psychopathology

The proposal that affect regulation can be considered as a functional domain underlying both healthy and maladaptive mental functioning is based on a profound reformulation experienced by psychiatry and mental health research in the past years. The categorical diagnostic systems (i.e., DSM/ICD) widely used until now to account for mental disorders are under intense criticism, inasmuch as they are based on the clinical presentation of a heterogeneous set of signs, symptoms, and syndromes with different physiopathological mechanisms involved, grouped in categories of doubtful validity (Jiménez & Altimir, 2019; Maj, 2012; Mann, 2010).

In view of this discussion, the National Institute of Mental Health (NIMH) has recently proposed the Research Domain Criteria Initiative (RDoC) with the aim of classifying mental disorders based on a dimensional, transdiagnostic, and multilevel approach that considers behavioral and neurobiological mechanisms organized along systems underlying basic psychological capacities, rather than on discrete categories, and including the full range of variation, from normal to abnormal (Cuthbert & Insel, 2013). These systems include social processes (affiliation and attachment), cognitive, arousal/regulatory, sensoriomotor, and positive and negative valence systems. From this perspective, mental disorders are considered disruptions of the normal-range operation of these systems (Cuthbert & Insel, 2013). At the same time, it assumes that the origins and pathways of psychopathology may operate at many levels, including the genetic/neural, the individual, the family environmental, and the social contextual, thus implying that interventions and treatments can be accommodated according to their suitability at these different levels (Bolton, 2013).

Meanwhile, affect regulation has evidenced a growing interest among several disciplines, including cognitive sciences (Gross, 2014; Taipale, 2016), neuroscience (Damasio, 1998; Gyurak & Etkin, 2014; Schore, 2012; Schuessler, 2003), developmental and attachment theories (Beebe & Lachmann, 2002; Bowlby, 1969; Fonagy, Gergely, Jurist, & Target, 2002; Tronick, 2007), and psychopathology, psychiatry, and psychotherapy (Fonagy et al., 2002; Schore, 2012; Taipale, 2016). This interest responds to the increasing acknowledgment of its central relevance for the operation of the human mind, the development of the self (Taipale, 2016), and the etiopathology and maintenance of several mental disorders (Berenbaum, Raghavan, Le, Vernon, & Gomez, 2003; Berking et al., 2019; Greenberg, 2002; Kring & Bachorowski, 1999; Mennin & Farach, 2007). In fact, over 75% of the categories of the Diagnostic and Statistical Manual of Mental Disorders (American Psychiatric Association, 2013) are characterized by problems with affect regulation, and emotion dysregulation has been described as underlying many of the most common forms of psychopathology (Barlow & Allen, 2004; Kring & Sloan, 2009; Gratz et al., 2015; Grecucci et al., 2015). This highlights the fact that although affect regulation is considered relevant for these fields of research, and perhaps precisely because of this, it still lacks a clear and unambiguous definition (Fonagy et al., 2002; Gross, 2014).

Given this conceptual diversity, the notion of affect regulation as a functional domain of mental operation gives an opportunity to understand it as a mechanism that lays at the crossroads of several of the systems proposed by the RDoC. Therefore, the different definitions and models of affect regulation can be organized based on the level of operation this mechanism is being evidenced. In this chapter, we attempt an overview of affect regulation as a mechanism involved in some constructs belonging to the different research domains (social processes systems – affiliation and attachment – positive/negative valence, cognitive and arousal/regulatory).

Particularly regarding depression, disruptions in affect regulation capacities have been associated with impaired social skills, poor quality of life, and poor capacity to label and identify affective states (Compare, Zarbo, Shonin, Van Gordon, & Marconi, 2014). At the same time, depressed individuals show negative biases in the recognition of emotion, which increases significantly according to diagnostic severity (Punkanen, Eerola, & Erkkilä, 2011), and difficulties in accepting and processing negative emotional material (Joormann & Gotlib, 2010), which in turn is associated with longer episodes of sadness and depressed mood (Teasdale, 1988; Nolen-Hoeksema, Wisco, & Lyubomirsky, 2008). These difficulties in emotion regulation (Campbell-Sills & Barlow, 2007; Gross & Munoz, 1995; Mennin, Holoway, Fresco, Moore, & Heimberg, 2007) are particularly evident in an inability to modify and adapt strategies to cope with negative emotions across different circumstances (Aldao, Nolen-Hoeksema, & Schweizer, 2010; Cole & Kaslow, 1988; Joorman, Siemer, & Gotlib, 2007). Thus, individuals who cannot manage their emotional responses to everyday events will have more periods of distress that may evolve into depressive symptoms (e.g., Mennin, Holoway, Fresco, Moore, & Heimberg, 2007; Nolen-Hoeksema, Wisco, & Lyubomirsky, 2008).

Meanwhile, personality disorders, and particularly borderline personality disorder (BPD), which is perhaps the most studied of these diagnostic categories (Bateman & Fonagy, 2006, 2012; Linehan, 1993; Lynch, Trost, Salsman, & Linehan, 2007), include emotion dysregulation among its most characteristic features (Fonagy, Luyten, & Strathearn, 2011; Linehan, 1993; Reisch, Ebner-Priemer, Tschacher, Bohus, & Linehan, 2008; Sanislow et al., 2002; Westen, 1991, 1998). This is reflected in the fact that several of the diagnostic criteria for BPD, such as self-harm, affective instability, and impulsivity, are a result of affect dysregulation (Conklin, Bradley, & Westen, 2006). Affect dysregulation associated with this disorder generally refers to an impairment in the capacity to modulate affect, resulting in a spiraling of increased emotional intensity and a sense of loss of control and of rapid changes in their quality, disrupting the capacity to reflect on this experience (Linehan & Heard, 1992; Westen, 1991, 1998). Underlying these difficulties in achieving affect self-regulation within BPD is a failure of mentalizing abilities in contexts of intense emotionality (Bateman & Fonagy, 2006, 2012, 2019).

We believe that in order to develop a better comprehension of how affect regulation as a functional domain is acquired and developed, and subsequently manifested in depression and personality disorders, we must try to integrate two different perspectives, which in turn account for different levels of mental operation. First, we review developmental perspectives, describing models where the object of regulation is the self, in order to understand how different affect regulatory mechanisms and styles are consolidated throughout development as a functional domain and influence personality and psychopathology. We then review emotional processing models where the object of regulation is emotion and its present experience and describe the specific processes involved in its appraisal and modulation. Finally, we discuss the contribution of understanding affect regulation in depression and personality disorders from a dimensional approach to the development of personality and psychopathology. The value of this approach resides in its coherence with the notion of functional domain, inasmuch as it underscores the understanding of psychopathology based on a continuum from normal to abnormal functioning along different levels of operation. Both perspectives, therefore, provide an opportunity to integrate knowledge from different disciplines in an attempt to contribute to the effort of achieving an "explanatory pluralism" of mental disorders (Kendler, 2005), at the same time that it highlights the richness involved in a person-centered approach rather than a disorder-centered perspective.

3.1 Developmental Perspective on Affect Regulation

The relevance of affect and affect regulation has grown largely associated with advances in the field of developmental psychology and neuroscience, as well as attachment research over the past five decades. These fields have gathered substantial evidence indicating the interactive nature of the development of the human mind and brain (Allen, 2013; Schore, 2003). Findings in developmental neuroscience have concluded that the infant brain is designed to be shaped by the social environment in which it develops (Thomas et al., 1997), and in that sense, it is considered to be a "social brain" (Brothers, 1990). The processes involved in the caregiver-infant interactions constitute a dialectical sequence of mutually driven behaviors, where the regulatory functions of the caregiver not only modulate the infant's internal states, favoring the emergence of socio-affective functions in the developing self, but also shape the emergent self's capacity for self-organization (Schore, 2016). This implies that the self develops within a relational matrix through processes that are organized dyadically between the infant and its caregiver (Lachmann, 2001; Schore, 2016). What this array of findings in the field of infant development and attachment conclude is that what is transacted within the infant-caregiver exchange is precisely affect, through a highly efficient and essentially nonverbal system of emotional communication (Allen, 2013; Schore, 2016). Affect regulation constitutes, then, a central mechanism in the process through which the infant moves from a state of co-regulation with its caregiver to self-regulation, in what is considered a developmental achievement (Fonagy et al., 2002; Taipale, 2016). This underscores the relevance that affect regulation plays in the constitution and development of the self (Beebe & Lachmann, 2002; Fonagy et al., 2002; Tronick, 1989). As Schore (2003) points out, research on these varying disciplines, as well as clinical data, are supporting the notion that in infancy and along the human life span, the regulation of affect is a central organizing principle of human development and motivation.

From this perspective, then, the object of regulation is the *self*, and the primary means through which it is achieved is affect. In the attempt to better define the domain of affect regulation, this conceptualization is paramount, as it constitutes the basic premise of the models that we will review in this section. These models allow to contextualize the functional domain of affect regulation as something human beings learn and develop early in infancy (Kopp & Neufeld, 2003), and that will influence the capacity for affect self and hetero-regulation by means of emotional interactive repertoires that will be put forward by the individual in subsequent relationships throughout the life span (Beebe & Lachmann, 2002; Fonagy et al., 2002; Schore, 2012; Tronick, 1989; Tronick & Cohn, 1989).

Throughout these models, affect regulation has been consistently linked to the attachment system, and therefore they are intimately related from their origin in early human development and subsequently remain strongly imbricated throughout the life of an individual (Bateman & Fonagy, 2004, 2012). Affect regulation is the primary function of the innate motivational attachment system. Throughout the continuous transactions between infant and caregiver, which seek to regulate the changing levels of arousal of the baby, and its emotional states, affect regulation emerges as one of the main human capacities. The specific forms of affect regulation that will be shaped and consolidated throughout development will be strongly influenced by the quality of these transactions along a range of time and behaviors, which will progressively become organized in configurations of actions and responses that will result in the individual's sense of self and of others (Allen, 2013). This will be at the core of the individual's capacity for self-regulation and for the regulation of the interactions with others (Beebe, Knoblauch, Rustin, & Sorter, 2005). Accordingly, early experiences of emotional neglect and of various types of abuse will strongly affect the individual's capacity for emotional regulation and ultimately for the development of a coherent sense of self (Allen, 2013; Fonagy & Target, 1997; Bateman & Fonagy, 2012; Ripoll, Snyder, Steele, & Siever, 2013).

We will now review the most relevant models of regulation of the self that have emerged from developmental and attachment research, pointing out the aspects that we consider most relevant for the understanding of affect regulation as a functional domain that shapes and consolidates throughout development.

3.1.1 Attachment Theory and Affect Regulation

Any attempt at describing the developmental bases of affect regulation must consider attachment theory as the primary theoretical model of reference (Bowlby, 1969; Schore, 2003). This is founded on the evidenced-based notion that the main function of the attachment system is affect regulation (Allen, 2013). Furthermore, Sroufe (1996) has pointed out that attachment can be defined as the dyadic regulation of emotion.

To understand this relationship, we must review the fundamental concepts developed by attachment theory. John Bowlby (1969) investigated the mechanisms by which the child forms a secure attachment of emotional communication with the mother, and how this early social-emotional learning is then internalized in the form of a lasting ability to regulate and thus generate and maintain states of emotional security (Schore, 2003). He described the attachment system as one that evolved not only to ensure physical protection but also to provide a sense of security and comfort in the face of distress or fear. This relationship develops since birth and involves a coordination of the child's attachment system (the way the infant seeks protection and proximity with its caregiver) with the parental care system (the way the caregiver responds to the infant's emotional needs) (Allen, 2013).

According to this model, it is within the framework of the innate motivational system of attachment that the process of affect regulation in early childhood is developed, by means of two primary channels. On the one hand, when faced with situations that threaten the availability or closeness of the attachment figure, the child experiences emotional distress and seeks proximity to its caregiver in order to restore the feeling of security that results from her protective and comforting presence (Meyer & Pilkonis, 2005). On the other hand, the caregiver who is sensitive and responsive is able to help the baby regulate his/her feelings of distress, allowing him/her to experience an emotional sense of "felt security" (Pietromonaco, Feldman Barrett, & Powers, 2006). Although physical protection is a fundamental aspect of the attachment system, research has placed more relevance to the reestablishment of the sense of security. In other words, the possibility of turning to a responsive and available caregiver for relief of pain or fear constitutes a safe haven. This is a process that takes place through multiple channels of interaction (nonverbal, verbal, vowel, neuroendocrine, kinesthetic, among others), generating different qualities of experience between the infant and the caregiver depending on the degree of responsiveness of the latter. Understood in this way, affect regulation is a process that is based on the strategies of approach or avoidance by the child towards the figure of the caregiver. The function of restoring a feeling of security – by the caregiver – when the attachment system of the infant activates, accounts for the central function of emotion regulation (Ainsworth, Blehar, Waters, & Wall, 1978; Bowlby, 1969; Fonagy et al., 2002).

Based on the experience of a responsive and sensitive parent that is capable of reading and comforting the infant, it gradually develops a secure or insecure attachment style (Allen, 2013). Secure attachment provides two fundamental experiences for the infant. It constitutes a safe haven where the infant feels comforted, and at the same a secure base, which allows the exploration of the world. This double function optimally balances the fundamental developmental dialectic of relatedness and autonomy. This means that the securely attached child or adult will be able of being dependent at the same time as independent (Allen, 2013).

The sustained experience of security or insecurity within the attachment relationship is maintained by what Bowlby (1969) called internal working models (IWM). As the particular interactions and regulatory behaviors and responses between the infant and its caregiver repeat over time, the child eventually begins to internalize his/her experiences with the caregiver in such a way that they become organized in mental representation, or a set of beliefs and feelings about oneself, the others, and the relationships (Allen, 2013; Luyten & Blatt, 2015). These, in turn, form prototypes for later relationships (Bartholomew & Horowitz, 1991). These internal representations include explicit autobiographical, episodic memories, beliefs and attitudes about self and relationship partners, and generic declarative knowledge about attachment interactions, but at the same time may be implicit, not conscious, and contain procedural knowledge about how to regulate emotions and behave affectively in close relationships (Allen, 2013; Mikulincer & Shaver, 2007).

Together, these contents constitute general beliefs about whether attachment figures will be available and responsive (view of others) and whether the self is worthy of love (view of self) (Pietromonaco et al., 2006). These relatively stable representations of oneself and others are the basis of the attachment styles developed by the infant and consolidated later on in adulthood (Allen, 2013). The seminal work by Mary Ainsworth (Ainsworth et al., 1978) and her study of infants' reactions to the Strange Situation, and decades of subsequent research, have yielded consistent descriptions of secure and insecure attachment styles in children.

Thus, secure attachment stems from the experience of a consistent emotional responsiveness from the caregiver. This pattern of attachment is associated with representations of others as available, reliable, caring, and loving in the face of emotional distress. In turn, these experiences consolidate into a representation of oneself as worthy of love and care and basically lovable (Main, Hesse, & Hesse, 2011; Main, Kaplan, & Cassidy, 1985). It should be noted that these representations do not imply an idealized vision of oneself and others, but allow the possibility of a balanced one, which tolerates failures and negative as well as positive aspects of self and others in a flexible way (Allen, 2013). Secure attachment, therefore, is the basis for the capacity for emotional regulation (Allen, 2013), and thus for helping the individual to keep fear and anxiety at bay, allowing him/her to maintain a fundamental state of emotional security throughout their lives (Van der Kolk, 2014).

Meanwhile, insecure attachment styles are the consequence of adaptive strategies displayed by the individual to maintain attachment (i.e., closeness to the figure of the caregiver), in the face of repeated experiences of suboptimal care (Allen, 2013). Ambivalent insecure attachment is based on IWM of attachment figures as being able to provide love and care, but in an inconsistent way, so they become unreliable. The ambivalence then lies in the fact that the infant expects his or her caregiver to be loving, but at the same time to fail or to show rejection. Therefore, representations of relationships with others are shaped by a mixture of hope and expectations of disappointment. Not knowing what to expect from their parents, and not being sure how to get love and affection, leads to the child making many efforts to get their caregiver's attention, often clinging and whining, and becoming demanding. The anxiety inherent to these conflicting expectations leads in turn to suspicion and hypervigilance, and to hypersensitivity, with a continued expectation of receiving signs of rejection and potential abandonment. This, in turn, often leads to misperceptions or overreactions to the usual failures in attunement or responsiveness that are characteristic of interpersonal relationships. In this way, the representation of oneself that takes shape throughout these experiences are that of being someone who is inadequate, weak, and unworthy of love, generating a feeling of insecurity in oneself and of self-criticism. In terms of affective regulation strategies in the face of emotional distress, the ambivalent pattern involves the hyperactivation of attachment needs in order to elicit the care of an inconsistent and nonresponsive figure (Allen, 2013; Main et al., 2011).

Avoidant attachment, on the other hand, is mainly associated with IWM of the main attachment figures as rejecting and unavailable, which convey to the child the idea that he/she is not important and, moreover, that he/she is a nuisance, so he/she will not be able to count on her caregiver to feel safe. In the face of this experience, the infant develops a sense of himself or herself as someone who is not worthy of care and affection, in contrast to which he or she must develop self-protective strategies. This is associated, therefore, with an attitude of distrust towards the figures of attachment, which leads to strategies of self-defense such as hostility and suspicion, and a defensive insufflation of oneself, as well as a tendency to attribute blame for problems to others. In this way, the individual is in a permanent attempt to remain in control in relationships. These defensive and hostile attitudes can turn into self-fulfilling prophecies, generating in others a rejecting and hostile response. In terms of affective regulation strategies in the face of suffering and pain, the avoidance pattern involves deactivation (hypoactivation) of attachment needs to avoid the experience of consistent rejection (Allen, 2013).

Based on Ainsworth's work, researchers on adult attachment have described how individual's internal working models based on childhood attachment patterns to caregivers are evident subsequently within romantic relationships and in self-reported descriptions of attachment to parents (Allen, 2013; Bartholomew & Horowitz, 1991; Wei, Russell, Mallinckrodt, & Vogel, 2007). This research has supported the notion that the particular quality and characteristics of these representations will have important consequences for the subsequent psychological functioning of the individual (Mikulincer & Shaver, 2007). Therefore, they are considered by several authors as the foundations of the development and functioning of the personality (Luyten & Blatt, 2015; Meyer & Pilkonis, 2005; Pietromonaco et al., 2006). Although these representations are more or less persistent throughout life, marking a trajectory in the child's emotional, social, and representational development, for Bowlby (1988) they were potentially flexible and modifiable in the context of subsequent relationships, showing a balance of stability and change throughout the life span (Allen, 2013).

3.1.2 Mentalization and Affect Regulation

Drawing on attachment theory and psychoanalysis, Fonagy and colleagues (Fonagy, 2015; Fonagy et al., 2002; Fonagy & Target, 2002, 2007) have refined a model that explores how the affective experiences between infant and caregiver contribute to the acquisition of self-regulation as a result of co-regulation, by means of mentalization (Fonagy et al., 2002). The mentalization model takes as its starting point the explanatory power of Bowlby's model based on the IWMs, which lies in the idea of cognitive models that encode interpersonal expectations based on representations of self and others and thus provide prototypes for subsequent relationships. Furthermore, they incorporate subsequent developments in attachment research and theory, with particular emphasis on the work of Mary Main and the notion of coherence proper of IWM associated with secure attachment patterns. Based on these formulations, Fonagy and colleagues develop the construct of mentalization as the capacity that secure attachment relationships provide the infant with (Fonagy, 2015). Mentalization is defined by the authors as the ability to conceive of oneself and others as possessing beliefs, feelings, attitudes, desires, and intentions and therefore to give meaning and predictability to the behavior of others (Allen, Fonagy, & Bateman, 2008).

The theory of mentalization is based on three assumptions about the development of the self: (1) the sense of self as an agent is based on the experience of attribution of mental states by a significant figure (i.e., the primary caregiver); (2) this capacity develops from interaction with the caregiver (often the mother) through a process of "contingent mirroring"; and (3) this capacity can be altered by traumatic experiences (Weinberg, 2006). Fonagy and Target (2002) argue that evolution would have selected attachment as the main training field for the development of regulation, adding that regulation – especially self-regulation – is the master key between genetic predisposition, early experience, and adult functioning.

The process by which the caregiver enables the infant to develop a second order system of representation for mental states, that is, mentalization, is described by the social biofeedback model (Fonagy & Target, 2002). Affect regulation lays at the heart of this process and therefore is inextricably linked to the regulation of the self (Fonagy et al., 2002). Thus, early affect regulation is carried out by the primary caregiver, who reads the baby's automatic emotional expressions and reacts with various expressions, as an affective mirroring, which allows the child's affects to be modulated (Gergely, 2007; Gergely & Watson, 1999; Watson, 2001). The quality of how affect is reflected impacts the development of the processes of emotional regulation and self-control, including mechanisms of attention and voluntary control.

In this process, the caregiver's ability to offer the baby an adequate and metabolized reflect of its affective experience is central. In the process of mirroring, the caregiver elaborates the emotional experience of the baby in her own internal world. Here the key mechanism is the caregiver's self-regulation of emotions (Fonagy & Target, 2002), expressed in the capacity to control the responses to stress, maintain the focus of attention, and interpret her own mental states as well as the infant's. The caregiver's sensitivity to the infants' emotional cues and her own emotional states is based on the ability to mentalize the child and herself (Fonagy, 2015; Fonagy & Bateman, 2006). Furthermore, Taipale (2016) makes the case for the relevance of considering that the caregiver *is in charge* of affect regulation at the onset: from pre-dyadic regulation, to dyadic regulation, to increasing self-regulation. The caregiver initially manages affect regulation and progressively "facilitates" it, because the infant is initially unskilled and unable to adjust its environment.

The extent to which the child is able to adequately attribute the caregiver's emotional reflection as belonging to the caregiver and distinguish it from its own emotional states will depend on two simultaneous responses by the caregiver: the degree to which the reflected affect is marked, that is, it constitutes an exaggerated version of the emotional expression that distinguishes it perceptually from the realistic expression of an emotion (therefore, it is not the mother's internal state), and the degree of contingency of the response, that is, the degree of relationship, whether temporal, sensory, or spatial, between the emotional behavior of the baby and the mother's affective reflection. This will allow the infant to attribute that emotion to him/herself (Fonagy et al., 2002; Gergely, 2007). Specifically, when the caregiver reflects the affects through certain ostensible keys, this induces in the child the corresponding interpretative attitude, activating his/her search for internal reference. As a result of this pointing out and using subtle but biologically coded indicators that the reflected affect is not the same as that of the person expressing it, the reflected emotion is separated from that of the caregiver and the child can search for the internal state to which that emotion refers (Bateman & Fonagy, 2012; Fonagy, Gergely, & Target, 2007). This contingent feedback forms the basis for the development in the baby of an understanding of the emotions and intentions not only of the other, but also of its own. These are fundamentally interdependent and parallel processes, involving a continuous back and forth between internal and external characteristics of the self and the other (Bateman & Fonagy, 2012). During the first three months of life, the child would be oriented to seek stimuli of perfect contingent response, to achieve a primary exploration and representation of his/her body, which would have an evolutionary function. It has been observed that from the age of three months onwards, he would show a preference for imperfect degrees of contingency, that is, for "necessary but less than perfect" responses by his attachment figures, in order to explore and represent the social world (Fonagy et al., 2002). Along these processes, Taipale (2016) highlights the way which infants modify their environment to deal with their own affects and emotions through hetero-regulation. This hetero-regulation is other-based, where significant others function as social mirrors for the child through their own subjectivities (Taipale, 2016).

These interactions within a secure relationship would be decisive in facilitating the development of psychophysiological and psychological self-regulation mechanisms (Fonagy & Target, 2002). The quality of the affect's mirroring impacts the development of emotional regulation and self-control processes, including attention and voluntary control mechanisms. On the contrary, when the relationships between the baby and its caregivers are insecure and unpredictable, the development of a sense of self is made difficult, affecting the possibility of predicting one's own and another's behavior, the capacity for emotional regulation, and the construction of appropriate mental representations for blurred, chaotic, and confusing internal states (de la Cerda, Martínez, & Tomicic, 2019; Fonagy & Target, 2007). Furthermore, experiences of a traumatic nature in the context of emotional deprivation and abuse of various kinds leave important cognitive and emotional traces in these regulatory capacities (Bateman & Fonagy, 2012; Ripoll et al., 2013). According to Taipale (2016), early interaction and the type of attachment developed in early infancy with the caregiver somehow sketch a developmental direction for subsequent self-regulation. This will be later manifest in developmental difficulties as well as difficulties in adult functioning and in different attachment patterns. If the child is not properly mirrored in the affect regulation process, or is mirrored ambiguously or negatively, there will be an insufficient capacity to learn to control one's own affect, and this will result in an impaired or distorted emotional development (Taipale, 2016).

Throughout the course of pre-dyadic and dyadic forms of early affect regulation, self-regulation becomes increasingly independent as the infant gradually internalizes the regulatory functions that are initially managed by the caregiver (Taipale, 2016). With this respect, the social biofeedback model proposes that, through this process, the infant internalizes the mother's empathic response, which generates a secondary representation of its own emotional state, modulating an emotional experience that can then be thought of as different to the primary experience. It is from this dyadic relationship that a gradual organization of self-states emerges and is finally cemented in intersubjectivity (Bateman, & Fonagy, 2004). For Fonagy et al. (2002), this process would be the basis of the development of mentalization. This will largely determine the child's ability to develop representations of him/herself and others as separate entities with different intentions, desires, and feelings (Fonagy et al., 2002; Gergely, 2007; Gergely & Watson, 1999; Watson, 2001), which will translate into particular characteristics of later psychological functioning (Fonagy et al., 2002), including affect regulation.

3.1.3 Coordination, Miscoordination, and Affect Regulation

Another model that contributes to the understanding of how affect regulation develops during early childhood is the Mutual Regulation Model proposed by Tronick and his collaborators (Tronick, 1989, 2001; Tronick et al., 1998). While the MRM has developed in parallel to that of Fonagy and colleagues described above, we believe it richly complements the understanding of the processes and mechanisms involved in the development of affect regulation in early childhood. This model is based on conceptualizations in attachment theory, as well as in relational and intersubjective approaches within the framework of psychoanalytic thought, at the same time that it informs on empirical research on mother-infant interactions. Its primary value is that it emphasizes the uniqueness of the attachment bond beyond the paradigmatic relational representations postulated by Bowlby (Fonagy, 2015; Stern et al., 1998; Tronick, 1989, 2001; Tronick et al., 1998). Specifically, it highlights the more subtle and dynamic processes of affect regulation that unfold in a bidirectional manner between mother and infant, giving rise to representations of relationships based on states of coherence and dyadic meaning-making (Cohn & Tronick, 1988). In that sense, it emphasizes the integration of self-regulation and interactive regulation processes within the framework of the attachment relationship, where each member of the dyad has the dual task of interacting with the environment (i.e., coordinating with the partner in the interaction), while regulating their own emotional states (Beebe & Lachmann, 2015; Tronick, 1989). This implies that both participants of the dyad negotiate moment by moment the state of the relationship, oscillating continuously between states of coordination and miscoordination (Tronick, 1989, 2001).

These states are the result of the ongoing mother-infant interaction, in which each member of the dyad communicates his/her affective evaluation of the state of what is taking place in the interaction and his/her relational intention, through "relational movements" (Tronick et al., 1998). The process of mutual regulation involves the ability of each member of the dyad – and particularly the caregiver – to understand the meaning of the other's affective display and communication, and to direct the actions of the partner so that both can achieve their objectives.

Emotions play a critical role in this evaluative process, motivating and organizing the infant's behavior. If the infant evaluates that his/her goal is being accomplished, a positive emotional state will be experienced, thus motivating further engagement (smiling and gazing at mother), whereas, if the infant's evaluation is that his/her goal is not being accomplished, he/she will experience negative affect, either anger which motivates the removal of the obstacle or sadness and disengagement, when the obstacle cannot be removed (Campos, Barrett, Lamb, Goldsmith, & Steinberg, 1983; Tronick, 2007).

The infant will make relational moves indicating his/her evaluations of whether he/she is succeeding in achieving a goal through affective displays. The caregiver's ability to read these moves will be used to guide his/her actions for facilitating the infant's achievement of these goals. Thus, through this affective communication system, the caregiver is responsible for the reparation of the infant's failure into success and the simultaneous transformation of his negative emotions into positive ones (Gianino & Tronick, 1988). However, the infant may also display several coping behaviors to shift his/her own attention away from a disturbing event (looking away) or to substitute positive for negative stimulation (self-comforting, self-stimulation), as means of controlling his/her own negative affective states (Rothbart & Derryberry, 1984). If this is successful, the infant shifts from a negative to a more positive emotional state (Gianino & Tronick, 1988; Tronick, 2007), in a process of self-regulation. Both types of interactions account for the process of mutual regulation (i.e., bidirectional regulation), inasmuch as the infant modifies his/her affective displays and behaviors on the basis of his/her appreciation of the caregiver's affective displays and behavior (Cohn & Tronick, 1987).

Miscoordination occurs when one of the participants fails to accurately perceive the meaning of the emotional display of the interactive partner and therefore reacts inappropriately to it (Tronick et al., 1998; Tronick & Cohn, 1989). Reparation consists of the behaviors aimed at remediating these interactive errors and is associated with positive affect. At the same time, the experience of reparation can promote the development of interactive skills and the learning of interaction rules in the child as elements of adaptive relational schemes (Tronick & Cohn, 1989). The normal and frequent miscoordinated states are understood as interactive errors, generating negative affect, whereas the transitions from miscoordinated to coordinated states are understood as interactive repairs, which in turn generate positive affect (Gianino & Tronick, 1988; Tronick, 2007). It is relevant to indicate that, according to this model, normal interactions contemplate the oscillation between periods of interactive success and interactive error, as well as frequent reparations of those errors, so the infant often experiences transformations from negative to positive affect, implying that experiences of negative emotion are brief. Thus, caregiver-infant interactions are successful when the process of self-regulation and interactive regulation is in balance, that is, when none of the members of the dyad are excessively involved in self-regulation processes, at the expense of mutual regulation (Tronick, 2007). As research on face-to-face mother-infant interactions developed by Beatrice Beebe and colleagues have indicated, excessive monitoring by one member of the dyad, at the expense of self-regulation, defines the pole of interactive surveillance, while concern for self-regulation, at the expense of interactive sensitivity, defines the pole of withdrawal or inhibition (Beebe et al., 2000, 2012; Beebe & Lachmann, 2002).

The infant's experience of interactive reparation and the transformation of negative affect into positive affect allow him/her to make a more effective use of his/her affective regulatory capacities both self-directed and those directed to the interactive partner (i.e., the environment). Repeated experiences of reparation enables the infant to establish clear boundaries between self and other, to develop a representation of him/herself as effective, of interactions as positive and reparable, and of the caregiver as reliable and trustworthy, contributing to the capacity of maintaining engagement with the external environment in the face of stress (Tronick, 2007).

The problem arises when interactions are characterized by the infant's experience of prolonged periods of interactive failure and negative affect, with scarce presence of interactive repairs, and therefore few experiences of transformations of negative to positive affect (Tronick, 2007). Infants who chronically experience miscoordinated interactions with their caregivers also experience few instances of mutually positive and contingent states. There is a chronic experience of failure, nonreparation, and negative affect, resulting in the establishment of a predominant self-directed style of regulatory behavior, disengaging from the interaction to devote his/her regulatory capacities to controlling negative affects. This regulatory pattern was observed by Tronick in infants of depressed mothers, who were preoccupied with self-comfort and self-directed regulatory behaviors (turning away, loss of postural control, oral self-comfort, self-clasping, and rocking), showing lowered interactive regulation (Beebe & Lachmann, 2015; Tronick, 1989). Ultimately, the infant develops a representation of self as ineffective and of the caregiver as unreliable. According to Tronick (2007), these regulatory patterns are often observed in psychopathology later on throughout development, manifested in relational-emotional repertoires displayed on later relationships.

In a similar vein as the abovementioned models have described, this model proposes that the impact of the specific quality of repeated early infant-caregiver transactions in adult functioning operates by means of representations. As mother-infant affective regulation interaction along the states of coordination and miscoordination, unfold and repeat over time, the child begins to recognize them, have expectations about how they proceed, and remember these recurring patterns, generalizing and organizing them along the dimensions of time, space, affect, and activation, into representations (Beebe et al., 2012; Beebe & Lachmann, 2002). The dyadic nature of these representations implies that the subject has expectations of relationship and of the roles that both members of the dyad must fulfill in the interaction and that they are activated in each new interactive encounter (Beebe & Lachmann, 2002).

What this model emphasizes is that, inasmuch as the child's strategies for relating to his/her caregiver are enacted prior to the availability of symbols, the most primary form of representation consists of enactive relational procedures that govern "how to do" with others or "implicit relational knowledge" (Lyons-Ruth et al., 1998). These enactive representations include skills and adaptive responses that are evident in behavior but remain unconscious, insofar as they are not represented in a symbolic way. Instead, these patterns are pre-symbolically represented as sequences of organized actions and stored in implicit procedural memory, which are mentally accessed in new social encounters (Beebe & Lachmann, 2002). These forms of representation operate throughout life, not just in childhood, and tend to persist into adolescence and adulthood in the absence of major changes in close relationships. This in turn affects the development of interactive repertoires of emotional exchange that are part of generalized regulatory procedures which are completed and made more complex through a life of subsequent significant relationships and determine, in a more or less stable way, the manner in which relationships are negotiated and maintained throughout life (Beebe, 2006; Beebe & Lachmann, 2002; Tronick, 1989; Tronick & Cohn, 1989). These repertoires contain the modes and styles of affect regulation, regarding both self-regulation strategies and interactive regulatory strategies, that is, when the environment –the interaction partner – is incorporated into the regulatory process.

So far we have made a review of the main developmental models that establish affect regulation as a central element of the development of the self during early childhood. In that respect, at this level of description, affect regulation is involved in the processes and mechanism of what the RDoC categories denominate social processes (i.e., attachment as a motivational system) and arousal/regulatory systems. As we have seen, development of the self cannot be understood without considering that it is mediated by the regulation of affects. At the same time, this provides an understanding of the way in which the process of affect regulation is developed in the context of primary attachment relationships and how the particular characteristics that it adopts will cement the repertoires and schemas of coping and regulating affects later in the life of the individual. This in turn allows an appreciation of the individual differences involved in the affect regulatory strategies displayed later in adulthood. Furthermore, it is relevant to consider not only how affect regulation as a mechanism for coping with relational stress originates but also how it may be susceptible to transformation in the context of subsequent significant interpersonal relationships, including the psychotherapeutic relationship. From this point of view, affect regulation as a functional domain that is undermined as a result of maladaptive coping styles can be approached from these comprehensive parameters of the social systems with a view to improving the repertoires available to the individual.

3.2 Emotion Processing Perspectives

An understanding of affect regulation as a functional domain can benefit from incorporating what research on emotion processing has contributed to the field. From this line of research, emotion is the object of regulation and therefore describes how human beings relate to their own emotions and regulate them by means of appraisal processes. We consider it relevant to review this model of emotions, since we cannot ignore the relevance it has to examine the cognitive, experiential, and physiological underpinnings that determine the phenomenology of emotion and the strategies employed to regulate them.

From this perspective, affect regulation is distinguished from emotion regulation, based on the differentiation between affect and emotion. The term *affect* is used to refer to the superordinate phenomena of emotion-related states that involve relatively quick good-bad discriminations (Scherer, 1984), including *emotions* (anger, sadness, etc.), *stress responses* (whole-body unspecified affective responses) to circumstances that exceed the person's ability to cope, and *moods*, such as depression or euphoria, which last longer and are more diffuse as to their trigger (Gross, 2014). Within this umbrella of affective phenomena, emotions are considered of much shorter duration (Ekman, 2007), are elicited by specific objects, and often give rise to behavioral response tendencies relevant to these objects (Gross, 2014). Emotions arise when an individual attends to and evaluates a certain situation as being psychologically relevant to a specific goal. Its relevance can be either external (a real threat to survival like a snake in the tent) or internal (fear of being fired). These specific goals may vary regarding their endurance, level of awareness, complexity, and idiosyncrasy. The important issue is that it is the specific meaning the situation has for achieving these goals that gives rise to emotions.

Based on these distinctions, affect regulation is then considered as a superordinate process that includes mechanisms such as coping, emotion regulation, mood regulation, and traditional ego-defensive processes (Gross, 1998). Meanwhile, emotion regulation refers to a functional process that shapes which emotions a person has, when he/she has them, and how he/she experiences or expresses them (Gross, 2014; Gross & Thompson, 2007). More specifically, Eisenberg, Fabes, Guthrie, and Reiser (2000) distinguish between regulation of internal processes or physiological states and the regulation of behavioral reactions associated with emotions. The first one describes the

> process of initiating, maintaining, modulating, or changing the occurrence, intensity, or duration of internal feeling states and emotion-related physiological processes, often in the service of accomplishing one's goals (…) emotion regulation is often achieved through effortful management of attention (e.g., attention shifting and focusing, distraction) and cognitions that affect the interpretation of situations (e.g., positive cognitive restructuring) as well as through neurophysiological processes" (p. 137).

Whereas emotion-related behavior regulation is defined as the process of initiating, maintaining, inhibiting, modulating, or changing the occurrence, form, and duration of behavioral concomitants of emotion. This includes observable facial and gestural responses and other behaviors associated with internal emotion-related psychological or physiological states and goals (Eisenberg et al., 2000). This type of regulation may involve the communication of emotion and inhibition or activation of behavior linked to emotion or attempts to modify the emotion-inducing environment. Emotion regulation and behavior regulation are intricately associated, particularly in infancy (Eisenberg et al., 2000).

According to Gross (2014), when an emotion is elicited and experienced, the situation is attended to, giving rise to appraisals, that is, to assessments of what the situation means or entails regarding the individual's relevant goals. The emotional responses generated by these unfolding appraisals involve changes in three simultaneous areas: subjective experience, behaviors, and physiology (neurobiological response system). Thus, emotions make the person feel and incline him/her to act, this last experience including changes in facial and body behavior, which in turn are associated with autonomic and neuroendocrine responses (Gross, 2014). These responses modify the ongoing person-situation transaction that gave rise to the response in the first place. An important implication of this model is the notion that emotional responses often lead to changes in the environment that alter the likelihood of the emergence of that emotion or of other emotions (Gross, 2014).

From this perspective, emotion regulation involves (a) the activation of a regulatory goal (what the individual is trying to accomplish), which can be an emotion in the self (intrinsic emotion regulation) or the emotion in other (extrinsic emotion regulation); (b) the engagement of regulatory processes responsible for altering the emotion trajectory (these strategies can be explicit or implicit, depending on the level of awareness); and (c) the modulation of the emotion trajectory or outcome, that is, the latency, rise time, magnitude, duration, and offset of responses in the behavioral, experiential, or physiological domains of experience (Gross, 1998, 2014). Emotion regulatory strategies can be distinguished according to the point along the emotion-generative process in which they impact. Thus, these regulatory strategies may be aimed at the situation selection, that is, taking actions that make it more or less likely that the situation that gave rise to the emotions will be present; the situation modification (directly modifying the situation in order to alter its emotional impact); attentional deployment, changing the focus of attention in order to influence emotion; and cognitive change (modification of appraisal to alter emotional significance, and response modulation, directly influencing the behavioral, experiential, or physiological components of the emotional response) (Gross, 2014).

However, the relationship between emotion and voluntary control and cognition can be seen with other subtleties. According to some authors, emotion regulatory processes can be understood as occurring along a continuum between explicit (conscious, effortful, and deliberate) regulation and implicit (unconscious, automatic) regulation (Gyurak & Etkin, 2014). Implicit emotion regulation operates without conscious supervision or does not involve explicit intentions and seeks to modify the quality, intensity, or duration of an emotional response. The distinctive characteristic of implicit emotion regulation is that it can be prompted without the individual's conscious awareness of engaging in this process nor the individual's conscious intention of regulating the emotion (Gyurak, Gross, & Etkin, 2011; Koole & Rothermund, 2011; Koole, Webb, & Sheeran, 2015). Explicit emotion regulation is based on self-insight and conscious emotion regulatory strategies and techniques and is therefore mediated by language. Some authors within this line of thought suggest that implicit emotion regulation relates to defense mechanisms, and therefore deficits in implicit emotion regulation, rather than explicit emotion regulation, may be accountable for psychopathology, including anxiety and mood disorders (Rice, & Hoffman, 2014).

A similar perspective is assumed by Schore (2003) when he describes how emotional dysregulation is expressed in defense mechanisms during psychotherapy. He proposes that patient-therapist mechanisms of interactive emotional transaction have a common element with the caregiver-infant relationship (Schore, 2003) in a remnant of nonverbal, prerational stream that binds throughout life, acting also between the therapeutic dyad (Schore, 2011). Several psychopathologies have associated symptoms of emotional dysregulation. In that sense, defense mechanisms can be understood as forms of emotional regulation strategies for avoiding, minimizing, or converting affects that are too difficult to tolerate (Cole, Michel, & O'Donnell, 1994). From this perspective, it is the transference-countertransference matrix the psychotherapeutic scenario in which these strategies of affect regulation and pathogenic schemas of dysregulation must be recognized and addressed. These analogical and visual latent schemas are stored in the visuospatial right hemisphere that contains an analogical representational system (Tucker, 1992) and a nonverbal processing mode that are inaccessible to the language centers (Joseph, 1982).

Finally, we take into consideration Greenberg's (Greenberg, Paivio, Mateu, & Blasco, 2000) proposition of an inverse relationship between emotion and voluntary control. Instead of the notion of emotion as a phenomenon subordinated to reason, Greenberg et al. (2000) suggests that emotions have an organizing role, functioning as guides that inform what is meaningful to human beings. He questions the predominance of consciousness as the top of the hierarchy of control of human behavior and instead postulates the notion of emotional schemes, a set of organizational principles that are built upon the repertoire of innate responses of the individual, as well as from his/her past experience. These emotional schemes act at a higher level of experiential processing that is at once emotional, motivational, and cognitive, which would guide both conscious thought and action. Such high-level tacit processing constitutes a high subjective integration of the biological and the existential, acting as a source of sophisticated information about ourselves and our relationship with those around us (Greenberg, Rice, & Elliot, 1993; Greenberg & Paivio, 2003). These emotional patterns interact with the situation at the instance and give rise to the present experience. They are personal and idiosyncratic, containing emotional memories, hopes, expectations, fears, and knowledge that have been gained from previous experiences. But they are not based only on emotion; they rather constitute a complex synthesis of affect, cognition, motivation, and action, which is responsible for giving each person an integrated sense of himself or herself and the world, as well as a subjectively felt meaning (Greenberg & Paivio, 2003; Greenberg & Safran, 1987; Greenberg et al., 1993, Pascual-Leone, 1991). From this perspective, the scheme generated in the subjective experience is not a representation of reality understood in its logical and rational sense. Rather, as Pascual-Leone (1991) points out, it is a recording of subjectively lived experience. Therefore, the affect-reason sequence also turns around, where self-consciousness becomes a result of emotions rather than of thought or rationality. Automatic emotional responses proceed and influence the conscious meanings an individual has about what happens to him/her, affecting his/her interpretations. It is then the intense emotional meanings that a person attributes to his/her experience that determine his/her cognitive responses. In order to read the relevant affective patterns of the environment, individuals make use of emotional schemata, and to be able to change this structure that, from this perspective, would operate in an implicit way, it is necessary that it be activated. When an individual is emotionally activated, he/she can experience his/her internal states and access the associated cognitions. Therefore, it would not be, from this interpretative framework, cognition that allows an individual to correct the emotion, but just the opposite, the awareness of the activated but accessible emotion would be the one that would allow a person, at least in theoretical terms, to access the way he/she is organizing the experience. In words of Pascual-Leone (2018) individuals change emotion with emotion, and there seems to be enough support to consider that the sequential emotional processing (emotion changing emotion) may be an important causal mechanism of change in psychotherapy.

The level of description of emotions and emotion regulation provided by the models described above contribute to an understanding of affect regulation as an operation belonging to the negative/positive, cognitive, and arousal/regulatory systems proposed by the RDoC initiative. As we have reviewed, regulation of emotions involves effortful management of attention focus and selection, as well as cognitions that affect the interpretation of situations associated with emotions. At the same time, the explicit appraisal process involves cognitive evaluations of the characteristics of the emotional experience, which in turn modify behavioral responses. Meanwhile, the positive or negative experiences that result from the modification of the ongoing person-situation transaction that gave rise to the emotional response, and therefore lead to changes in the environment, altering the likelihood of generating that or other emotions, relate to the operations of the reward system (positive/negative valuation). The arousal system is also described within this model, through the physiological components of the emotional response and its modification.

In synthesis, we review two important perspectives in the understanding of affect regulation that are associated with distinct operative levels in terms of RDoC systems. One group considers affect regulation as a key process for the regulation of the self, whereas another group place affect, and particularly emotion, as the object of regulation. The reviewed perspectives can be understood as referring to different domains of operation regarding affect, and therefore proposing different ways to conceptualize and understand its regulation.

3.3 Affect Regulation Within a Dimensional Perspective of Psychopathology

Categorical diagnostic classifications of mental disorders such as the Diagnostic and Statistical Manual of Mental Disorders (DSM, APA, 2013) and the International Classification of Diseases (ICD-11, WHO, 2018) have been subject to criticism in the last couple of decades, as they have failed in their attempt to identify and articulate distinct psychopathological categories (Borges & Naugle, 2017). This situation has been well documented by many authors (Clark, 2007; Krueger & Markon, 2006; Widiger & Clark, 2000; Widiger & Samuel, 2005). One of these criticisms regard the consistent findings of high rates of co-occurrence among categorically defined disorders such as depression and personality and the lack of clear boundaries between them (Krueger & Tackett, 2003; Widiger & Clark, 2000). This is consistently supported by research that indicates that personality functioning and psychopathology are intimately intertwined, inasmuch as there is evidence of patterns of comorbidities between DSM Axis I and Axis II (Clarkin & Huprich, 2011; Krueger, 1999, 2005; Westen, Gabbard, & Blagov, 2006). Several other studies confirm this and suggest that the differentiation between DSM Axis I and Axis II is arbitrary and counterproductive (Blatt, Besser, & Ford, 2007; Blatt & Ford, 1994; Blatt & Levy, 1998; Krueger et al., 2005; Kupfer, First, & Regier, 2002; Westen, Novotny, & Thompson-Brenner, 2004). There is evidence that supports the notion that personality can serve both as a buffer in face of stress or psychological challenge, or as a vulnerability factor, which can contribute to varying periods of psychiatric distress (Johnson et al., 2000; Johnson, Rabkin, Williams, Remien, & Gorman, 2000; Mervielde, De Clercq, Fruyt, & Van Leeuwen, 2005).

Particularly regarding the relationship between depression and personality disorders, in an extensive review of the literature, Klein, Kotov, and Bufferd (2011) found different possible explanations for their commonality: both disorders may have common causes, both belong to a continuous spectrum, personality would constitute a precursor or predisposition for the development of depression, personality exerts a pathoplastic effect on depression, personality is a state-dependent phenomena, or personality is a consequence of depressive episodes (Klein et al., 2011). This multiplicity of possible relationships between depression and personality, together with the fact that the DSM and ICD categories lack coherence with emerging findings from genetics, neuroscience, and behavioral sciences (Cuthbert & Insel, 2013), confirms the need for a revision of the validity of categorical definitions of mental disorders.

A second criticism refers to the lack of specificity among a single psychopathological disorder. Most taxonomic categories are based on the clinical presentation of a heterogeneous set of signs and symptoms, with different physiopathological mechanisms involved, grouped in a single disorder (Jiménez & Altimir, 2019; Maj, 2012; Mann, 2010). Additionally, these systems often assume a relatively unique etiopathogenesis of each discrete disorder (Blatt & Luyten, 2009, 2010; Clark, 2005; De Clercq et al., 2006; Krueger et al., 2007; Livesley, 2008; Watson, 2005). Furthermore, this does not allow to identify intra- and inter-patient variability. For example, there is currently no doubt that depression is a heterogeneous syndrome (Hassler, 2010). This heterogeneity is given to an important extent by the clear relations between personality functioning and depression which are difficult to disentangle (Gunderson et al., 2014), and many models have been proposed to explain this association (Klein et al., 2011).

Therefore, contemporary formulations on psychopathology have emphasized the importance of having a broad and dimensional approach compared to more categorical, disorder-center propositions (Blatt & Luyten, 2010; Clark, 2007; Krueger & Markon, 2006; Widiger & Clark, 2000; Widiger & Samuel, 2005). There are clear examples of how the field is currently shifting from a categorical identification of personality disorders to a dimensional view of them (Zimmermann, et al., 2019). Some examples are the DSM-5 Alternative Model for PD (AMPD) in DSM-5 section III (APA 2013) and the chapter on personality disorders and related traits in the recent version of ICD-11 (WHO, 2018). Both of them aim to identify personality disorders as impairments in personality functioning and maladaptive personality traits.

Particularly relevant are theory-driven and developmental person-centered approaches to personality and psychopathology that assume a fundamental continuity between normal personality features and psychopathology (Allen, 2013; Luyten, & Blatt, 2011). They incorporate, among others, attachment theory, contributing with a dynamic developmental standpoint (Fonagy, 2000). From this perspective, there is an emphasis in considering the developmental pathways of psychopathology that include genetic, temperament, and personality dimensions, and their interaction with the environment, in the conformation and consolidation of disrupted cognitive-affective schemas of self and others across the life span (Blatt & Luyten, 2009, 2010; Clark, 2005; De Clercq et al., 2006; Krueger et al., 2007; Livesley, 2008; Watson, 2005). In doing this, they allow a focus on the patient's particularities.

As Luyten and Blatt (2011) point out, there is increasing consensus within the personality and psychopathology developmental fields that the dimensions for understanding these pathways should be based on contemporary theories of personality development and personality organization. This approach has the advantage of incorporating a fundamental change in perspective, from a focus on the disorder and the set of symptoms to a person-centered approach, which considers a comprehension based on the expression of subjectivity and not only symptomatology and which understands this expression as a complex psychological process that results from a specific trajectory (Allen, 2013; Luyten & Fonagy, 2019).

From this perspective, the RDoC proposal for understanding mental phenomena based on functional domains may contribute to better define these pathways, considering the different levels of operation involved in them. One of these domain is affect regulation and its emergence, development, and maintenance along these dimensions. This perspective allows to establish connections between the reviewed developmental models of affect regulation and the psychological and neuroscientific models, with the manifestation of this functional domain in adulthood and across the experience of depression and personality dysfunction.

Here, we take as a starting point the growing empirical evidence that indicates that interpersonal relatedness and self-definition are the key psychological coordinates of human functioning as well as of normal and disrupted personality development (Luyten & Blatt, 2011, 2013; Sibley & Overall, 2007; Skodol et al., 2011) and somehow underlie all interpersonal circumplex conceptualizations of personality (Safran & Muran, 2000). These dimensions, and particularly their related disturbances in self and other representations, constitute the central axes for organizing, classifying, and treating psychological disorders (Luyten & Blatt, 2011, 2015). More specifically, they may allow a comprehension of the impairments that underlie depression and personality dysfunction (Morey et al., 2011; Verheul et al., 2008; Livesley, 2006).

3.3.1 Affect Regulation Within the Relatedness-Self-Definition Continuum

Among the existing validated dimensional theory-driven models of personality, we consider that Blatt's two polarities model of relatedness and self-definition (Blatt, 2008; Blatt & Shichman, 1983), together with current adult attachment models (e.g., Mikulincer & Shaver, 2007), can provide a comprehensive conceptualization for discussing affect regulation as a functional domain of healthy as well as psychopathological operations of human psychism. At the same time, they provide a coherent template for integrating both developmental and psychological models of affect and emotion regulation into the understanding of depression and personality dysfunction. The dimensional approach to understanding personality and psychopathology, and particularly depression and personality disorders, may take advantage of the notion of affect regulation as a functional domain along the individual's trajectory throughout development from early childhood to adulthood.

In an exhaustive integration of the advances in knowledge derived from attachment theory (Mikulincer & Shaver, 2007; Sibley & Overall, 2007), as well as from research and theory-driven models of personality (Benjamin, 2005; Leary, 1957; Pincus, 2005), Sydney Blatt (2008; Blatt, & Luyten, 2009) has developed a comprehensive conceptualization that postulates that personality develops across the life span through a continuous interaction between the capacity of relatedness and self-definition. These two dimensions are based on underlying cognitive-affective interpersonal schemas, or what attachment theory has called internal working models, of self and others. These schemas can range from relatively broad representations applicable to various situations, to more relationship-specific representations of self and others (Luyten, & Blatt, 2011). Thus, these two dimensions would be involved in the capacity to establish and maintain reciprocal, meaningful, and personally satisfying interpersonal relationships with others and at the same time establish a coherent, realistic, differentiated, and essentially positive sense of agency and identity (Luyten, & Blatt, 2011; 2013). This conceptualization emphasizes the dialectical and synergistic interaction between these two human tendencies, inasmuch as, during development, the individual needs to experience a sense of security (i.e., safe haven) in order to explore the world and develop a sense of agency, whereas he/she needs to develop an increasing differentiated sense of self, in order to maintain a healthy intimate relationship. Thus, higher levels of self-definition are associated with more mature levels of interpersonal relatedness and, in a dialectical manner, more mature levels of interpersonal relatedness foster further differentiation and integration in the development of the self (Luyten & Blatt, 2011).

As we can see, the dialectic among these polarities intimately relates to the interactive processes involved in early attachment relationships and that consolidate differing levels of the development and regulation of the self (Allen, 2013). This model assumes that attachment styles developed during early infancy and consolidated in adulthood would constitute distal antecedents of adult functioning and specifically of its psychopathological manifestation (Blatt, 2004). From this perspective, psychopathology is seen as distorted attempts to maintain a balance, although maladaptive, between the tendency for relatedness and for self-definition, resulting in an excessive emphasis on one line of development at the expense of the other (Blatt, 2008; Luyten & Blatt, 2011; Meyer & Pilkonis, 2005; Mikulincer & Shaver, 2007). These can manifest either through an intense distorted preoccupation with the quality of interpersonal relationships or exaggerated defensive efforts to try to consolidate and stabilize the sense of self (Blatt, Auerbach, & Behrends, 2008; Blatt et al., 2007; Blatt & Ford, 1994). There is enough empirical support that relates the dependency-self-relatedness dimensions as central elements of human development with current formulations of attachment theory, implying that these two dimensions underlie anxious and avoidant attachment styles, respectively (Luyten & Blatt, 2011; Meyer & Pilkonis, 2005; Mikulincer & Shaver, 2007, Roisman et al., 2007). Thus, in a meta-analysis, Sibley & Overall (2007) found a high correlation between autonomy (self-determination) and avoidant attachment, and between sociotropy (relatedness) and anxious attachment.

Blatt (Blatt & Luyten, 2009) proposes that the severe disruptions among the dependency-self-definition dimensions described above characterizes two primary configurations of general psychopathology, which have been extensively described previously in this volume: (1) an anaclitic type that involves, at different developmental levels, a distorted polarized emphasis on interpersonal relatedness and (2) an introjective type that involves a distorted and polarized emphasis on self-definition. As it has been mentioned in previous chapters, this fundamental polarity between self-definition and relatedness may constitute a specific vulnerability for developing depression, either through alterations in interpersonal relationships (anaclitic – loss, abandonment, or need for closeness) or through alterations in self-esteem (introjective – feelings of failure, guilt, or low self-esteem) (Dagnino et al., 2017; Luyten & Blatt, 2011).

Both configurations can also be found on personality disorders. For example, research has indicated that individuals with dependent, histrionic, and borderline personality disorder traits (according to the Diagnostic and Statistical Manual of Mental Disorders – DSM) tend to have greater concerns with interpersonal relationship issues than with self-definition issues. In contrast, individuals with features of antisocial, narcissistic, paranoid schizoid, schizotypal, avoidant, and obsessive-compulsive disorders show more concern with self-definition issues (Blatt & Luyten, 2010; Luyten & Blatt, 2011). A possible explanation for the profound disorganization of the structure of the self in BPD patients can be found in the failure of mentalization and, therefore, in the capacity for affect regulation, both self-regulation and the regulation in interpersonal relationships. Given that the individual's difficulties in achieving self-regulation involve a greater sensitivity toward any kind of emotional cue (Lynch et al., 2006; Bateman & Fonagy, 2019), the loss of the capacity to mentalize is more severe in contexts of intense emotionality. It has been proposed that in these contexts, modes of thinking about subjective experiences that precedes complete mentalization reemerge, generating a re-externalization of internal disorganized, intolerable, and painful states (Bateman & Fonagy, 2012).

3.3.2 Affect Regulation Within the Adult Attachment Spectrum

In line with the two-polarity personality model, contemporary attachment theory and research has underscored the notion that different forms of psychopathology are dynamic conflict-defense constellations that reflect different attempts to find a balance between relatedness and self-definition. They have also emphasized that these processes are central issues in normal individuals (Mikulincer & Shaver, 2007; Sibley & Overall, 2007), thus supporting the continuum between normal and maladaptive psychological functioning (Luyten, & Blatt, 2011). Specifically, this approach conceptualizes adaptive personality functioning as a balance between relationship and self-definition, expressed in low or moderate levels of anxiety and avoidance of attachment typical of individuals with secure attachment (Mikulincer & Shaver, 2007). The dimension of avoidant attachment (discomfort with the relational proximity and dependency within relationships) is conceptually and empirically superimposed with the dimension of self-definition. In turn, the dimension of anxious attachment, expressed in internal working models characterized by fear of rejection and concern about abandonment, overlaps with the dimension of relatedness (Luyten & Blatt, 2011). Within this framework, research on adult attachment (Meyer & Pilkonis, 2005; Mikulincer & Shaver, 2007; Pietromonaco et al., 2006) has highlighted the association between attachment and emotional regulation in close relationships. They point out that, like children, when an adult is distressed by an emotional threat, he or she may seek an attachment figure in an attempt to regain a sense of security. In the case of adults, however, conflicting interactions are the ones that usually induce emotional distress, and they are likely to trigger attachment behaviors since they often raise concerns about the availability and emotional responsiveness of the interactive partner (Simpson, Rholes, & Phillips, 1996).

Bartholomew and Horowitz (1991) propose four categories of adult attachment according to the possible combinations of positive and negative models of self and others. On the continuum of self-representation, which has also been interpreted as the degree of attachment anxiety, people with positive valence would experience low levels of anxiety, and their sense of self-worth would not be easily compromised by inadequate external validation. Meanwhile, people with negative valence tend to be very anxious about potential rejection and depend on the approval of others to maintain their sense of self-esteem. On the continuum of representing others, or the degree of avoidance of attachment, individuals with positive valence show motivation to approach and trust others in difficult situations and to value and seek intimacy in relationships. On the other hand, people with a negative value in this dimension show a motivation to avoid closeness, to prefer a safe distance from others and to value situations of loneliness over those involving intimacy. The four types of adult attachments resulting from these combinations are secure attachment (low avoidance and low anxiety), concerned attachment (low avoidance and high anxiety), fearful attachment (high avoidance and high anxiety), and indifferent attachment (high avoidance and low anxiety).

The attachment system activates in an automatic manner in front of either external threats or internal sources of distress related to the attachment system. When it works properly, it generates in the individual the experience of emotional security, resulting in effective strategies to cope with difficult situations that are present in life (Shaver & Mikulincer, 2014). Research indicates that during moments of stress, people automatically seek internal representations of attachment figures that promote the sense of security. Thus, the mental activation of these representations generates positive emotions, including relief, satisfaction, gratitude, and love. These emotions, in turn, enable the effective coping of the stressful event and restore emotional equilibrium, by accelerating emotional recovery and the reduction of negative thoughts (Shaver & Mikulincer, 2014; Selcuk, Zayas, Günaydin, Hazan, & Kross, 2012). Experimental evidence has indicated that this activation takes place even when the threats to the attachment systems are unconscious (Mikulincer, Gillath, & Shaver, 2002). This implies that either real or symbolic interactions with available and supportive attachment figures, and the resulting feeling of security, can be seen as psychological resources for dealing with adverse situations, fostering sustained well-being and mental health (Shaver & Mikulincer, 2014).

Disturbances in the sense of security regarding attachment are considered risk factors for emotional problems and for psychopathology. As we have reviewed earlier with respect to affect regulation during early attachment interactions between infant and caregiver, secondary attachment strategies (anxious hyperactivation and avoidant deactivation) are initially adaptive, as they constitute the child's adjusted response to the caregiver's sensibility (i.e., inconsistent availability or consistent unavailability) (Allen, 2013; Shaver & Mikulincer, 2014). However, these strategies become maladaptive when implemented in later relationships in which support seeking and relational interdependence may be satisfactory and help the person maintain a sense of well-being in the face of stressful situations. If we consider that these maladaptive attachment strategies depend on distorted representations of self and others, a self-preserving loop can be observed as they encourage the repeated activation or suppression of negative emotions, which in turn promotes the continued dependence on these distorted representations. Progressively, these patterns of affect and relational regulation become detrimental for mental health (Mikulincer & Shaver, 2007; Shaver & Mikulincer, 2014).

Empirical data indicates that individuals with high degrees of anxious attachment resort to hyperactivation strategies to regulate the activation of their attachment system, meaning that they show greater emotional reactivity than others across a wider range of situations, because they would tend to perceive these events as threatening (Pietromonaco et al., 2006). Several studies confirm that this hyperactivation involves the activation of negative affective states, and the search for others to help regulate them, through strategies such as clinging, controlling and coercive behaviors, cognitive and behavioral efforts to establish physical contact, and attempts to get a sense of oneness with the other (Collins & Feeney, 2000; Mikulincer, 1998; Shaver & Mikulincer, 2014; Simpson, Rholes, & Nelligan, 1992).

Research supports the notion that anxious individuals tend to perceive negative emotions as congruent with the goals of attachment proximity, thus generating attempts to maintain and even exaggerate the experience of these emotions. Several strategies have been observed which tend to intensify the presence and the severity of threats and to overemphasize their sense of vulnerability and helplessness, as these cues may elicit attention and care from attachment figures. Attempts at augmenting negative emotions can be achieved by distortions in the appraisal of threatening situations, such as perceptually intensifying the threatening aspects of relatively benign events, holding pessimistic beliefs about their own abilities to handle distress, or attributing these events to uncontrollable causes or an overall personal inability (Mikulincer & Shaver, 2007). Other strategies include attentional focus on internal indicators of distress (Cassidy & Kobak, 1988), with specific hypervigilance to physiological correlates of emotional states, an intensification of memories of threat-related experiences, and rumination referred to real or potential threats. Exposure to threatening situations or self-destructive behaviors also contributes to the intensification of negative emotions. Eventually, the activation of these strategies generates an amplified cycle of distress even after the threat objectively disappears (Mikulincer & Shaver, 2007; Shaver & Mikulincer, 2014).

Meanwhile, deactivation strategies employed by avoidant individuals in the face of stressful attachment events involve the inhibition of tendencies or actions that seek proximity to others (Mikulincer & Shaver, 2007) (i.e., the activation of the attachment system) and instead generate attempts to distance themselves from these figures (Collins & Feeney, 2000; Mikulincer, 1998; Simpson et al., 1992). Avoidant strategies also include suppressing or dismissing any threat that might activate the attachment system (i.e., any experience that is associated with the feeling of need for others), as well as downregulating both negative and positive affects. Specifically, regarding negative affect, the inhibitory efforts are directed towards emotions such as fear, anxiety, anger (inasmuch as it also implies relational involvement), sadness, shame, guilt, and distress, since they are associated with the experience of threat and sense of vulnerability. Additional strategies include denying or suppressing thoughts and memories associated with emotions, diverting attention from content associated with emotions, suppressing behavioral tendencies related to emotions, and masking or inhibiting the verbal and nonverbal expression of emotions. These deactivation strategies serve the function of avoiding the recognition of the individual's own emotional reactions. These individuals seem determined to manage stressors on their own (i.e., "compulsive self-sufficiency"), maximizing autonomy and distance from relationships (i.e., distorted attempts towards the pole of self-definition), as they experience discomfort in the face of relational intimacy (Mikulincer & Shaver, 2007). The ultimate consequence of these avoidant affect regulatory approaches is a decreased tendency to integrate emotional experience in cognitive structures and therefore to use them effectively in information processing and social behavior (Shaver & Mikulincer, 2014).

Shaver and Mikulincer (2014) propose that the relationship between attachment and affect regulation in adult functioning allows a comprehension of prototypical modes of operating of human beings in the face of the experience of threat to the attachment motivational system. But, at the same time, it allows an understanding of the individual differences reflected in patterns of coping with stressful events that are both relevant and irrelevant to the attachment system. Several studies provide evidence that differences in attachment styles influence the ways individuals assess, cope with, and react emotionally and physiologically to both attachment-relevant and non-attachment-relevant stressful events, that is, to events that have no direct implications for close relationships (Mikulincer & Shaver, 2007). Moreover, even though attachment style is often measured as a single global orientation to close relationships, attachment orientation is rooted in a complex cognitive and affective neural network that includes episodic and semantic memories, as well as both secure and insecure mental representations (Mikulincer & Shaver, 2007). Furthermore, Bateman and Fonagy (2012) underscore the fact that the individual differences in terms of the activation or deactivation of their attachment strategies describe a paradoxical relationship between attachment, stress, mentalization, and affect regulation. Studies have shown that activation of the attachment system is associated with the activation of the mesocorticolimbic dopaminergic system, which plays a central role in the cerebral reward system (Insel & Young, 2001) and is associated with increase in sensibility to social signals and a decrease in levels of stress and of social avoidance (Fonagy & Luyten, 2009; Luyten & Blatt, 2011; Bateman & Fonagy, 2012). At the same time, activation of this system is associated with a relative deactivation of arousal and the emotional regulation system, like that of the neurocognitive systems involved in mentalization, including the cortex (Bateman & Fonagy, 2012).

3.4 Conclusions

This chapter has reviewed the concept of affect regulation from the perspective of the functional domain criteria, in an attempt to understand and describe its role for psychopathology, and specifically for depression and personality dysfunction. In doing so, we have incorporated the ongoing discussions within the fields of psychiatry, psychology, and psychopathology research that call for a reformulation of diagnostic systems that account for both healthy and maladaptive mental functioning. This has meant a critic to the traditional categorical diagnostic systems and to the limitations they present for a valid and comprehensive understanding of mental disorders. In the face of such limitations, the Research Domain Criteria Initiative (RDoC) proposed by the NIMH has meant a valuable approach, inasmuch as it is based on a dimensional, transdiagnostic, and multilevel perspective that considers behavioral and neurobiological mechanisms organized along systems underlying basic psychological capacities, rather than on discrete categories of disorders. Perhaps its particular value for the comprehension of affect regulation resides in the fact that it assumes that the origins and pathways of psychopathology may operate at many levels, including the genetic/neural, the individual, the family environmental, and the social contextual. This is of particular interest when attempting a review and integration of affect regulation into the comprehension of mental functioning, since, as we have seen, it is a very broad field that has yielded a diversity of definitions and approaches.

In that sense, RDoC is a transdiagnostic and multilevel approach that recognizes "bottom-up," as well as "top-down" causation, allowing the integration of epistemological, methodological, and empirical perspectives that make possible the observation and systematization of a phenomenon as complex as affect regulation (Jiménez, de la Cerda & Altimir, 2017; Jiménez & Altimir, 2019). Therefore, inasmuch as it is understood as a functional domain that can operate in multiple and synchronic levels of mental phenomena, RDoC opens a window of opportunity for collaboration between different approaches from various disciplines to the understanding of affect regulation, under the spirit of an explanatory pluralism (Kendler, 2005).

In this integrative attempt, we have proposed to complement two main approaches to defining and understanding affect regulation. One of them is a developmental perspective that bases psychic development in the matrix of early significant affect relationships. As we have seen, attachment constitutes a cornerstone for the understanding of healthy and maladaptive self and other representations and subsequently for the human dialectic between relatedness and self-definition. Secure attachment, therefore, is the basis for the capacity for affect regulation (Allen, 2013) and for helping the individual to keep fear and anxiety at bay, allowing him/her to maintain a fundamental state of emotional security throughout his/her life (Van der Kolk, 2014). Insecure attachment experiences, instead, will result in distorted images of self and others and polarized attempts at self-definition or relatedness that involve impaired affect regulatory capacities. On another level of comprehension, we can draw on emotion processing models to make sense of how individual's idiosyncratic attachment-related repertoires of affective experience and regulation concretely unfold in the immediate management of emotions at the experiential, behavioral, and physiological domains.

Finally, we have discussed the contribution of understanding affect regulation, at these two levels, in depression and personality disorders based on a dimensional framework for understanding the development of personality and psychopathology. We have reviewed two models that focus on relatedness and self-definition as the central coordinates of human mental development and that, in doing so, highlight a person-centered approach that can contribute to the formulation of treatments that adapt to each patient's specific particularities and needs. The value of this approach resides in its coherence with the notion of functional domain, inasmuch as it underscores the understanding of psychopathology based on a continuum from normal to abnormal functioning along different levels of operation.

References

Ainsworth, M. D. S., Blehar, M. C., Waters, E., & Wall, S. (1978). *Patterns of attachment: A psychological study of the strange situation*. Hillside, NJ: Lawrence Erlbaum Associates.

Aldao, A., Nolen-Hoeksema, S., & Schweizer, S. (2010). Emotion-regulation strategies across psychopathology: A meta-analytic review. *Clinical Psychology Review, 30*(2), 217–237. https://doi.org/10.1016/j.cpr.2009.11.004

Allen, J., Fonagy, P., & Bateman, A. (2008). *Mentalizing in clinical practice*. Washington, DC: American Psychiatric Press.

Allen, J. G. (2013). *Restoring mentalizing in attachment relationships. Treating trauma with plain old therapy*. Washington, DC: American Psychiatric Publishing.

American Psychiatric Association. (2013). Diagnostic and statistical manual of mental disorders (5th ed.). https://doi.org/10.1176/appi.books.9780890425596

Barlow, L. B., & Allen, M. L. (2004). Choate Toward a unified treatment for emotional disorders. *Behavior Therapy, 35*(2), 205–230. https://doi.org/10.1016/S0005-7894(04)80036-4

Bartholomew, K., & Horowitz, L. M. (1991). Attachment styles among young adults: A test of a four-category model. *Journal of Personality and Social Psychology, 61*(2), 226–244. https://doi.org/10.1037/0022-3514.61.2.226

Bateman, A. y Fonagy, P. (2004). *Psychotherapy for Borderline Personality Disorder: mentalization-based treatment*. Nueva York: Oxford University Press.

Bateman, A.W., & Fonagy, P. (2006). *Mentalization based treatment for borderline personality disorder: A practical guide*. Oxford: Oxford University Press.

Bateman, A., & Fonagy, P. (2012). *Handbook of mentalizing in mental health practice*. Washington, DC: American Psychiatric Pub.

Bateman, A., & Fonagy, P. (2019). *Handbook of mentalizing in mental health practice* (2nd ed.). Washington, DC: American Psychiatric Pub.

Beebe, B., Knoblauch, S., Rustin, J., & Sorter, D. (2005). *Forms of intersubjectivity and infant research and adult treatment*. New York, NY: Other Press.

Beebe, B., Jaffe, J., Lachmann, F., Feldstein, S., Crown, C. and Jasnow, M. (2000), Systems models in development and psychoanalysis: The case of vocal rhythm coordination and attachment. *Infant Mental Health Journal, 21*, 99–122. https://doi.org/10.1002/(SICI)1097-0355(200001/04)21:1/2<99::AID-IMHJ11>3.0.CO;2-#

Beebe, B., & Lachmann, F. (2002). *Infant research and adult treatment: Co-constructing interactions*. Hillsdale, NJ: The Analytic Press.

Beebe, B., Lachmann, F., Markese, S., Buck, K. A., Bahrick, L. E., Chen, H., Cohen, P., Andrews, H., Feldstein, S., & Jaffe, J. (2012). On the Origins of Disorganized Attachment and Internal Working Models: Paper II. An Empirical Microanalysis of 4-Month Mother-Infant Interaction. *Psychoanalytic Dialogues, 22*(3), 352–374. https://doi.org/10.1080/10481885.2012.679606

Beebe, B., & Lachmann, F. M. (2015). The expanding world of Edward Tronick. *Psychoanalytic Inquiry, 35*(4), 328–336. https://doi.org/10.1080/07351690.2015.1022476

Benjamin, L. T., Jr. (2005). A history of clinical psychology as a profession in America (and a glimpse at its future). *Annual Review of Clinical Psychology, 1*(1), 1–30. https://doi.org/10.1146/annurev.clinpsy.1.102803.143758

Berenbaum, H., Raghavan, C., Le, H. N., Vernon, L. L., & Gomez, J. J. (2003). A taxonomy of emotional disturbances. *Clinical Psychology: Science and Practice, 10*(2), 206–226. https://doi.org/10.1093/clipsy/bpg011

Berking, M., Eichler, E., Luhmann, M., Diedrich, A., Hiller, W., & Rief, W. (2019). Affect regulation training reduces symptom severity in depression – A randomized controlled trial. *PloS One, 14(*8), e0220436. https://doi.org/10.1371/journal.pone.0220436

Blatt, S. J. (2004). Experiences of depression: Theoretical, clinical, and research perspectives. *American Psychological Association*. https://doi.org/10.1037/10749-000

Blatt, S. J. (2008). Polarities of experience: Relatedness and self-definition in personality development, psychopathology, and the therapeutic process. *American Psychological Association*. https://doi.org/10.1037/11749-000

Blatt, S. J., Auerbach, J. S., & Behrends, R. S. (2008). Changes in the representation of self and significant others in the treatment process: Links between representation, internalization, and mentalization. In E. L. Jurist, A. Slade, & S. Bergner (Eds.), *Mind to mind: Infant research, neuroscience, and psychoanalysis* (pp. 225–263). Other Press.

Blatt, S. J., Besser, A., & Ford, R. Q. (2007). Two primary configurations of psychopathology and change in thought disorder in long-term, intensive, inpatient treatment of seriously disturbed young adults. *American Journal of Psychiatry, 164*(10), 1561–1567. https://doi.org/10.1176/appi.ajp.2007.05111853

Blatt, S. J., & Ford, R. (1994). *Therapeutic change: An object relations perspective*. New York, NY: Plenum Press.

Blatt, S. J., & Levy K. N. (1998). A psychodynamic approach to the diagnosis of psychopathology. In Making Diagnosis Meaningful, ed. J.W. Barron. Washington, DC: American Psychological Association, pp. 73–109

Blatt, S. J., & Luyten, P. A. (2009). A structural-developmental psychodynamic approach to psychopathology: Two polarities of experience across the life span. *Development and Psychopathology, 21*(3), 793–814. https://doi.org/10.1017/S0954579409000431

Blatt, S. J., & Luyten, P. A. (2010). Reactivating the psychodynamic approach to classify psychopathology. In T. Millon, R. F. Krueger, & E. Simonsen (Eds.), *Contemporary directions in psychopathology: Scientific foundations of the DSM-V and ICD-11* (pp. 483–514). New York, NY: Guilford Press.

Blatt, S. J., & Shichman, S. (1983). Two primary configurations of psychopathology. *Psychoanalysis & Contemporary Thought, 6*(2), 187–254.

Bolton, D. (2013). *What is Mental Disorder?: An essay in philosophy, science, and values* (online ed.). Oxford University Press.

Borges, L. M., & Naugle, A. E. (2017). The role of emotion regulation in predicting personality dimensions. *Personality and Mental Health, 11*(4), 314–334. https://doi.org/10.1002/pmh.1390

Bowlby, J. (1969). *Attachment and loss* (Vol. 1: Attachment). London, UK: Hogarth Press and the Institute of Psycho-Analysis.

Bowlby, J. (1988). *A secure base* (2nd ed.). New York, NY: Basic.

Brothers, L. (1990). The social brain: A project for integrating primate behavior and neurophysiology in a new domain. *Concepts in Neuroscience, 1*, 27–51.

Campbell-Sills, L., & Barlow, D. H. (2007). Incorporating emotion regulation into conceptualizations and treatments of anxiety and mood disorders. In J. J. Gross (Ed.), *Handbook of emotion regulation* (pp. 542–559). New York, NY: Guilford Press.

Campos, J. J., Barrett, K. C., Lamb, M. E., Goldsmith, H. H., & Steinberg, C. (1983). Socioemotional development. In M. M. Haith & J. J. Campos (Eds.), *Handbook of child psychology* (Infancy and developmental psychobiology) (Vol. 2, pp. 783–915). New York, NY: Wiley.

Cassidy, J., & Kobak, R. R. (1988). Avoidance and its relationship with other defensive processes. In J. Belsky & T. Nezworski (Eds.), *Clinical implications of attachment* (pp. 300–323). Hillsdale, NJ: Erlbaum.

Clark, L. A. (2005). Temperament as a unifying basis for personality and psychopathology. *Journal of Abnormal Psychology, 114*(4), 505–521. https://doi.org/10.1037/0021-843X.114.4.505

Clark, L. A. (2007). Assessment and diagnosis of personality disorder: perennial issues and an emerging reconceptualization. *Annual Review of Psychology, 58*, 227–257. https://doi.org/10.1146/annurev.psych.57.102904.190200

Clarkin, J. F., & Huprich, S. K. (2011). Do DSM-5 personality disorder proposals meet criteria for clinical utility? *Journal of Personality Disorders, 25*(2), 192–205. https://doi.org/10.1521/pedi.2011.25.2.192

Cohn, J. F., & Tronick, E. Z. (1988). Mother-infant face-to-face interaction: Influence is bidirectional and unrelated to periodic cycles in either partner's behavior. *Developmental Psychology, 24*(3), 386–392. https://doi.org/10.1037/0012-1649.24.3.386

Cole, P. M., & Kaslow, N. J. (1988). Interactional and cognitive strategies for affect regulation: Developmental perspective on childhood depression. In L. B. Alloy (Ed.), *Cognitive processes in depression* (pp. 310–343). New York, NY: The Guilford Press.

Cole, P. M., Michel, M. K., & O'Donnell, L.T. (1994). The development of emotional regulation and dysregulation: A clinical perspective. *Monographs of the Society for Research in Child Development, 59*(2–3), 73–100. https://doi.org/10.2307/1166139

Collins, N. L., & Feeney, B. C. (2000). A safe haven: An attachment theory perspective on support seeking and caregiving in intimate relationships. *Journal of Personality and Social Psychology, 78*(6), 1053–1073. https://doi.org/10.1037/0022-3514.78.6.1053

Compare, A., Zarbo, C., Shonin, E., Van Gordon, W., & Marconi, C. (2014). Emotional regulation and depression: A potential mediator between heart and mind. *Cardiovascular Psychiatry and Neurology, 2014*, 1–10.

Conklin, C. Z., Bradley, R., & Westen, D. (2006). Affect regulation in borderline personality disorder. *The Journal of Nervous and Mental Disease, 194*(2), 69–77. https://doi.org/10.1097/01.nmd.0000198138.41709.4f

Cuthbert, B. N., & Insel, T. R. (2013). Toward the future of psychiatric diagnosis: The seven pillars of RDoC. *BMC Medicine, 11*(126), 1–8. https://doi.org/10.1186/1741-7015-11-126

Dagnino, P., Pérez, C., Gómez, A., Gloger, S., & Krause, M. (2017). Depression and attachment: How do personality styles and social support influence this relation? *Research in Psychotherapy: Psychopathology. Process and Outcome, 20*(1), 53–62. https://doi.org/10.4081/ripppo.2017.237

Damasio, A. R. (1998). Emotion in the perspective of an integrated nervous system. *Brain Research Reviews, 26*(2–3), 83–86. https://doi.org/10.1016/s0165-0173(97)00064-7

de la Cerda, C., Martínez, C., & Tomicic, A. (2019). La función reflexiva como aprendizaje procedural en la interacción terapéutica: El funcionamiento reflexivo-relacional [Mentalization as procedural learning in psychotherapeutic interaction: a relational reflective functioning]. *Revista Argentina de Clínica Psicológica, 28*(3), 285–294. https://doi.org/10.24205/03276716.2019.1142

Eisenberg, N., Fabes, R. A., Guthrie, I. K., & Reiser, M. (2000). Dispositional emotionality and regulation: Their role in predicting quality of social functioning. *Journal pf Personality and Social Psychology, 78*(1), 136–157. https://doi.org/10.1037/0022-3514.78.1.136

Ekman, P. (2007). *Emotions revealed*. New York, NY: St. Martin's Griffin.

Fonagy, P. (2015). Mutual regulation, mentalization, and therapeutic action: A reflection on the contributions of Ed Tronick to developmental and psychotherapeutic thinking. *Psychoanalytic Inquiry, 35*(4), 355–369. https://doi.org/10.1080/07351690.2015.1022481

Fonagy, P., & Bateman, A. (2006). Mechanisms of change in mentalization-based treatment of BPD. *Journal of Clinical Psychology, 62*(4), 411–430. https://doi.org/10.1002/jclp.20241

Fonagy, P., Gergely, G., Jurist, E., & Target, M. (2002). *Affect regulation, Mentalization and the development of the self*. New York, NY: Other Press.

Fonagy, P., Gergely, G., & Target, M. (2007). The parent-infant dyad and the construction of the subjective self. *Journal of Child Psychology and Psychiatry, 48*(3–4), 288–328. https://doi.org/10.1111/j.1469-7610.2007.01727.x

Fonagy, P., Luyten, P., & Strathearn, L. (2011). Borderline personality disorder, mentalization, and the neurobiology of attachment. *Infant Mental Health Journal, 32*(1), 47–69. https://doi.org/10.1002/imhj.20283

Fonagy, P., & Luyten, P. (2009) A developmental, mentalization-based approach to the understanding and treatment of borderline personality disorder. *Development and Psychopathology, 21*(4), 1355–1381. https://doi.org/10.1017/S0954579409990198

Fonagy, P., & Target, M. (1997). Attachment and reflective function: Their role in self-organization. *Development and Psychopathology, 9*(4), 679–700. https://doi.org/10.1017/S0954579497001399

Fonagy, P., & Target, M. (2002). Early intervention and the development of self–regulation. *Psychoanalytic Inquiry, 22*(3), 307–335. https://doi.org/10.1080/07351692209348990

Fonagy, P., & Target, M. (2007). The rooting of the mind in the body: New links between attachment theory and psychoanalytic thought. *Journal of the American Psychoanalytic Association, 55*(2), 411–456.

Gergely, G. (2007). The social construction of the subjective self: The role of affect-mirroring, markedness, and ostensive communication in self development. In L. Mayes, P. Fonagy, & M. Target (Eds.), *Developmental science and psychoanalysis*. London, UK: Karnac.

Gergely, G., & Watson, J. S. (1999). Early socio-emotional development: Contingency perception and the social-biofeedback model. In P. Rochat (Ed.), *Early socialization* (pp. 101–136). Mahwah, NJ: Lawrence Erlbaum Associates.

Gianino, A., & Tronick, E. Z. (1988). The mutual regulation model: The infant's self and interactive regulation, coping, and defensive capacities. In T. Field, P. McCabe, & N. Schneiderman (Eds.), *Stress and coping* (pp. 47–68). Hillsdale, MI: Erlbaum.

Gratz, K. L., Bardeen, J. R., Levy, R., Dixon-Gordon, K. L., & Tull, M. T. (2015). Mechanisms of change in an emotion regulation group therapy for deliberate self-harm among women with borderline personality disorder. *Behaviour Research and Therapy, 65*, 29–35. https://doi.org/10.1016/j.brat.2014.12.005

Greenberg, L. S. (2002). *Emotion-focused therapy: Coaching clients to work through their feelings*. Washington, DC: APA.

Greenberg, L. S., & Paivio, S. C. (2003). *Working with emotions in psychotherapy* (Vol. 13). Guilford Press.

Grecucci, A., Pappaianni, E., Siugzdaite, R., Theuninck, A. & Job, R. (2015). Mindful Emotion Regulation: Exploring the Neurocognitive Mechanisms behind Mindfulness. *Journal of Biomedicine and Biotechnology*. https://doi.org/10.1155/2015/670724

Greenberg, L. S., Paivio, S., Mateu, C., & Blasco, M. (2000). *Trabajar con las emociones en la psicoterapia* [Working with emotions in psychotherapy]. Barcelona, Spain: Ediciones Paidós Ibérica, SA.

Greenberg, L. S., Rice, L., & Elliot, R. (1993). *Facilitating emotional change: A process experiential approach*. New York, NY: Guilford.

Greenberg, L. S., & Safran, J. D. (1987). The Guilford clinical psychology and psychotherapy series. In *Emotion in psychotherapy: Affect, cognition, and the process of change*. New York, NY: Guilford Press.

Gross, J. J. (1998). The emerging field of emotion regulation: An integrative review. *Review of General Psychology, 2*(3), 271–299. https://doi.org/10.1037/1089-2680.2.3.271

Gross, J. J. (2014). Emotion regulation: Conceptual and empirical foundations. In J. J. Gross (Ed.), *Handbook of emotion regulation* (pp. 3–20). New York, NY: The Guilford Press.

Gross, J. J., & Munoz, R. F. (1995). Emotion regulation and mental health. *Clinical Psychology: Science and Practice, 2*(2), 151–164. https://doi.org/10.1111/j.1468-2850.1995.tb00036.x

Gross, J. J., & Thompson, R. A. (2007). Emotion regulation: Conceptual foundations. In J. J. Gross (Ed.), *Handbook of emotion regulation* (pp. 3–24). New York, NY: Guilford Press.

Gunderson, J. G., Stout, R. L., Shea, M. T., Grilo, C. M., Markowitz, J. C., Morey, L. C., et al. (2014). Interactions of borderline personality disorder and mood disorders over 10 years. *Journal of Clinical Psychiatry, 75*(8), 829–834. https://doi.org/10.4088/JCP.13m08972

Gyurak, A., & Etkin, A. (2014). A neurobiological model of implicit and explicit emotion regulation. In J. J. Gross (Ed.), *Handbook of emotion regulation* (pp. 76–90). New York, NY: The Guilford Press.

Gyurak, A., Gross, J. J., & Etkin, A. (2011). Explicit and implicit emotion regulation: A dual-process framework. *Cognition and Emotion, 25*(3), 400–412. https://doi.org/10.1080/02699931.2010.544160

Hassler, G. (2010). Pathophysiology of depression: Do we have any solid evidence of interest to clinicians? *World Psychiatry, 9*(3), 155–161. https://doi.org/10.1002/j.2051-5545.2010.tb00298.x

Insel, T. R., & Young, L. J. (2001). The neurobiology of attachment. Nature reviews. *Neuroscience, 2*(2), 129–136. https://doi.org/10.1038/35053579

Jiménez, J. P., & Altimir, C. (2019). Beyond the hermeneutic/scientific controversy: A case for a clinically sensitive empirical research paradigm in psychoanalysis. *The International Journal of Psychoanalysis, 100*(5), 940–961. https://doi.org/10.1080/00207578.2019.1636253

Jiménez, J. P., de la Cerda, C., & Altimir, C. (2017). Un enfoque novedoso, científico y clínicamente sensible para investigar el proceso psicoanalítico. Manuscrito, presentado en el panel "Investigación y Psicoanálisis" 60° Congreso Internacional de Psicoanálisis IPA, Argentina [A new, scientific and clinically sensitive approach to investigate the psychoanalytic process. Manuscript presented at the "Research and Psychoanalysis" panel of the 60th International Congress of Psychoanalysis IPA, Argentina].

Johnson, J. G., Cohen, P., Kasen, S., Skodol, A. E., Hamagami, F., & Brook, J. S. (2000). Age-related change in personality disorder trait levels between early adolescence and adulthood: a community-based longitudinal investigation. *Acta Psychiatrica Scandinavica, 102*(4), 265–275. https://doi.org/10.1034/j.1600-0447.2000.102004265.x

Johnson, J. G., Rabkin, J. G., Williams, J. B. W., Remien, R. H., & Gorman, J. M. (2000). Difficulties in interpersonal relationships associated with personality disorders and Axis I disorders: A community-based longitudinal investigation. *Journal of Personality Disorders, 14*(1), 42–56. https://doi.org/10.1521/pedi.2000.14.1.42

Joormann, J., & Gotlib, I. H. (2010). Emotion regulation in depression: Relation to cognitive inhibition. *Cognition and Emotion, 24*(2), 281–298. https://doi.org/10.1080/02699930903407948

Joorman, J., Siemer, M., & Gotlib, I. H. (2007). Mood regulation in depression: Differential effects of distraction and recall of happy memories on sad mood. *Journal of Abnormal Psychology, 116*(3), 484–490. https://doi.org/10.1037/0021-843X.116.3.484

Joseph, R. (1982). The neuropsychology of development: Hemispheric laterality, limbic language, and the origin of thought. *Journal of Clinical Psychology, 38*(1), 4–33. https://doi.org/10.1002/1097-4679(198201)38:1<4::AID-JCLP2270380102>3.0.CO;2-J

Kendler, K. S. (2005). Toward a philosophical structure for psychiatry. *The American Journal of Psychiatry, 162*(3), 433–440. https://doi.org/10.1176/appi.ajp.162.3.433

Klein, D. N., Kotov, R., & Bufferd, S. J. (2011). Personality and depression: Explanatory models and review of the evidence. *Annual Review of Clinical Psychology, 7*, 269–295. https://doi.org/10.1146/annurev-clinpsy-032210-104540

Koole, S. L., & Rothermund, K. (2011). I feel better but I don't know why: The psychology of implicit emotion regulation. *Cognition and Emotion, 25*(3), 389–399. https://doi.org/10.1080/02699931.2010.550505

Koole, S. L., Webb, T. L., & Sheeran, P. L. (2015). Implicit emotion regulation: Feeling better without knowing why. *Current Opinion in Psychology, 3*, 6–10. https://doi.org/10.1016/j.copsyc.2014.12.027

Kopp, C. B., & Neufeld, S. J. (2003). Emotional development during infancy. In R. J. Davidson, K. R. Scherer, & H. H. Goldsmith (Eds.), *Handbook of affective sciences* (pp. 347–374). New York, NY: Oxford University Press.

Kring, A. M., & Bachorowski, J. A. (1999). Emotions and psychopathology. *Cognition and Emotion, 13*(5), 575–599. https://doi.org/10.1080/026999399379195

Kring, A. M., & Sloan, D. M. (2009). *Emotion regulation and psychopathology: A transdiagnostic approach to etiology and treatment*. The Guilford Press.

Krueger R. F. (1999). The structure of common mental disorders. *Archives of General Psychiatry, 56*(10), 921–926. https://doi.org/10.1001/archpsyc.56.10.921

Krueger R. F. (2005). Continuity of axes I and II: toward a unified model of personality, personality disorders, and clinical disorders. *Journal of Personality Disorders, 19*(3), 233–261. https://doi.org/10.1521/pedi.2005.19.3.233

Krueger, R. F., & Markon, K. E. (2006). Reinterpreting comorbidity: A model-based approach to understanding and classifying psychopathology. *Annual Review of Clinical Psychology, 2*, 111–133. https://doi.org/10.1146/annurev.clinpsy.2.022305.095213

Krueger, R. F., & Tackett, J. L. (2003). Personality and psychopathology: Working toward the bigger picture. *Journal of Personality Disorders, 17*(2), 109–128. https://doi.org/10.1521/pedi.17.2.109.23986

Krueger, R. F., Markon, K. E., Patrick, C. J., & Iacono, W. G. (2005). Externalizing psychopathology in adulthood: a dimensional-spectrum conceptualization and its implications for DSM-V. *Journal of Abnormal Psychology, 114*(4), 537–550. https://doi.org/10.1037/0021-843X.114.4.537

Krueger, R. F., Markon, K. E., Patrick, C. J., Benning, S. D., & Kramer, M. D. (2007). Linking antisocial behavior, substance use, and personality: an integrative quantitative model of the adult externalizing spectrum. *Journal of Abnormal Psychology, 116*(4), 645–666. https://doi.org/10.1037/0021-843X.116.4.645

Kupfer, D. J., First, M. B., & Regier, D. A. (2002). A research agenda for DSM—V. American Psychiatric Association.

Lachmann, F. (2001). Some contributions of empirical infant research to adult psychoanalysis: What have we learned? How can we apply it? *Psychoanalytic Dialogues, 11*(2), 167–185. https://doi.org/10.1080/10481881109348605

Leary, T. (1957). Interpersonal diagnosis of personality; a functional theory and methodology for personality evaluation. Ronald Press

Linehan, M. (1993). *Skills-training manual for treatment of borderline personality disorder*. New York, NY: Guilford.

Linehan, M. M., & Heard, H. L. (1992). Dialectical behavior therapy for borderline personality disorder. In J. F. Clarkin, E. Marziali, & H. Munroe-Blum (Eds.), *Borderline personality disorder: Clinical and empirical perspectives* (pp. 248–267). New York, NY: Guilford Press.

Livesley, W. J. (2006). General assessment of personality disorder (GAPD). Unpublished manuscript, Department of Psychiatry, University of British Columbia.

Livesley J. (2008). Integrated therapy for complex cases of personality disorder. *Journal of Clinical Psychology, 64*(2), 207–221. https://doi.org/10.1002/jclp.20453

Luyten, P., & Blatt, S. J. (2011). Integrating theory-driven and empirically-derived models of personality development and psychopathology: a proposal for DSM V. *Clinical Psychology Review, 31*(1), 52–68. https://doi.org/10.1016/j.cpr.2010.09.003

Luyten, P., & Blatt, S. J. (2013). Interpersonal relatedness and self-definition in normal and disrupted personality development: Retrospect and prospect. *American Psychologist, 68*(3), 172–183. https://doi.org/10.1037/a0032243

Luyten, P., & Blatt, S. J. (2015). A hierarchical multiple-level approach to the assessment of interpersonal relatedness and self-definition: Implications for research, clinical practice, and DSM planning. *Journal of Personality Assessment, 98*(1), 5–13. https://doi.org/10.1080/00223891.2015.1091773

Luyten, P, & Fonagy, P. (2019). Mentalizing and trauma. In A. Bateman & P. Fonagy (Eds.) Handbook of mentalizing in mental health practice (pp 79–99). Second Edition. Washington, DC: American Psychiatric Publishing

Lyons-Ruth, K., Bruschweiler-Stern, N., Harrison, A. M., Morgan, A. C., Nahum, J. P., Sander., et al. (1998). Implicit relational knowing: Its roles in development and psychoanalytic treatment. *Infant Mental Health Journal, 19*, 282–289.

Lynch, T. R., Chapman, A. L., Rosenthal, M. Z., Kuo, J. R., & Linehan, M. M. (2006). Mechanisms of change in dialectical behavior therapy: theoretical and empirical observations. *Journal of Clinical Psychology, 62*(4), 459–480. https://doi.org/10.1002/jclp.20243

Lynch, T. R., Trost, W. T., Salsman, N., & Linehan, M. M. (2007). Dialectical behavior therapy for borderline personality disorder. *Annual Review of Clinical Psychology, 3*, 181–205. https://doi.org/10.1146/annurev.clinpsy.2.022305.095229

Main, M., Hesse, E., & Hesse, S. (2011). Attachment theory and research: Overview with suggested applications to child custody. *Family Court Review, 49*(3), 426–463. https://doi.org/10.1111/j.1744-1617.2011.01383.x

Main, M., Kaplan, N., & Cassidy, J. (1985). Security in infancy, childhood, and adulthood: A move to the level of representation. *Monographs of the Society for Research in Child Development, 50*(1/2), 66–104. https://doi.org/10.2307/3333827

Maj, M. (2012). Development and validation of the current concept of major depression. *Psychopathology, 45*(3), 135–146. https://doi.org/10.1159/000329100

Mann, J. J. (2010). Clinical Pleomorphism of major depression as a challenge to the study of its pathophysiology. *World Psychiatry, 9*(3), 167–168. https://doi.org/10.1002/j.2051-5545.2010.tb00304.x

Mennin, D. S., & Farach, F. J. (2007). Emotion and evolving treatments for adult psychopathology. *Clinical Psychology: Science and Practice, 14*(4), 329–352. https://doi.org/10.1111/j.1468-2850.2007.00094.x

Mennin, D. S., Holoway, R. M., Fresco, D. M., Moore, M. T., & Heimberg, R. G. (2007). Delineating components of emotion and its dysregulation in anxiety and mood psychopathology. *Behavior Therapy, 38*(3), 284–302. https://doi.org/10.1016/j.beth.2006.09.001

Mervielde, I., De Clercq, B., De Fruyt, F., & Van Leeuwen, K. (2005). Temperament, personality, and developmental psychopathology as childhood antecedents of personality disorders. *Journal of Personality Disorders, 19*(2), 171–201. https://doi.org/10.1521/pedi.19.2.171.62627

Meyer, B., & Pilkonis, P. A. (2005). An attachment model of personality disorder. In M. F. Lenzenweger & J. F. Clarkin (Eds.), *Major theories of personality disorder* (pp. 231–281). New York, NY: The Guilford Press.

Mikulincer, M. (1998). Adult attachment style and affect regulation: Strategic variations in self-appraisals. *Journal of Personality and Social Psychology, 75*(2), 420–435. https://doi.org/10.1037/0022-3514.75.2.420

Mikulincer, M., Gillath, O., & Shaver, P. R. (2002). Activation of the attachment system in adulthood: Threat-related primes increase the accessibility of mental representations of attachment figures. *Journal of Personality and Social Psychology, 83*(4), 881–895. https://doi.org/10.1037/0022-3514.83.4.881

Mikulincer, M., & Shaver, P. R. (2003). The attachment behavioral system in adulthood: Activation, psychodynamics, and interpersonal processes. In M. P. Zanna (Ed.), *Advances in experimental social psychology* (pp. 53–152). New York, NY: Academic Press.

Mikulincer, M., & Shaver, P. R. (2007). *Attachment in adulthood: Structure, dynamics and change*. New York, NY: The Guilford Press.

Morey, L. C., Berghuis, H., Bender, D. S., Verheul, R., Krueger, R. F., & Skodol, A. E. (2011). Toward a model for assessing level of personality functioning in DSM-5, part II: Empirical articulation of a core dimension of personality pathology. *Journal of Personality Assessment, 93*(4), 347–353. https://doi.org/10.1080/00223891.2011.577853

Nolen-Hoeksema, S., Wisco, B. E., & Lyubomirsky, S. (2008). Rethinking Rumination. *Perspectives on Psychological Science, 3*(5), 400–424. https://doi.org/10.1111/j.1745-6924.2008.00088.x

Pascual-Leone, A. (1991). The psychological unit and its role in task analysis: A reinter pretation of object permanence. In M. Chapman y M. Chandler (Eds), Criteria for Competence. Controverse in the Conceptualization and Assessment of children's Abilities. Hillsdale

Pascual-Leone, A. (2018). How clients "change emotion with emotion": A programme of research on emotional processing. *Psychotherapy Research, 28*(2), 165–182. https://doi.org/10.1080/10503307.2017.1349350

Pietromonaco, P. R., Feldman Barrett, L., & Powers, S. I. (2006). Adult attachment theory and affective reactivity and regulation. In D. K. Snyder, J. Simpson, & J. N. Hughes (Eds.), *Emotion regulation in couples and families: Pathways to dysfunctions and health* (pp. 57–74). Washington, DC: American Psychological Association.

Pincus, A. L. (2005). A Contemporary integrative interpersonal theory of personality disorders. In M. F. Lenzenweger & J. F. Clarkin (Eds.), *Major Theories of Personality Disorder* (p. 282–331). Guilford Press.

Punkanen, M., Eerola, T., & Erkkilä, J. (2011). Biased emotional recognition in depression: Perception of emotions in music by depressed patients. *Journal of Affective Disorders, 130*(1–2), 118–126. https://doi.org/10.1016/j.jad.2010.10.034

Reisch, T., Ebner-Priemer, U. W., Tschacher, W., Bohus, M., & Linehan, M. M. (2008). Sequences of emotions in patients with borderline personality disorder. *Acta Psychiatrica Scandinavica, 118*(1), 42–48. https://doi.org/10.1111/j.1600-0447.2008.01222.x

Rice, T. R., & Hoffman, L. (2014). Defense mechanisms and implicit emotion regulation: A comparison of a psychodynamic construct with one from contemporary neuroscience. *Journal of the American Psychoanalytic Association, 62*(4), 693–708. https://doi.org/10.1177/0003065114546746.

Ripoll, L. H., Snyder, R., Steele, H., & Siever, L. J. (2013). The neurobiology of empathy in borderline personality disorder. *Current Psychiatry Reports, 15*(3), 344. https://doi.org/10.1007/s11920-012-0344-1

Roisman, G. I., Holland, A., Fortuna, K., Fraley, R. C., Clausell, E., & Clarke, A. (2007). The Adult Attachment Interview and self-reports of attachment style: an empirical rapprochement. *Journal of Personality and Social Psychology, 92*(4), 678–697. https://doi.org/10.1037/0022-3514.92.4.678

Rothbart, M., & Derryberry, D. (1984). Emotion, attention and temperament. In C. Izard, J. Kagan, & R. Zajonc (Eds.), *Emotion, cognition and behavior* (pp. 133–156). New York, NY: Cambridge University Press.

Sanislow, C. A., Morey, L. C., Grilo, C. M., Gunderson, J. G., Shea, M., Skodol, A. E, et al. (2002) Confirmatory factor analysis of DSM-IV borderline, schizotypal, avoidant and obsessive-compulsive personality disorders: Findings from the collaborative longitudinal personality disorders study. *Acta Psychiatrica Scandinavica, 105*(1), 28–36. https://doi.org/10.1034/j.1600-0447.2002.0_479.x

Safran, J., & Muran, C. (2000). *Negotiating the therapeutic alliance. A relational treatment guide.* New York: The Guilford Press.

Schore, A. N. (2011). The right brain implicit self lies at the core of psychoanalysis. *Psychoanalytic Dialogues, 21*(1), 75–100. https://doi.org/10.1080/10481885.2011.545329

Schore, A. N. (2016). Affect Regulation and the Origin of the Self. The Neurobiology of Emotional Development. Lawrence Erlbaum Associates, Inc.

Scherer, K. R. (1984). On the nature and function of emotion: A component process approach. In K. R. Scherer & P. E. Ekman (Eds.), *Approaches to emotion* (pp. 293–317). Hillsdale, NJ: Erlbaum.

Schore, A. N. (2003). *Affect dysregulation and disorders of the self.* New York, NY: W.W. Norton & Company.

Schore, A. N. (2012). *The science of the art of psychotherapy*. New York, NY: W. W. Norton & Company.

Schuessler, G. (2003). Neurobiology and psychotherapy. Expanded version of the lecture given at the congress in Innsbruck on 'neurobiology and psychotherapy'.

Selcuk, E., Zayas, V., Günaydin, G., Hazan, C., & Kross, E. (2012). Mental representations of attachment figures facilitate recovery following upsetting autobiographical memory recall. *Journal of Personality and Social Psychology, 103*(2), 362–378. https://doi.org/10.1037/a0028125

Shaver, P. R., & Mikulincer, M. (2014). Adult attachment and emotion regulation. In J. J. Gross (Ed.), *Handbook of emotion regulation* (pp. 157–172). New York, NY: The Guilford Press.

Sibley, C. G., & Overall, N. C. (2007). The boundaries between attachment and personality: Associations across three levels of the attachment network. *Journal of Research in Personality, 41*(4), 960–967. https://doi.org/10.1016/j.jrp.2006.10.002

Simpson, J. A., Rholes, W. S., & Nelligan, J. S. (1992). Support seeking and support giving within couples in an anxiety-provoking situation: The role of attachment styles. *Journal of Personality and Social Psychology, 62*(3), 434–446. https://doi.org/10.1037/0022-3514.62.3.434

Simpson, J. A., Rholes, W. S., & Phillips, D. (1996). Conflict in close relationships: An attachment perspective. *Journal of Personality and Social Psychology, 71*(5), 899–914. https://doi.org/10.1037/0022-3514.71.5.899

Skodol, A. E., Bender, D. S., Morey, L. C., Clark, L. A., Oldham, J. M., Alarcon, R. D., et al. (2011). Personality disorder types proposed for DSM-5. *Journal of Personality Disorders, 25*(2), 136–169. https://doi.org/10.1521/pedi.2011.25.2.136

Sroufe, L. A. (1996). *Emotional development: The organization of emotional life in the early years*. New York, NY: Cambridge University Press.

Stern, D. N., Sander, L. W., Nahum, J. P., Harrison, A. M., Lyons-Ruth, K., Morgan, A. C., et al. (1998). Non-interpretive mechanisms in psychoanalytic therapy. The 'something more' than interpretation. *International Journal of Psychoanalysis, 79*(5), 903–921.

Taipale, J. (2016). Self-regulation and beyond: Affect regulation and the infant-caregiver dyad. *Frontiers in Psychology, 7*(889), 1–13. https://doi.org/10.3389/fpsyg.2016.00889

Teasdale, J. D. (1988). Cognitive vulnerability to persistent depression. *Cognition and Emotion, 2*(3), 247–274. https://doi.org/10.1080/02699938808410927

Thomas, D. G., Whitaker, E., Crow, C. D., Little, V., Love, L., Lykins, M. S., et al. (1997). Event-related potential variability as a measure of information storage in infant development. *Developmental Neuropsychology, 13*(2), 205–232. https://doi.org/10.1080/87565649709540678

Tronick, E. (1989). Emotions and emotional communication in infants. *American Psychologist, 44*(2), 112–119. https://doi.org/10.1037//0003-066X.44.2.112

Tronick, E. (2001). Emotional connections and dyadic consciousness in infant-mother and patient-therapist interactions. *Psychoanalytic Dialogues, 11*(2), 187–194. https://doi.org/10.1080/10481881109348606

Tronick, E. (2007). *The neurobehavioral and social-emotional development of infants and children*. New York, NY: W. W. Norton & Company.

Tronick, E., Bruschweiler-Stern, N., Harrison, A. C., Lyons-Ruth, K., Morgan, A. C., Nahum, J. P., et al. (1998). Dyadically expanded states of consciousness and the process of therapeutic change. *Infant Mental Health Journal, 19*(3), 290–299.

Tronick, E., & Cohn, J. F. (1989). Infant-mother face-to-face interaction: Age and gender differences in coordination and the occurrence of miscoordination. *Child Development, 60*(1), 85–92. https://doi.org/10.2307/1131074

Tucker, D. M. (1992). Developing emotions and cortical networks. In M. R. Gunnar & C. A. Nelson (Eds.), *Minnesota symposium on child psychology* (*Developmental behavioral neuroscience*) (Vol. 24, pp. 75–128). Hillsdale, NJ: Erlbaum.

Van der Kolk, B. (2014). The body keeps the score. In *Brain, mind, and body in the healing of trauma*. New York, NY: Penguin Group.

Verheul, R., Andrea, H., Berghout, C., Dolan, C. C., van Busschbach, J. J., Van Der Kroft, P. J. A., et al. (2008). Severity indices of personality problems (SIPP-18): Development, factor structure, reliability, and validity. *Psychological Assessment, 20*(1), 23–34. https://doi.org/10.1037/1040-3590.20.1.23

Watson, J. S. (2001). Contingency perception and misperception in infancy: Some potential implications for attachment. *Bulletin of the Menninger Clinic, 65*(3), 296–320. https://doi.org/10.1521/bumc.65.3.296.19848

Watson, D. (2005). Rethinking the mood and anxiety disorders: a quantitative hierarchical model for DSM-V. *Journal of Abnormal Psychology, 114*(4), 522–536. https://doi.org/10.1037/0021-843X.114.4.522

Wei, M., Russell, D. W., Mallinckrodt, B., & Vogel, D. L. (2007). The experiences in close relationship scale (ECR)-short form: Reliability, validity, and factor structure. *Journal of Personality Assessment, 88*(2), 187–204. https://doi.org/10.1080/00223890701268041

Weinberg, E. (2006). Mentalization, affect regulation, and development of the self. *Journal of the American Psychoanalytic Association, 54*(1), 251–269. https://doi.org/10.1177/00030651060540012501

Westen, D. (1991). Cognitive-behavioral interventions in the psychoanalytic psychotherapy of borderline personality disorders. *Clinical Psychology Review, 11*(3), 211–230. https://doi.org/10.1016/0272-7358(91)90101-Y

Westen, D. (1998). Affect regulation and psychopathology: Applications to depression and borderline personality disorder. In W. Flack & J. Laird (Eds.), *Affect and Psychopathology* (pp. 394–406). New York, NY: Oxford University Press.

Westen, D., Novotny, C. M., & Thompson-Brenner, H. (2004). The empirical status of empirically supported psychotherapies: assumptions, findings, and reporting in controlled clinical trials. *Psychological Bulletin, 130*(4), 631–663. https://doi.org/10.1037/0033-2909.130.4.631

Westen, D., Gabbard, G. O., & Blagov, P. (2006). Back to the Future: Personality Structure as a Context for Psychopathology. In R. F. Krueger & J. L. Tackett (Eds.), *Personality and psychopathology* (p. 335–384). The Guilford Press.

Widiger, T. A., & Clark, L. A. (2000). Toward DSM-V and the classification of psychopathology. *Psychological Bulletin, 126*(6), 946–963. https://doi.org/10.1037/0033-2909.126.6.946

Widiger, T. A., & Samuel, D. B. (2005). Diagnostic categories or dimensions? A question for the Diagnostic And Statistical Manual Of Mental Disorders–fifth edition. *Journal of Abnormal Psychology, 114*(4), 494–504. https://doi.org/10.1037/0021-843X.114.4.494

World Health Organization. (2018). ICD-11: international statistical classification of diseases and related health problems: eleven revision (2nd ed). https://apps.who.int/iris/handle/10665/42980

Zimmermann, J., Woods, W. C., Ritter, S., Happel, M., Masuhr, O., Jaeger, U., Spitzer, C., & Wright, A. G. C. (2019). Integrating structure and dynamics in personality assessment: First steps toward the development and validation of a personality dynamics diary. *Psychological Assessment, 31*(4), 516–531. https://doi.org/10.1037/pas0000625

Chapter 4
The Functional Domain of Self-Other Regulation

Nicolas Lorenzini, Peter Fonagy, and Patrick Luyten

Abstract Depression and personality disorder, in particular borderline personality disorder as defined by DSM and ICD classifications, are characterized by great phenomenological heterogeneity, and high comorbidity with each other and with other psychiatric disorders. These characteristics suggest that several domains of mental functioning are differentially affected, to give rise to one or another diagnosis and their comorbidities. This chapter reviews and links the evidence related to the impairments in functioning of the self-other domain, particularly in adult depression, through advancing a model based on three of its main component systems: stress regulation (negative valence and arousal/regulatory systems), reward (positive valence systems), and mentalizing (system for social processes or social cognition) systems, which we see as interconnected. For each of these systems, we review and link the evidence arising from genetic, neurophysiological and behavioral domains. The chapter follows a developmental psychopathology perspective, which highlights the developmental cascades that give rise to such psychopathology. Finally, we propose an understanding of comorbidity and heterogeneity, future lines for research and for the development of evidence-based interventions.

Keywords Depression · Personality disorders · Stress regulation · Reward system · Mentalizing

---

N. Lorenzini (✉)
Research Department of Clinical, Educational and Health Psychology, University College London, London, UK

P. Fonagy
Research Department of Clinical, Educational and Health Psychology, University College London, London, UK

Millennium Institute for Research in Depression and Personality (MIDAP), Santiago, Chile

P. Luyten
Research Department of Clinical, Educational and Health Psychology, University College London, London, UK

Millennium Institute for Research in Depression and Personality (MIDAP), Santiago, Chile

Faculty of Psychology and Educational Sciences, KU Leuven (University of Leuven), Leuven, Belgium

G. de la Parra et al. (eds.), *Depression and Personality Dysfunction*, Depression and Personality, https://doi.org/10.1007/978-3-030-70699-9_4

4.1 Introduction

The matrix of domains and levels related to diverse psychopathologies and behavioral problems which comprise the Research Domain Criteria (RDoC) model proposed by the US National Institute of Mental Health Research (NIMH) is a much-needed change in the approach to the study of vulnerability factors implicated in mental disorders. Its shift from categorical and disease-oriented models towards a dimensional approach focusing on the underlying systems and mechanisms implicated in psychopathology is promising in its potential to further our insights into the nature of psychopathology and its treatment, elements that are missing in other classification systems (Cuthbert & Insel, 2013).

In the particular case of depression and borderline personality disorder (BPD), other classification systems yield diagnoses which are characterized by both a wide phenomenological heterogeneity and a high level of comorbidity. These characteristics suggest that several underlying systems or domains of mental functioning are differently affected in order to give rise to the various presentations of these disorders. This chapter aims at presenting a comprehensive approach based on the RDoC methodology to these disorders, specifically focusing on the impairments of the regulation of the relationship between the self and others. Although these impairments could be solely ascribed to the Domain of Systems for Social Processing, they in fact emerge from a three-pronged series of interacting impairment in a) the stress regulation system, b) reward, and c) the mentalizing systems (or social cognition systems). These impairments relate to each of the five proposed research domains and must be considered from a developmental perspective. In fact, the most prevalent age of onset for these disorders, the transition implied in the end of adolescence and beginning of adulthood, illustrates that the developmental perspective is unavoidable, given that the three interacting impairments we propose as central for the development of these disorders increase the risk for psychopathology especially during developmental transitions. This is especially true for the transition between adolescence and adulthood, when the establishment of new and more complex relationships and the achievement of an individuated sense of agency rely heavily on self-regulatory, reward (and the incentive value of attachment and agency/autonomy in particular), and mentalizing functions. For this reason, the main objective of this chapter is to present a novel approach for the emergence of these psychopathologies and, from it, to shed light on the issue of mental and somatic comorbidity, the development of interventions and prevention, which ultimately illustrates the heuristic power of the RDoC.

4.2 The Useful Potential of Dimensional and Developmental Perspectives in the Conception of Psychopathology

Depression is one of the world-leading causes of disability, morbidity, and mortality (Collins et al., 2011) and a major risk factor for suicide (Han, Compton, Gfroerer, & McKeon, 2015). Epidemiological studies place the 12-month prevalence of depression between 7.5% and 11.3% in older adolescents and 9.6% in young adults, with several studies presenting even higher figures (Avenevoli, Swendsen, He, Burstein, & Merikangas, 2015; Ibrahim, Kelly, Adams, & Glazebrook, 2013; Kessler et al., 2003; Mojtabai, Olfson, & Han, 2016). Particularly for depression, similar figures have been found for children and adolescents (Nock et al., 2013; Wilkinson, Kelvin, Roberts, Dubicka, & Goodyer, 2011), and the mean age of onset is gradually moving to earlier ages (Kessler et al., 2003; Kessler et al., 2005). Indeed, a meta-analysis by Costello, Erkanli, and Angold (2006) estimated that 2.8% of children under the age of 13 and 5.6% of 13–18-year-olds suffer from depressive disorders. Studies which focus only on major depressive disorder (MDD) as defined in the fifth edition of the Diagnostic and Statistical Manual of Mental Disorders (DSM-5; American Psychiatric Association, 2013) have found a prevalence of approximately 2% in children and 4–8% in adolescents. Lifetime estimates range between 15% and 20% (Birmaher, Ryan, Williamson, Brent, & Kaufman, 1996). For dysthymic disorder, epidemiological studies suggest prevalences between 0.6% and 1.7% for children and between 1.6% and 8.0% for adolescents (Birmaher et al., 1996). It is noteworthy that, until adolescence, depressive disorders are equally prevalent in boys and girls, but from age 14 the female:male ratio changes to approximately 2:1, and this ratio persists throughout adulthood (Angold, Erkanli, Silberg, Eaves, & Costello, 2002; Birmaher, Brent, & Issues, 2007). Therefore, it is crucial for any theoretical approach to depression to provide an explanation for the emergence of these gender differences in development. It is also important to consider that while the phenomenological (symptomatic) expression of depression in children and adolescents resembles that in adults in many respects, there are also some significant differences: children and adolescents typically show more anxiety and anger, fewer vegetative symptoms, and less verbalization of hopelessness than adults (American Psychiatric Association, 2013). Also, depression in young age is accompanied with comorbidities of both internalizing and externalizing symptomatology (Lee & Stone, 2012), which puts into question the neat distinction made between depression and other disorders and behavioral problems. This questioning is in line with the RDoC approach, which focuses dimensionally on neural circuits that cut across descriptive diagnoses, leading to blurred boundaries between different "disorders" and thus, correspondingly, between factors implicated in vulnerability for depression and other disorders.

In the case of BPD, epidemiological studies have only late-adolescent and adult samples. The latest edition of the DSM specifies that the criteria for diagnosis should be traced to at least the end of adolescence or the beginning of adulthood (American Psychiatric Association, 2013). For that reason, clinicians and researchers are careful in ascribing this diagnostic label to children or younger adolescents. Prevalence varies depending on the study: point prevalence in BPD ranges between 1 and 2 percent of the general population, with lifetime prevalence of 5.9%, with higher prevalences in females (Torgensen, 2014; Ullrich & Coid, 2009). In college student samples, the prevalence of BPD ranges from 0.5% to 32.1%, with lifetime prevalence of 9.7%, according to a meta-analysis (Meaney, Hasking, & Reupert, 2016). For a very complete view on personality pathology in adolescents, see the work of Carla Sharp, arguably the most important author on this topic (Sharp, 2020;

Sharp, Penner, & Ensink, 2019; Sharp, Vanwoerden, & Wall, 2018; Sharp & Wall, 2018).

In spite of the status of personality disorder as an adult diagnosis, there is a myriad of evidence which finds borderline-like features in adolescence and, more importantly, strong connections between early adversity and receiving the BPD diagnosis later in life (Fonagy & Bateman, 2016). In the case of adolescents, available epidemiological studies suggest that the prevalence of BPD in the general population of adolescents is around 3%, and in the clinical population it ranges from 11% in adolescent outpatients clinic to 78% in adolescents attending an emergency department because of suicidal behavior (Guilé, Boissel, Alaux-Cantin, & de La Rivière, 2018; Zanarini et al., 2017). In younger children, a diagnosis of BPD is rarely made, but some authors have observed that certain psychopathological manifestations during childhood (12 years old or younger) resemble borderline features, like affective instability, relationship difficulties, negative self-concept, increased risk of suicidal ideation, suicidal behavior, and development of psychopathology (Rogosch & Cicchetti, 2005). Moreover, a systematic review showed that children with borderline-like features are more likely to have a history of maltreatment and that children who had been maltreated were more likely to present with borderline-like features (Ibrahim, Cosgrave, & Woolgar, 2018). From a neuroscientific perspective, children who presented borderline-like features also showed a less efficient processing in attention networks related to conflict, comparable to that in adult BPD patients, independently from the presence of a history of maltreatment. There are wider similarities: children whose sleeping problems were followed between ages 2.5 and 6.8 years were at significantly higher risk of later BPD symptomatology if they had persistent nightmares, which is a symptom commonly reported by adult BPD patients (Lereya, Winsper, Tang, & Wolke, 2017).

Besides the correspondence or similarity that some researchers have been able to find between the manifestations of adult BPD and those presented by certain children and adolescents, it is the relationship between early adversity and later development of BPD which suggests the value of a developmental approach to understanding this disorder. Adolescents with emerging BPD are more likely to report adverse experiences in childhood than their nonclinical peers, and these experiences are greater in frequency and type. This same sample, however, reported less severity of these experiences than adult BPD patients (Temes et al., 2017).

A prospective study following 500 individuals with documented cases of childhood neglect and physical and sexual abuse, together with 396 demographically matched control children, found that significantly more children who suffered physical or emotional abuse or neglect met criteria for BPD as adults in comparison to controls. Other results emerged: having a parent with substance use problems and not being employed full-time, not being a school graduate, and having a diagnosis of drug abuse, MDD, or post-traumatic stress disorder (PTSD) were predictors of later BPD and in fact moderated the relationship between abuse and neglect, and adult development of BPD (Widom, Czaja, & Paris, 2009).

A meta-analysis of 97 studies comparing BPD patients to nonclinical controls found that individuals with BPD are almost 14 times more likely to report childhood adversity (Porter et al., 2019).

Indeed, severity of BPD symptomatology appears to be related to particular characteristics of early adversity. For example, young adults diagnosed with BPD showed significantly less non-suicidal self-injury if they did not report early abuse than BPD youth with early abuse. Moreover, the occurrence of childhood abuse in this BPD sample was associated with a fivefold increase in the rate of lifetime suicide attempts in comparison with the BPD youths who did not report early abuse (Kaplan et al., 2016). Indeed, exposure to trauma, specifically sexual abuse prior to and during puberty, has been consistently related to the risk for the emergence of BPD (Newnham & Janca, 2014), as with its severity (e.g., cumulative exposure to sexual abuse throughout childhood increases the risk of psychotic experiences in BPD) (Shirley, 2017).

A developmental approach to psychopathology is further supported by evidence that a general psychopathology (or "p") factor underlies all psychopathology and provides a comprehensive explanation for the extensive comorbidity among disorders, as well as many of other features denoting severity in individuals who we traditionally consider to be "hard to reach" or "treatment resistant." In the words of Caspi and colleagues, "one underlying dimension that summarized individuals' propensity to develop any and all forms of common psychopathologies" (Caspi et al., 2014, p. 13). Analyzing the Dunedin longitudinal study, Caspi et al. examined the structure of psychopathology from adolescence to midlife, considering dimensionality, persistence, current, and sequential comorbidity. They found that vulnerability to mental disorder is better described by one general psychopathology factor – labelled the "p" (for psychopathology) factor – than by three higher-order (spectral) factors (internalizing, externalizing, and thought disorder). A higher p factor score was associated with "more life impairment, greater family antecedents, worse developmental histories, and more compromised early-life brain function" (Caspi et al., 2014, p. 13). Several studies have replicated this p factor structure, which appears to be the overarching factor of psychopathology at different developmental stages (Carragher et al., 2016; Laceulle, Vollebergh, & Ormel, 2015; Lahey et al., 2015; Martel et al., 2017; Patalay et al., 2015). Importantly, the p factor concept explains in part why discovering isolated causes, consequences, or biomarkers and specific, tailored treatments for psychiatric disorders has proved so elusive, further supporting a dimensional conceptualization of psychopathology as that proposed by the RDoC (Fonagy & Campbell, 2015).

The evidence backing the developmental nature of psychopathology and the high prevalence of comorbidity guides our conception of depression and personality disorders, in addition to the dimensional view conveyed by the RDoC. Indeed, the RDoC approach, which focuses on neural circuits that cut across descriptive diagnoses, will necessarily challenge distinctions between the various disorders described in categorical diagnostic manuals and therefore between the factors implicated in the vulnerability for mental disorders.

The focus of the RDoC is on neural circuitry, with levels of analysis progressing "upward" to behavior and "downward" to genetic and molecular levels (Insel et al., 2010). In this chapter we take a similar approach, focusing on the domains of neural circuits/physiology, behavior, and genes.

4.3 A Stress-Reward-Mentalizing Model of Depression and Personality Pathology

There are several theories, both in personality pathology and in depression, which have described impairments in the area of neurology, behavior, and genes, but they have tended, with some exceptions (Auerbach, Admon, & Pizzagalli, 2014; Bogdan, Nikolova, & Pizzagalli, 2013; Davey, Yücel, & Allen, 2008; Dillon et al., 2014; Lawrence, Allen, & Chanen, 2010; Panksepp & Watt, 2011; Pizzagalli, 2014), to direct research towards a single one of these three systems. This chapter attempts to integrate the evidence found for each of these biobehavioral systems, arguing that they have evolved in response to the continuing need of adaptation to constantly changing circumstances, namely, a) a system that deals with stress following threat (the stress/threat system); b) a system that produces rewarding effects associated with positive environmental features, including the formation of interpersonal relationships involved in infant–mother, mother–infant, pair-bonding, and other attachment relationships, and experiences of agency and autonomy (the reward system); and c) a mentalizing or social cognitive system, which subserves the capacity to understand oneself and others in terms of intentional mental states such as feelings, desires, wishes, attitudes, and values and delivers the necessary computational power human beings need to navigate their complex interpersonal world and to acquire a sense of agency and autonomy.

Both internal and contextual factors might disrupt their highly interrelated and coordinated functions, disruption that might take the form of depression and/or personality disorders. With an evolutionary perspective in mind, it is important to clarify that what we know is that mental health disorders, including depression and personality disorders, are not in themselves maladaptive. For example, the genetic predisposition to depression may have been maintained in the human genome because depression is a mechanism that attempts to minimize or terminate distress associated with separation and loss (Davey et al., 2008; Gilbert, 2006; Panksepp & Watt, 2011), and BPD might develop as a reaction to an insecure and threatening environment where basic trust towards the social world might be fended off, to avoid falling victim to the hostility of such environment (Fonagy, Bateman, Lorenzini, Luyten, & Campbell, 2021; Fonagy, Luyten, & Allison, 2015; Fonagy, Luyten, Allison, & Campbell, 2017b).

Our proposed model argues that excessive or age-inappropriate stress during development, in combination with genetically increased stress sensitivity, leads to impairments in reward sensitivity, and in turn in the capacity for mentalizing and social cognition. As mentioned above, when considering the typical ages of onset of these disorders (late adolescence and young adulthood), among the main normative developmental tasks, we find the establishment of mature and differentiated relationships and of autonomous agency. We argue that these developmental tasks are central sources of further stress and therefore set the stage for the emergence of psychopathology. This is because they put mentalizing capacities (perhaps already somewhat impaired; Sharp et al., 2019) under considerable pressure, in spite of their function as key sources of reward.

4.4 Stress (RDoC Negative Valence and Arousal/Regulatory Systems)

4.4.1 Neural Circuits and Physiology

Systems whose function is to regulate stress are discussed in the RDoC under what is called negative valence and arousal/regulatory systems, and their relevance has been abundantly demonstrated when it comes to the understanding of the vulnerability and emergence of depression (Heim & Binder, 2012) and BPD (Bourvis, Aouidad, Cabelguen, Cohen, & Xavier, 2017).

We can see depression as a developmental, stress-related disorder with elevated levels of stress, most likely in combination with increased stress sensitivity, leading to increased vulnerability for depression and other stress-related disorders. Similarly, we see BPD in relation to stress as also developmentally determined (Carvalho Fernando et al., 2014; Ehrenthal, Levy, Scott, & Granger, 2018; McLean & Gallop, 2003). From this perspective, it is imperative to understand the developmental origins of the capacity for stress regulation, including the hypothalamic-pituitary-adrenal (HPA) axis and other sympathetic neural structures of the stress system, are involved in detecting, integrating, and responding to threats and other sources of stress. Also included in this system are the amygdala and hippocampus, and areas in the prefrontal cortex (PFC), most notably the anterior cingulate cortex, orbitofrontal cortex, and medial PFC (MPFC), as key players in this network (Arnsten, 2011; Hastings, Parsey, Oquendo, Arango, & Mann, 2004; McEwen, 2007; Pervanidou & Chrousos, 2012; Siegle, Konecky, Thase, & Carter, 2003). These interconnected structures serve allostasis, understood as the capacity to continuously adapt to changing circumstances (McEwen, 2007), and the failure of attempts to establish allostasis is known as allostatic load. Therefore, there is a series of closely interrelated physiological systems responsible for establishing and maintaining allostasis, serving the fight/flight/freeze response when faced with acute stress, and a broader set of regulatory responses associated with the stress response more generally (Bourvis et al., 2017; Gold, Machado-Vieira, & Pavlatou, 2015; Gunnar & Quevedo, 2007; McEwen, 2007; Pervanidou & Chrousos, 2012). These include the HPA axis and the autonomic nervous system, as well as the metabolic system, gut, kidneys, and immune system, each with their relatively distinct mediators (e.g., cortisol, sympathetic and parasympathetic transmitters, metabolic hormones, and cytokines, respectively). This demonstrates the close intertwining of the stress system with several other bodily systems, which interact in complex ways. This assumption has important implications for the emergence of comorbidity and heterogeneity of clinical presentations in both depression and BPD.

It is important to note that while the functioning of the HPA axis both in depression and in BPD is abnormal, the literature yields conflicting results regarding the nature of such abnormality.

In depression, HPA hyperactivity, correlated to greater stress sensitivity, is particularly present in patients with depression who have suffered adverse experiences during childhood. But not all depressive presentations have a history of childhood stress, and other risk factors for hyperactivity, such as female gender, are significant in predicting hyperactivity of the HPA axis (Heim & Binder, 2012; Heim, Newport, Mletzko, Miller, & Nemeroff, 2008). However, there is some evidence in adults, children, and adolescents which suggests that while acute stress may initially lead to HPA hyperactivity, chronic stress may progressively lead to a switch to hypoactivity of the HPA axis, given the wear and tear in physiological system (Miller, Chen, & Zhou, 2007; Raabe & Spengler, 2013). These empirical inconsistencies indeed may be behind the great variety of presentations and subtypes in depression. They also lend further support to a developmental perspective in the understanding of depression, through identifying critical periods for the development and reorganization of the stress system: core structures of this system, such as the hippocampus, have the largest increase in volume during infant/toddler years and then steadily decline, while the prefrontal cortex develops slower with peaks in maturation and plasticity during adolescence, approximately between 8 and 15 years (Andersen & Teicher, 2008; Giedd et al., 2009; Heim & Binder, 2012). Specifically, frontal cortical control of the amygdala seems to increase from adolescence to adulthood: adolescents show increased amygdala response and decreased habituation to repeated laboratory emotional tasks in comparison to adults, associated with less functional connectivity between prefrontal regions and the amygdala (Yurgelun-Todd & Killgore, 2006). Furthermore, while both adolescents and adults recruit the dorsal anterior cingulate cortex and the dorsolateral prefrontal cortex in response to stress, adults additionally recruit the anterior insula, which is related to decreased autonomic stress response (Strang, Pruessner, & Pollak, 2011). Moreover, the PFC is subject to cortical thinning during adolescence, due in part to synaptic pruning and programmed cell death (Mutlu et al., 2013; Shaw et al., 2008). In conclusion, abnormalities in the stress system related to depression vary depending on developmental challenges, with immediate and often lasting effects on these and associated systems such as the immune, metabolic, and cardiovascular systems (Lupien, McEwen, Gunnar, & Heim, 2009; Pervanidou & Chrousos, 2012).

In the case of BPD, functional abnormalities of the HPA axis show dysregulated feedback inhibition (lowering of cortisol levels): at times suppressed (particularly with comorbid depression), and at times enhanced with self-harm behavior and PTSD comorbidity (Carvalho Fernando et al., 2012; Dixon-Gordon, Gratz, & Tull,

2013; Wingenfeld, Hill, Adam, & Driessen, 2007; Zimmerman & Choi-Kain, 2009). While for BPD patients, basal cortisol is higher than in controls (Lieb, Zanarini, Schmahl, Linehan, & Bohus, 2004), after psychosocial stress, alpha amylase and cortisol responses seem to be attenuated despite greater subjective stress experience (Nater et al., 2010; Scott, Levy, & Granger, 2013).

From an anatomical point of view, reduced gray matter volume (GMV) of the (chiefly on the right) hippocampus has been reported in BPD (Bøen et al., 2014; Krause-Utz, Winter, Niedtfeld, & Schmahl, 2014; Schulze, Schmahl, & Niedtfeld, 2016). This finding is similarly found in patients suffering from PTSD, and in healthy adults with traumatic histories, which might imply that the thinning of the hippocampus is not necessarily specific to BPD, but a response to trauma in general. Conversely, reduction in the volume of the amygdala has been consistently shown in BPD patients, regardless of PTSD comorbidity. As stated before, the amygdala develops early in life, which, taken together with the fact that the difference in amygdala volume between adolescent BPD patients and healthy controls has not been observed, suggests that the loss in volume of the amygdala is a consequence of the disorder (Chanen et al., 2008; Niedtfeld et al., 2013; Wingenfeld, Spitzer, Rullkötter, & Löwe, 2010). When it comes to anatomical specificities of frontal regions in BPD, the evidence is not as clear. While some studies show a reduced GMV of the orbitofrontal cortex (OFC) and anterior cingulate cortex (ACC; Krause-Utz et al., 2014; Wingenfeld et al., 2010), other studies find no difference with healthy controls (Kuhlmann, Bertsch, Schmidinger, Thomann, & Herpertz, 2013). Other studies have found greater GMV in BPD patients in cortical areas, including bilateral volume increases in the middle cingulate cortex (MCC) and the posterior cingulate cortex (PCC; Jin et al., 2016), and the right middle frontal gyrus, which is part of the dorsolateral prefrontal cortex (dlPFC) and is involved in the inhibition of emotions and unwanted memories (Kluetsch et al., 2012). These anatomical observations, taken together and in spite of their inconsistencies, seem to suggest a decrease in the volume of structures devoted to stress and emotion processing and an increase in the volume of areas involved in inhibition and regulation processing.

In terms of brain connectivity, experimental paradigms using stressful stimuli show greater and prolonged activation of the right amygdala and hippocampus and decreased activity in the bilateral dlPFC and ACC in BPD patients (Hazlett et al., 2012; Koenigsberg et al., 2009; Minzenberg, Fan, New, Tang, & Siever, 2007; Nicol, Pope, Romaniuk, & Hall, 2015; Schulze et al., 2011; van Zutphen, Siep, Jacob, Goebel, & Arntz, 2015). Interestingly, the overactivation of the amygdala in BPD patients faced with stressful situations is reversed by both non-suicidal self-injury (NSSI) and dissociation, which are both considered common maladaptive strategies to deal with stress in BPD (Reitz et al., 2015; Stiglmayr et al., 2008).

It has been consistently found that BPD patients show lower serum levels of oxytocin (OXT), a key hormonal messenger for early infant/caregiver interaction, impact of early stress, attachment patterns, future response to acute stress, and non-genetic transmission of behavioral traits (Bourvis et al., 2017). The heightened response of BPD patients to threatening stimuli is significantly attenuated after administration of intranasal OXT, as well as decreased dysphoric stress-induced feelings in BPD patients compared to controls (Bertsch et al., 2013; Simeon et al., 2011). Evidence also shows neurovegetative imbalances in BPD patients when faced with stressful situations, with an increased sympathetic response and a decreased parasympathetic response. This could account for the frequent disruptive behaviors observed in BPD, such as the arousal of the "flight or fight response," impulsivity, emotional liability, and even heart rate response (Koenig, Kemp, Feeling, Thayer, & Kaess, 2016; Kuo, Fitzpatrick, Metcalfe, & McMain, 2016; Weinberg, Klonsky, & Hajcak, 2009).

Notwithstanding the RDoC's proposition that the stress and arousal/regulatory systems are different domains, it does link the latter system to homeostatic regulation, which is also a core task of the stress system (McEwen, 2006). Further research is needed to ascertain whether the arousal and regulatory systems are really different systems. At least in depression, being one of the disorders most closely associated with sleep problems and circadian rhythm, the distinction between these two systems is unclear: stress and disturbances of circadian rhythm have mutually reinforcing effects, as sleep deprivation is a powerful stressor that itself contributes to allostatic load (McEwen, 2006; Tsuno, Besset, & Ritchie, 2005). There is a similar difficulty in differentiating these two regulatory systems in the case of BPD (Bourvis et al., 2017).

4.4.2 Genetics

In adult depression, heritability has been extensively studied, with robust estimates of about 30%–40% (Sullivan, Neale, & Kendler, 2000). There is increasing evidence for the role of gene–environment (GxE) correlations and interactions in depression, with much research focusing on candidate genes involved in the stress system, such as the serotonin transporter gene-linked polymorphic region (5-HTTLPR, arguably the most researched genetic variant in psychology, psychiatry, and neuroscience). Specifically, it has been found that individuals carrying one or two copies of the relatively low-expressing short (S) allele of this polymorphic region show increased neuroticism, a personality trait known to be involved in the propensity to depression and sensitivity to stress. Carriers of the S allele also show amygdala reactivity to threats, depressive symptoms, diagnosable depression, and suicidality, experiencing stressful life events and childhood maltreatment (Caspi, Hariri, Holmes, Uher, & Moffitt, 2010). In spite of the volume of research that this particular GxE interaction has produced, it continues to be controversial given the many methodological limitations of existing research (Dick et al., 2015). However, the fact that genetic polymorphisms related to the system for stress regulation may be involved in depression necessarily leads to the promising field of epigenetics, which refers not to the genetic makeup which marks a propensity for depression within a stressful environment, but to the often-enduring effects of environmental factors on gene expression. Epigenetic mechanisms are indeed a convincing explanation for the high heritability of depression, but not its complete heritability. For example, epigenetic modifications of cytosine–guanine dinucleotide sites in DNA as a result of early adversity have been prospectively demonstrated in a community sample of 109 15-year-olds (Essex et al., 2013). In mice, chronic social defeat produces a sustained reduction in the expression of the protein RAC1 in the nucleus accumbens, which in turn is associated with depressive-like behaviors. Those behaviors are reversed after overexpression of the genetically regulated protein in the nucleus accumbens (Golden et al., 2013). Especially for depression, epigenetic models in both animals and human adults have focused on the differential between acute adult stress and early chronic stress, finding that adversity suffered during various developmental stages has distinct consequences for subsequent susceptibility to stress. These susceptibilities are the result of epigenetic effects in different areas of the nervous system, such as histone posttranslational modifications and gene expression, acetylation, and methylation, which are at the base of the decreased neuronal plasticity, aberrant behavioral responses to stress, depressive behaviors, and even response to antidepressants (for reviews, see Bagot, Labonté, Peña, & Nestler, 2014; Champagne & Curley, 2009; Uchida, Yamagata, Seki, & Watanabe, 2018). In connection with the last section of this chapter, circadian rhythms, for example, are able to modify metabolic functions at an epigenetic level, increasing the risk for and chronicity of depression (Sato & Sassone-Corsi, 2019). Moreover, the developmental epigenetically driven compromise of neuronal plasticity implies increased difficulties to adapt to the continual changes in the environment, including different sources of stress, not only by stiffening the response of the stress regulation system and other related biological systems such as the immune system, pain regulation systems, metabolic system, and reproductive system (McEwen, 2007), as argued by the Developmental Origins of Health and Disease (DOHaD) paradigm (Gluckman et al., 2009).

Even considering the novelty and therefore inevitable limitations of current research on GxE transactions, these models imply a distancing from the mere diathesis-stress models of depression to a broader model of differential susceptibility, that is, the idea that individuals show marked differences in terms of sensitivity to the environment, whether it is a benign environment or a protective one (Ellis, Boyce, Belsky, Bakermans-Kranenburg, & Van IJzendoorn, 2011).

In sum, mounting evidence that the environment has an important influence on phenotypic variation, particularly under poor environmental conditions (to which individuals with a history of trauma and neglect have often been exposed), leads us to consider the role of the broader environment in depression. Indeed, most types of adversity do not occur in isolation but are part of so-called risky families and environments (Repetti, Taylor, & Seeman, 2002) or "pathogenic relational environments" (Cicchetti & Toth, 2005, p. 414). The role of the environment in depression is still poorly understood, despite major findings demonstrating that such a link exists. Ethnic and sexual minority status, for instance, is an important but relatively neglected area in research on depression (Smith & Silva, 2011).

In BPD, the picture of genetic endowment and GxE interactions, including epigenetic phenomena, on the development of the stress system are not too different than those reviewed in this chapter for depression. Indeed, the symptom overlap observed between BPD and other disorders, including depression, hints to the various commonalities between the environmental, neurological, and genetic basis for BPD, depression, and other Axis I and II disorders (Cattane, Rossi, Lanfredi, & Cattaneo, 2017; Clark, Nuzum, & Ro, 2018; MacIntosh, Godbout, & Dubash, 2015; Tomko, Trull, Wood, & Sher, 2014). For example, genome-wide investigations show genetic overlap between BPD, bipolar disorder, schizophrenia, and MDD (Witt et al., 2017). Heritability of BPD is also similar to that of depression, with studies showing heritability figures ranging between 35% and 65%, with higher heritability estimates being obtained with self-ratings (Distel et al., 2010; Kendler, Myers, & Reichborn-Kjennerud, 2011; Reichborn-Kjennerud et al., 2013). A large multinational twin study found that genetic factors that influence individual differences in high neuroticism, low agreeableness, low conscientiousness, and low extraversion (as part of the five-factor model of personality) account for all genetic liability to borderline personality in people showing these traits, particularly high neuroticism (which is associated with stress regulation, as stated above). However, unique environmental effects on borderline personality were not shared with this five-factor model profile (33%; Distel et al., 2009). A similar study, with an extended twin design, found a 54.9% of unique environmental effects on BPD, while genetic effects explained 21.3% (additive effects) and 23.9% (dominant effect) of the variance in the disorder's presence (Distel et al., 2009). In any case, while factorial analyses of these heritability factors seem to be significant, most studies show that the biggest predictor of BPD is environmental (Reichborn-Kjennerud et al., 2013). Specific studies on genetic polymorphisms at the base of BPD have been unable to find associations between genetic variants and BPD risk, as shown in a meta-analysis looking at the serotonin transporter gene (SLC6A4), the promoter insertion/deletion (5-HTTLPR) and the intron 2 VNTR (STin2 VNTR), and the rs1800532 (A218C) polymorphism of the tryptophan hydroxylase 1 gene (TPH1; Calati, Gressier, Balestri, & Serretti, 2013).

Thus, the picture of the genetics of BPD has further complexity than mere heritability, even more than with depression. To obtain a clearer picture on the risk and emergence of this disorder, it is necessary to look at it from an epigenetic point of view. Indeed, many studies indicate that childhood maltreatment and other early adverse experiences are commonly reported in and strongly associated with BPD, and its symptoms, such as derealization or dysphoria (Charoensook, 2017; Machizawa-Summers, 2007; Zanarini et al., 2002). And indeed, at the level of general epigenetic processes, it has been found that BPD patients present increased levels of DNA methylation in several neuropsychiatrically relevant genes (Calati et al., 2013; Dammann et al., 2011), including those coding for serotonin receptors (HTR2A), glucocorticoid receptors (NR3C1, a major component of endocrine influence, specifically the stress response, upon the brain), monoaminoxidase A (MAO-A, an enzyme related to the functioning of several neurotransmitters and whose methylation is also related to depression, suicide, and antisocial behavior when childhood adverse experiences are present, and aggression in the face of social rejection), monoaminoxidase B (MAO-B, associated among other effects, to negative emotionality and cognitive decline), and soluble catechol-O-methyltransferase (S-COMT, relevant for emotional processing, as it seems to influence the interaction between prefrontal and limbic regions, and associated with subjective experience of well-being and neuroticism).

Evidence shows that some allelic variants (rs53576) of the gene coding for OXT receptors in BPD in a large sample of 20-year-olds under the influence of family environment (depressed or nondepressed mothers), in particular the allele A, experience a massive influence from family functioning. This result also shows a differential susceptibility pattern, where the individual carrying the A allele is affected by both normative and adverse family functioning with differential outcomes (Bourvis et al., 2017; Hammen, Bower, & Cole, 2015). The impact of genetic factors in conjunction with environmental effects on the development of BPD has been further highlighted by family and twin studies, which have found a polymorphism (Val158Met) of the gene coding for catechol-O-methyltransferase is associated with past traumatic events and impulsive tendencies in individuals with BPD (Leichsenring, Leibing, Kruse, New, & Leweke, 2011; Wagner et al., 2010). An epigenetic study on the HPA axis functioning in BPD patients showed significant associations between BPD patients with a history of trauma and polymorphism of FKBP5, a gene known to be involved in post-traumatic vulnerability, anxiety, and depression (Martín-Blanco et al., 2015) and in the regulation of stress by the HPA axis (Martín-Blanco et al., 2016).

Therefore, both in depression and BPD, genetic considerations are an important contributor in the understanding of psychopathology. However, it seems that the most fruitful way to address these contributors is the epigenetic perspective, which highlights the reciprocal interaction between biology and environment during development.

4.4.3 Behavior

The link between stress and depression is well studied at a behavioral level. Consistent with the neurobiological and genetic research reviewed so far, results are robust in showing that individuals with increased stress sensitivity seem to be particularly at risk for both depression and BPD.

Early adversity plays a key role in the emergence, severity, and chronicity of depression, given its potential effects on the programming of subsequent stress responses, particularly in individuals carrying genetic vulnerabilities (McCrory, De Brito, & Viding, 2012). In fact, population attributable fractions (the proportion of psychiatric disorders and suicide that could be explained by early adversity) range from 20% to 80% (Afifi et al., 2008; Dube et al., 2001). Congruent with the broad programming effects of early adversity and the interrelationship between stress and other neurobiological systems, it seems that multifinality is the rule rather than the exception, with studies typically finding a dose-response relationship between early adversity and the number of psychiatric disorders, functional somatic disorders, somatic diseases, and general indices of maladaptive intrapersonal and interpersonal functioning (Anda et al., 2006; Roseboom, Painter, van Abeelen, Veenendaal, & de Rooij, 2011).

In the case of depression, the relationship between stress and depression onset has been found to remain stable across the life span, even when controlling for the onset of previous episodes, consistent with the notion of programming effects (McLaughlin et al., 2010). But later-life stress is also important, with minor and major life stressors, particularly in interaction with personality features that confer vulnerability to depression (e.g., neuroticism and self-critical perfectionism) and with genetic vulnerability, being causally related to the onset of this disorder (Kendler & Gardner, 2014; Kendler, Kuhn, & Prescott, 2004; Luyten, Blatt, Van Houdenhove, & Corveleyn, 2006). This makes sense when we think of the nefarious effects of stress on individuals with an increased sensitivity to stress, in turn associated with vulnerability for depression. It is known that stressful events often precede the onset of depressive episodes (for a comprehensive review, see Mazure, 1998). In any case, it seems that current stressors act as a mediator between vulnerability to stress (and the presence of early stress) and the emergence of depressive symptomatology (Bakusic, Schaufeli, Claes, & Godderis, 2017; Vogt, Waeldin, Hellhammer, & Meinlschmidt, 2016). Consistent with hypotheses of stress sensitization (and the workings of the HPA axis), it has been observed that recurrent depressive episodes need less intensity and frequency in order to provoke new depressive episodes (Monroe, Anderson, & Harkness, 2019; Monroe & Harkness, 2005).

Maladaptive behaviors (such as smoking and drinking) and current environmental stressors (low income, lack of companionship) are also important contributors for both stress and depression (Morrissey, Ball, & Pandal, 2020).

However, it is noteworthy that several views on the generation and sustained risk for psychopathology propose that individuals who are vulnerable for depression also tend to generate their own stressful environments. Views like stress-generation perspectives, active vulnerability, or dynamic interactionism are backed by good experimental evidence to support this assumption, in large clinical, epidemiological, and twin studies (Hammen, 2005; Kendler et al., 2004; Luyten et al., 2006; Shahar, 2006). In line with these hypotheses, studies suggest that stress may play an even greater role in explaining the onset of depression in childhood and adolescence than in adulthood, with interpersonal stressors in particular (which are especially salient during these developmental stages) predicting the onset of depression in childhood and adolescence (Auerbach et al., 2014).

There is some evidence that gender differences in the prevalence of depression emerge around adolescence. This time in development is associated with the greater valuing, at least within Western societies, of agency, autonomy, and self-definition in men, while women tend to place greater emphasis on relatedness and attachment (for a review, see Blatt, 2008). Social stress in adolescence may affect women more because of their greater social orientation (Eiland & Romeo, 2013); consequently, they are more prone to internalizing disorders such as so-called somatic depression (i.e., depression characterized by anxious and somatic concerns) and other stress-related disorders involving preoccupation with issues of relatedness (such as pain and exhaustion syndromes; Kendler & Gardner, 2014).

In the case of BPD, the response to acute stress is enhanced, particularly for psychosocial sources of stress. Experimental paradigms aiming at provoking social stress response trigger increased negative emotions and cognitions in BPD subjects compared to healthy controls, but the patients' physiological responses to stress are attenuated (Deckers et al., 2015).

Moreover, in BPD patients, behavioral responses to acute stress are marked by impulsivity. The difference between borderline impulsivity and other disorders (such as attention-deficit hyperactivity disorder, ADHD) is that deficits in impulse control occur in BPD only under stressful conditions (Krause-Utz et al., 2016). As we have already reviewed in relation to the amygdala's activation in BPD patients facing acute stress, another widespread reaction to stress in BPD individuals is NSSI, present in 60–90% of patients. Patients tend to report NSSI spontaneously, together with the relief in stress experienced following self-injurious behaviors (Bourvis et al., 2017). This result seems to be at odds with the idea that physical pain is in itself a source of stress, but it has been demonstrated that it is the nociceptive effect of pain (and not tissue damage or sighting of blood) that acts as a stress reliever (Naoum et al., 2016; Willis et al., 2017).

But the presence of stress, even if not acute, is widespread among BPD patients, to the extent that the differences between the diagnoses of BPD and PTSD have been the subject of considerable attention (Amad, Ramoz, Thomas, & Gorwood, 2016; Gunderson & Sabo, 1993; Lewis & Grenyer, 2009; New, Perez-Rodriguez, & Ripoll, 2012). Comorbidity between these disorders has been reported to be as high as 68% (Golier et al., 2003; Heffernan & Cloitre, 2000; Pagura et al., 2010; Reich et al., 1997; Zlotnick, Franklin, & Zimmerman, 2002). Traumatic events have more severe features in comorbid patients than in PTSD-only patients (Clarke, Rizvi, & Resick, 2008), and the comorbidity correlates with deeper impairment of quality of life, more Axis I comorbidities, and increased risk for suicide attempts (Bolton, Mueser, & Rosenberg, 2006; Pagura et al., 2010).

What is important to bear in mind is that BPD individuals are especially reactive to acute stress stemming from social sources. This consideration will become important to understand impairments in the RDoC's social cognition system. Indeed, research has amply shown an inverse relationship between stress or arousal and mentalizing (Arnsten, 1998; Mayes, 2000). As stress and arousal increase, there is a switch from relatively slow, controlled, and nuanced mentalizing, mainly underpinned by prefrontal executive functions, to more rapid, automatic, and typically biased mentalizing mediated by posterior cortical and limbic structures (Luyten & Fonagy, 2015a).

Before we shift our focus to the mentalizing system, we will describe the contribution of the positive valence system (or reward system) in depression and BPD.

4.5 Reward (RDoC Positive Valence Systems)

4.5.1 Neural Circuits and Physiology

Adversity, early and later in life, leads to a downward spiral marked by the presence of distress and negative affect and the absence of positive affect, which brings us to the RDoC domains of positive valence and, specifically, reward. Just as for dysfunctions in stress regulation, evidence is growing for the role of altered reward sensitivity, particularly in depression.

The reward system itself is relatively well described and consists of mesolimbic and mesocortical pathways. Mesolimbic pathways originate from the ventral tegmental area and project mainly to ventral striatal regions and the nucleus accumbens in particular, as well as the hippocampus and amygdala. The mesocortical pathways involve projections to the PFC and ACC (Naranjo, Tremblay, & Busto, 2001; Pizzagalli, 2014; Russo & Nestler, 2013; Spear, 2000). Recent research has mainly focused on dopamine and OXT as key biological mediators involved in this system. Opioid and cannabinoid systems seem to be equally relevant, particularly as they have been related to the pain associated with social loss and rejection, which is increased in adolescence, particularly in females (Hsu et al., 2015; Panksepp & Watt, 2011; Spear, 2000). From the developmental perspective which guides our approach in this chapter, it is important to realize that the attachment system plays a key role in the development and regulation of the stress system through activation of the reward system, as suggested by studies in animals (including higher primates) and a growing body of research in humans (Hostinar, Sullivan, & Gunnar, 2014; Strathearn, 2011; Swain et al., 2014). Studies in normatively developing children have shown that secure attachment experiences typically buffer the effects of stress in early development, resulting in so-called adaptive hypoactivity of the HPA axis in early development (Gunnar & Quevedo, 2007). By contrast, insecure attachment experiences typically lead to increased vulnerability for stress, as expressed in dysfunctions of the HPA axis as well as the reward system (Auerbach et al., 2014; Pizzagalli, 2014; Strathearn, 2011).

Impairments in reward and incentive motivation in particular have been implicated in depression (particularly in typical features such as anhedonia) in adults, adolescents, and children (Auerbach et al., 2014; Bogdan et al., 2013; Bress, Smith, Foti, Klein, & Hajcak, 2012; Davey et al., 2008; Forbes, 2009; Forbes & Dahl, 2012; Heshmati & Russo, 2015; Hulvershorn, Cullen, & Anand, 2011; Kerestes, Davey, Stephanou, Whittle, & Harrison, 2014; Matthews & Robbins, 2003; Nestler & Carlezon 2006).

From the perspective of both evolutionary (Gilbert, 2006) and social science (Beck, 2009; Blatt, 2008), there seem to be two key areas of reward particularly relevant for depression, especially as they overlap with areas of stress associated with depression: social/attachment relationships and agency/autonomy.

The RDoC has included problems with reward in the positive valence systems domain, while affiliation and attachment are categorized in the systems for the social processing domain. Evidence suggests, however, that there is a substantial overlap between the behavioral and neurobiological systems involved in reward and attachment (Insel & Young, 2001; Panksepp & Watt, 2011; Rutherford, Williams, Moy, Mayes, & Johns, 2011; Swain, Lorberbaum, Kose, & Strathearn, 2007). Indeed, attachment cues (such as infant faces, infant cries, proximity of and interaction with attachment figures) are associated with the activation of neural circuits that are typically considered to be central to the reward system (such as the ventral tegmental area and nucleus accumbens). Individual differences in attachment styles and history, in turn, are associated with differential activation of brain regions that are part of the reward circuit (Fonagy & Luyten, 2016; Leckman et al., 2005; Vrticka & Vuilleumier, 2012). Social cognition or mentalizing seems to involve related, but different, capacities and behavioral and neurobiological systems (Luyten & Fonagy, 2015a). Therefore, as we have done in the past, we also prefer the notion of social cognition or mentalizing systems for this latter domain, rather than systems for social processes.

Therefore, in spite of the paucity of research about the relationship between agency/autonomy and the neurological reward system, behavioral research has abundantly demonstrated the rewarding nature of experiences of agency, autonomy, and autonomous motivation more generally (Ryan, Deci, & Vansteenkiste, 2016). This clearly reflects a gap in the literature, and future efforts should concentrate on the relationship between the reward system and the development of feelings of agency, autonomy, and achievement (Murayama, Matsumoto, Izuma, & Matsumoto, 2010).

Further emphasizing the links between attachment and the reward system, neuropeptides such as OXT and vasopressin have been shown to be key modulators in this context. Particularly for securely attached individuals, and in relation to in-group members, OXT has been shown to increase affiliative behavior when faced with distress; this optimizes the opportunities for effective co-regulation of stress with others and reduces behavioral and neuroendocrinological responses to stress (Neumann, 2008). Generally, mothers with higher serum levels of OXT tend to make more affectionate contact with their infants, are more likely to follow the infant's gaze with an affectionate touch, and generally present themselves to their infant with increased social salience (Apter-Levi, Zagoory-Sharon, & Feldman, 2014; Kim, Fonagy, Koos, Dorsett, & Strathearn, 2014). Oxytocin has also been associated with direct anxiolytic and anti-stress effects in community samples via downregulation of the HPA system (Feldman, Vengrober, & Ebstein, 2014). Furthermore, OXT has been shown to enhance mentalizing and trust in others, again increasing opportunities for effective downregulation of distress and exploration (Bartz, Zaki, Bolger, & Ochsner, 2011; Neumann, 2008) and leading to so-called broaden-and-build cycles associated with secure attachment and effective stress regulation (Fredrickson, 2001; Mikulincer & Shaver, 2007). However, these effects seem to be limited to enhancing existing positive affiliations (with in-group members); in fact, studies have reported that OXT administration leads to increased distrust, more bias in attributing intentions, and decreases in cooperative behavior in relation to out-group members, even in normatively developing individuals (Bartz et al., 2011). Furthermore, in individuals with an insecure attachment history, decreased basal OXT levels, negative effects of OXT administration on social behavior, and an increased cortisol response to stress have been reported (Bartz et al., 2011). Oxytocin therefore seems to increase the salience of attachment issues.

From a developmental perspective, the reorganization of the reward system (at the same time as the stress and mentalizing systems undergo major reorganization), in combination with the major changes in sociocultural expectations that occur in adolescence, seems to play an important role in explaining the emergence of depression in adolescence (Auerbach et al., 2014; Davey et al., 2008; Forbes & Dahl, 2012; Luciana, 2013; Spear, 2000). Adolescence is marked by major changes with regard to both relatedness and agency/autonomy because of the entry into a complex world of peer and romantic relationships (expressed in increased rejection sensitivity) as well as increasing demands for achievement (reflected in increased sensitivity to failure). Yet, both animal and human research suggests that adolescence is characterized by the lowest levels of dopamine in striatal regions and the highest levels of dopamine in prefrontal regions, possibly leading to a so-called mini-reward deficiency syndrome (Spear, 2007). This may also lead to compensatory behaviors such as risk taking and drug abuse, explaining the high comorbidity between depression and externalizing psychopathology in adolescence and depression and BPD in early adulthood (Hüpen et al., 2020). It may also explain why disappointment and/or frustration around the need for relationships, belongingness, and achievement/status (which are often intertwined) may lead to a downward spiral marked by suppression of the reward system, increased levels of stress, and impairments in mentalizing.

Considering the implication of the reward system in attachment, it is the inevitable to draw conclusions about the repercussions of anomalous functioning and connectivity of these brain structures and BPD functioning. As we have reviewed above, the reward system plays a central role in bonding and attachment. According to fMRI studies, romantic love is associated with an activation of the right ventral tegmental area (VTA) and the right posterior dorsal body and medial caudate nucleus (Aron et al., 2005). Besides the role of dopamine, endogenous opioid binding to μ-opioid peptide receptors has been proposed to be the basis of infant attachment. It has been established for decades that opioids, particularly β-endorphins, play a central role in forming social bonds (Bandelow, Schmahl, Falkai, & Wedekind, 2010; Panksepp, Herman, Conner, Bishop, & Scott, 1978). The endogenous opioid system (EOS) and the dopaminergic reward system are closely linked, with evidence suggesting that brain dopamine tends to code for the preparatory aspects of reward behavior, whereas brain opioids seem to mediate the perception of the hedonic properties of rewards (Barbano & Cador, 2007; Russ, 1992).

It is well established that BPD patients belong chiefly to insecure attachment groups (particularly disorganized attachment) and that many of them have suffered attachment trauma during early life (Fonagy, 2000; Fonagy, Target, & Gergely, 2000; Lorenzini & Fonagy, 2013). Aberrant functioning of the dopaminergic reward system as well as hindered EOS function and lower levels of OXT are likely to be at the base of many attachment issues observed in BPD.

In fact, evidence is consistent in showing anomalous functioning of the reward system in BPD, including reduced volumes of brain areas implicated in reward, decreased baseline metabolism of the reward system, abnormal activity in response to social and nonsocial reward/loss stimuli, and even differential brain functioning with regard to physical pain (in itself an important signal of negative reward), in the hippocampus, amygdala, ACC, medial temporal lobe, OFC, and several substructures of the PFC. Several of these anomalous structures are not exclusive to BPD: smaller hippocampal volumes are shared with PTSD and history of previous trauma, and differential amygdala volume is more likely to be found in BPD patients with comorbid of depression (New et al., 2012; Schmahl & Bremner, 2006). Neurobiological findings also support the diminished activity of the EOS in BPD, where frantic efforts to avoid abandonment, frequent and risky sexual contacts, and attention-seeking behaviors may be explained by attempts to make use of the rewarding effects of human attachment mediated by the EOS (Bandelow et al., 2010).

Moreover, reduced levels of OXT are another likely cause of BPD patients' perception of other people as more threatening and less trustworthy, and also the experience of social interactions as less rewarding. While OXT seems to increase the perceived attractiveness of and positive communication with intimate partners, which may be associated with increased activations in brain reward regions, in BPD patients, low oxytocin concentrations may increase the risk of poor social reciprocity in adult life, which in turn contributes to threat hypersensitivity, and may impede affect regulation capacities and experiences of social reward and support (Herpertz & Bertsch, 2015).

But the effects of the reward system's anomalies in BPD are not restricted to attachment and social behavior (Gagnon, 2017). Anhedonia and feelings of emptiness may be an expression of reduced activity of the EOS. Patients with BPD tend to abuse substances that target μ-opioid receptors. Self-injury, food restriction, aggressive behavior, and sensation seeking may be interpreted as desperate attempts to artificially set the body to survival mode in order to mobilize the last reserves of the EOS. BPD-associated symptoms such as substance abuse, anorexia, self-injury, depersonalization, and sexual overstimulation can be treated successfully with opioid receptor antagonists (Bandelow et al., 2010). BPD patients are less able to differentiate potentially rewarding and not rewarding when, in laboratory models, they are presented with emotional pictures, while showing functional anomalies in the bilateral pregenual anterior cingulate cortex, which highlights the interconnection between regulatory and reward systems (Enzi et al., 2013; Sarkheil, Ibrahim, Schneider, Mathiak, & Klasen, 2019; Sharp & Sieswerda, 2013).

Importantly, functioning anomalies of the dopaminergic reward system and the EOS are a main neural correlate of impulsivity and, in turn, of NSSI. Self-destructive behaviors can be understood as attempts to stimulate the EOS and the dopaminergic reward system, regardless of harmful consequences. Functional imaging studies have revealed the absence of prefrontal responses and reduced functioning in the subcortical reward systems (in the ventral striatum) during nonsocial positive (rewarding) reinforcement, which correlates with impulsivity levels in BPD (Völlm et al., 2007). This attenuated neural response to positive feedback and its correlation with impulsivity (and also with BPD symptom severity, particularly emotional arousal and dissociation) have been replicated in EEG studies (Schauer, Rauh, Leicht, Andreou, & Mulert, 2019; Seres, Unoka, & Keri, 2009; Stewart et al., 2019). Impulsivity is also correlated to enhanced neural responses to positive feedback in cortical areas of the brain (dorsomedial PCF and OFC), supporting the hypothesis about the existence of two distinct systems for the processing of positive and negative feedback, which might be differentially affected in BPD (Andreou et al., 2015). This differential impairment in neural responses of the reward system to positive or negative rewards might be reflecting subtypes of BPD according to the presence of NSSI, where BPD patients with NSSI demonstrate impairments in the ability to update reward associations after feedback. It is possible that the presence of NSSI involves alterations in the reward system independently of BPD and thus could be considered as a possible phenotype for reward-related alterations. In sum, this suggests that BPD patients with self-harming behavior correctly learn the association between self-injury and its immediate consequences (e.g., relief of emotional distress), but they fail in the representation of possible long-term (negative) results of this type of behavior (Vega et al., 2018). The impairment of BPD patients in anticipating aversive results from their actions, giving rise to impulsivity, is further reflected in attenuated anticipation responses in the ventral striatum and nucleus accumbens (Herbort et al., 2016). All these results lend further support to the idea that NSSI acts stimulate the (hypoactive) opioid endogenous system in BPD patients, resulting in immediately decreased negative affectivity (Bresin & Gordon, 2013).

4.5.2 Genetics

Whereas earlier studies of the genetics of depression focused mainly on the stress system, as reviewed earlier, there is an increasing interest in the role of genes associated with key neuromodulators of the reward system, such as dopamine (Auerbach et al., 2014) and oxytocin (McQuaid, McInnis, Abizaid, & Anisman, 2014). This interest has increased as a result of evidence for epigenetic modification of these neuromodulators through environmental and parental factors (Feldman et al., 2014) and the growing evidence for relationships between neuromodulators of the stress system (such as serotonin) and the reward system (Spear, 2000). For example, early insecure attachment experiences have been related to polymorphisms in the oxytocin receptor gene in adult patients with unipolar depression (Costa et al., 2009), which is in line with studies reporting dysregulated peripheral oxytocin release in women with depression (Cyranowski et al., 2008; McQuaid et al., 2014) and decreased activation of the reward system (Gotlib et al., 2010). A community-based study with a large sample of youths reported that the rs53576 oxytocin receptor gene polymorphism moderates the association between maternal depression in early childhood and depressive symptoms at age 15, and it is believed to be one of the genetic determinants of early parenting leading to adult BPD (Herpertz &

Bertsch, 2015; Thompson, Hammen, Starr, & Najman, 2014). Importantly, while behavioral genetic studies support the conclusion that genetic influences on individual differences in the capacity to form attachment relationships are negligible during early childhood (Bokhorst et al., 2003), one study found that in adolescence they predict 38% of security and 35% of insecurity, implying a more important contribution of genetic endowment in adult attachment, depression, and personality disorders (Fearon, Shmueli-Goetz, Viding, Fonagy, & Plomin, 2014). The continuity of attachment from infancy to adulthood may also be moderated by the presence of the oxytocin receptor coding gene (OXTR) G/G phenotype (Lee Raby, Cicchetti, Carlson, Egeland, & Andrew Collins, 2013).

It is interesting to note here that, genetically speaking, BPD and depression show significant overlap in heritability and moderate nonshared environmental influences, and indeed patients with more severe BPD symptoms will also show more severe depressive symptomatology (Bornovalova et al., 2018). Highlighting this overlap is necessary when referring to the reward system, especially in relation to attachment and social reward, given that most research of genetic levels exclusive to BPD focuses mainly on impulsivity, as seen in the previous section of this chapter. In fact, the so-called reward deficiency syndrome found in BPD, depression, and other psychiatric disorders (Comings & Blum, 2000) has been related with regard to the former disorder as associated with a polymorphic promoter dinucleotide repeat length variation of the NOS1 gene. This same polymorphism is related to both impulsiveness and empathy (Retz, Reif, Freitag, Retz-Junginger, & Rösler, 2010), which lends further evidence to the close relationship between reward and social-cognitive systems. Moreover, polymorphisms in the μ-opioid receptor gene in rhesus macaques are associated with higher levels of attachment during early infancy, which suggests, on the one hand, increased reward during maternal contact, but, on the other hand, greater persistence of separation distress (Barr et al., 2008). Preliminary evidence has nevertheless found that polymorphic variations in the OXTR gene interact with testosterone, serotonin, and dopamine in various ways, impacting the processing of social reward (Dölen, Darvishzadeh, Huang, & Malenka, 2013).

The relationship between reward and impulsivity has been extensively studied in both healthy and pathological behavior and refers to the decision to forgo better long-term outcomes in the face of immediate temptations, a phenomenon known experimentally as "delay discounting" (Arce & Santisteban, 2006; Martin & Potts, 2004; Rung & Madden, 2018). However, research on genetic and epigenetic correlates of impulsivity have been difficult to replicate: while some studies show that ventral striatal hyperactivity is associated to dopamine transporter polymorphisms in the community and BPD patients, other studies find no significant associations, so results remain controversial and more research in the epigenesis of dopamine and its relationship with impulsivity and the reward system is needed (Forbes et al., 2009; Joyce et al., 2006; Nemoda et al., 2010). There are more consistent results in the study of polymorphisms of the o-methyltransferase (COMT) and the 5-HTTPLR ss/sl polymorphism as mediating the effect of stressful life events on impulsivity in

BPD (Archer, Oscar-Berman, Blum, & Gold, 2012; Wagner et al., 2010; Wagner, Baskaya, Lieb, Dahmen, & Tadić, 2009).

Even when reward dysfunction is indeed observed in the brain functioning of BPD patients, as reviewed in the previous section, and in patients' behavior, as described below, genetic studies have in many cases not yielded significant results (MacKillop et al., 2019). The paucity of genetic research in the reward system of BPD, and the few robust results of such research together with the vast knowledge obtained by neuroimaging studies, suggests that biologically and behaviorally observable impairments in reward in the context of BPD are in an important part, instigated by adverse environmental conditions in development. The genetic influence might be stronger in the development of the system of reward processing through the exposure to harsh environments that seems to be associated with genes that directly influence other BPD features (Archer et al., 2012; Chanen & Kaess, 2012).

4.5.3 Behavioral Level

Most behavioral research on reward in BPD is related to impulsivity explained by delay discounting. But while healthy controls show a preference for immediate gratification only when they are under stress, BPD patients display such a preference regardless of stress, and it is generally to a greater degree than healthy controls (Fertuck, Lenzenweger, Clarkin, Hoermann, & Stanley, 2006; Lawrence et al., 2010). Usually, BPD patients show these impulsive decisions, but do not report impulsivity themselves, most of them reporting impulsivity only under stress conditions or due to a lack of premeditation (Berg, Latzman, Bliwise, & Lilienfeld, 2015; McCloskey et al., 2009). Interestingly, BPD patients who have had early trauma also show greater discounting depending not only on the delay, but on the probability of payoff. These patients choose the more certain and/or immediate rewards, irrespective of the value (Barker et al., 2015), and show blunted learning from reward, regardless of whether the rewards are social or nonsocial (Fineberg et al., 2018). This is in line with the conception of BPD patients, particularly those with childhood adverse experiences, as individuals who are consistently expecting negative outcomes and thus have difficulties with trusting the world around them (Fertuck, Fischer, & Beeney, 2018; Fonagy et al., 2015; Fonagy et al., 2017b; Fonagy, Luyten, Allison, & Campbell, 2017a; Vega et al., 2013).

There is a well-documented relationship between impairments related to the rewarding features of agency and attachment, vulnerability for depression and BPD, poor prognosis, and negative treatment response (Berenson et al., 2016; Kulacaoglu & Kose, 2018; Luyten & Blatt, 2013). Problems with agency/autonomy, in particular, as expressed in, for instance, high levels of self-criticism, have been related to increased vulnerability for depression, a more negative course of treatment, and poor response to treatment across a number of therapeutic modalities (Blatt, Zuroff, Hawley, & Auerbach, 2010; Shahar, 2015).

With regard to the rewarding nature of affiliation, insecure attachment has similarly been related to vulnerability for depression and BPD in children, adolescents, and adults (Fonagy et al., 2021; Grunebaum et al., 2010; Lee & Hankin, 2009; Lorenzini & Fonagy, 2013) and has been shown to negatively influence the course of these disorders (Agerup, Lydersen, Wallander, & Sund, 2015; Fonagy et al., 1996; Grassetti, 2011). Insecure attachment has also been related to the intergenerational transmission of vulnerability for psychopathology in both animal and human studies (Fonagy, Lorenzini, & Campbell, 2014; Luyten, Blatt, & Fonagy, 2013; Moutsiana et al., 2014; Moutsiana et al., 2015; Murray et al., 2011).

As mentioned in the previous section, studies have provided evidence for a relationship between disruptions in the attachment/reward systems and adversity. Insecure attachment has been shown to mediate the relationship between early adversity and later vulnerability for depression through impaired affect regulation, stress responsivity, and impairments in social problem-solving skills, in a number of longitudinal studies (Bifulco et al., 2006; Carlson, Egeland, & Sroufe, 2009; Sroufe, 2005; Styron & Janoff-Bulman, 1997).

There is no evidence for a specific association between particular attachment categories and vulnerability for depression. Both individuals who predominantly use attachment hyperactivating strategies (strategies that reflect desperate attempts to find security, rooted in the belief that others are not there to provide security and support, typical of individuals with anxious-preoccupied attachment styles) and those who predominantly use attachment deactivating strategies (i.e., strategies involving denying attachment needs and asserting one's own autonomy and independence in an attempt to downregulate stress, based on the conviction that others cannot provide support and comfort, correlating with anxious-avoidant and dismissive attachment styles) are at increased risk for depression. However, parental avoidant/dismissive attachment might be associated with greater vulnerability for a hostile/aggressive subtype of depression (MacGregor et al., 2014). In the case of BPD, 50–80% of diagnosed patients present with either preoccupied and/or disorganised attachment styles (Fonagy & Luyten, 2016; Lorenzini & Fonagy, 2013). Furthermore, there is some evidence that individuals with unresolved and disorganized attachment, that is, individuals who interchangeably use attachment hyperactivating and deactivating strategies, are at increased risk for a subtype of depression associated with BPD, marked by greater severity of depression, feelings of emptiness, anger, shame, and identity diffusion (Lecompte, Moss, Cyr, & Pascuzzo, 2014; Luyten & Fonagy, 2015b).

Evolutionarily, it has been speculated that insecure attachment strategies reflect different strategies to deal with (perceived) unavailability, non-responsiveness, or intrusiveness of attachment figures (Ein-Dor, Mikulincer, Doron, & Shaver, 2010). Different insecure attachment strategies have been related to different psychosocial and biological profiles in youth and in adults, which may shed important light on the vexing question of the heterogeneity of both depression and BPD. Indeed, studies in community samples suggest that attachment deactivating strategies and associated personality styles such as self-criticism are related to downregulation of the reward and threat detection system very early in information processing. Attachment hyperactivating strategies and related personality styles such as interpersonal dependency have been related to upregulation of the stress and threat detection systems and a failure to downregulate threat, leading to increasing hypervigilance (Luyten & Fonagy, 2015a; Vrticka & Vuilleumier, 2012).

When reviewing both the stress system and the reward system in both depression and BPD, the connection of these systems with the system of social cognition (which in this chapter we refer to as mentalizing) becomes apparent. It is in the interrelation of these systems that the symptomatology of these disorders arises, as well as evidence for their comorbidity and determinants of their severity. We will now review the findings addressing the structure, antecedents, and functioning of the mentalizing system in depression and BPD.

4.6 Mentalizing (RDoC Social Cognition and Cognitive Systems)

4.6.1 Neural Circuits and Physiology

With the domain of self-other regulation being the main interest of this chapter, it was unavoidable to refer to the RDoC domains above. It is indeed essential to bear in mind that the functional domain of self-other regulation is not found simply within social cognition, but that it deeply depends on stress regulation and reward, particularly when referring to depression and personality disorders in the borderline spectrum. We will discuss the RDoC social processes and cognitive systems domains together in this section because, although the neural circuits involved in mentalizing are somewhat distinct from those involved in attention and general (cognitive) reasoning and other cognitive systems such as planning, memory, and executive functioning (Adolphs, 2015; Van Overwalle, 2011), mentalizing is partly dependent on these capacities and, in turn, fosters them. Moreover, we are aware that the RDoC domain of social cognition is wider than mentalizing abilities per se. The former refers to a capacity for many mammals, while mentalizing is exclusive to humans. It also relies on brain systems that can be found in animal models and basic human research, but when referring to clinical constructs, mentalizing appears as a richer construct. In this chapter, social cognition and mentalizing are used somewhat interchangeably.

The human capacity for social cognition or mentalizing represents a major leap in evolution that conferred substantial survival value, as it enabled new and complex forms of collaboration and learning far beyond conditioning and imitative learning (Humphrey, 1976). This capacity accounts to a large extent for other major differences between humans and other animals, which lack this ability. These include: (a) the capacity for self-awareness and self-consciousness, (b) the human striving to transcend physical reality, and (c) the human capacity for complex forms of collaboration and relatedness.

However, these same capacities also appear to confer increased risk for the development of depression, BPD, and other disorders (Fonagy et al., 2017a, 2017b; Luyten, Fonagy, Lemma, & Target, 2012).

In the case of depression, first, the emergence of self-awareness and self-consciousness as a path to emulation brought with it social emotions, such as embarrassment, regret, shame, and guilt, which are commonly implicated in depression. Second, the species-specific striving to achieve something in life brings with it not only visions of an ideal state but also the awareness of being unable to achieve one's goals and desires, leading to feelings of distress, emotional pain, and, ultimately, helplessness and hopelessness. Finally, humans' strong emphasis on relatedness (the basis for social learning and the transgenerational transmission of culture and knowledge) brought with it a need to feel validated and recognized by others; this translates to social experience of oneself as worthy of being loved, cared for, respected, and admired – but also creates a risk for feelings of depression when these needs are chronically frustrated or thwarted (Luyten et al., 2012).

These three aspects of social cognition are at the forefront of development, particularly in adolescence (Crone & Dahl, 2012), which might explain the increase in prevalence of depression in this age period. Studies of normatively developing youth suggest that the mature capacity for perspective-taking develops by late adolescence, and the medial PFC and temporoparietal junction – key areas recruited during mentalizing – change radically in their relative weighting over the course of adolescence (Blakemore & Mills, 2014). In adults, impairments in the neural circuits implicated in mentalizing have been consistently reported. These include the mPFC, amygdala, hippocampus, and ventromedial parts of the basal ganglia (Cusi, Nazarov, Holshausen, MacQueen, & McKinnon, 2012; Drevets, Price, & Furey, 2008). These findings suggest that depression may be related to a failure to reappraise and regulate negative affect, reflecting a failure of controlled mentalizing more generally, which gives rise to more automatic, biased, and affect-driven mentalizing (i.e., based on nonreflective assumptions about the self and others).

Automatic and controlled mentalizing seem to be subserved by two different neural circuits. Phylogenetically older brain circuits relying primarily on sensory information appear to underlie automatic mentalizing, including the amygdala, basal ganglia, ventromedial prefrontal cortex (vmPFC), lateral temporal cortex (LTC), and dorsal anterior cingulate cortex (dACC) (Satpute & Lieberman, 2006). These brain areas are primarily involved in the rapid detection of threat and the fast and automatic modulation and processing of (social) information. It also relies on external features of self and others, like facial expression, posture, movement, etc. (Lieberman, 2007). The amygdala is linked to processing of the biological "value" of information and is particularly reactive to facial emotional expressions, which highlights its central role in the rapid processing of social information in the context of a rapid and automatic fight/flight response. The vmPFC plays a key role in the modulation of the amygdala and basal ganglia, and both the vmPFC and basal ganglia are involved in automatic intuition. The basal ganglia are also involved in reward-related implicit emotion processing. The ACC is implicated in nonreflective emotional distress related to both physical and social (i.e., exclusion) pain. The

LTC – in particular the superior temporal sulcus region – plays a role in fast and automatic processing of biological motion, face recognition, and attribution of intentions. Hence, all these regions are involved in fast and implicit processing of social information.

Conversely, controlled mentalizing involves phylogenetically newer brain circuits that rely more on linguistic/symbolic processing. Many of these circuits are also involved in executive functioning. It involves the lateral prefrontal cortex (LPFC), medial prefrontal cortex (mPFC), lateral parietal cortex (LPAC), medial parietal cortex (MPAC), medial temporal lobe (MTL), and rostral anterior cingulate cortex (rACC) (Lieberman, 2007; Satpute & Lieberman, 2006; Uddin, Iacoboni, Lange, & Keenan, 2007). The LPFC is activated by tasks requiring asymmetrical reasoning (e.g., X is causing Y, but this does not imply that Y causes X), requiring effortful control and involving considerable computational resources. The LPAC is also involved in tasks requiring reasoning, and the MPAC is involved in explicit perspective taking. The rACC is involved in explicit, reflected-upon conflict processing; the MTL has been implicated in explicit, declarative memory. The mPFC seems to be one of the core structures involved in mentalizing, but it is not clear whether this structure primarily belongs to the automatic or the controlled circuit, or both. Because the mPFC is larger in humans than in other primates, and because cognitive load decreases its performance, it is considered to belong to the controlled system. Controlled mentalizing tends also to prefer internal cues, that is to say, a properly reflective activity on mental states, one's own and those of others (Lieberman, 2007; Satpute & Lieberman, 2006; Uddin et al., 2007).

With regard to the self-other dimension, the same neural networks tend to be activated whenever we reflect on ourselves and others, involving the medial prefrontal cortex, temporal poles, and the posterior superior temporal sulcus/temporo-parietal junction in the LTC (Frith & Frith, 2006; Lieberman, 2007; Uddin et al., 2007; Van Overwalle, 2009). This common network underlying mentalizing with regard to both self and others in part explains the centrality of both identity problems and problems with mentalizing about others in most individuals with personality disorders, particularly BPD.

People who predominantly use attachment hyperactivating strategies most closely match the pattern of affect-driven mentalizing explained above as a result of hypervigilance for social rejection and exclusion. Attachment deactivating strategies, by contrast, have been related to downregulation of reward circuitry, but relative hyperactivation in the mPFC and ventral anterior cingulate cortex, areas that are involved in controlled mentalizing, social rejection, and emotion suppression; this suggests a pattern of cognitive overcontrol and overregulation (Luyten & Fonagy, 2015a; Vrticka & Vuilleumier, 2012). Attachment hyperactivating and deactivating strategies are assumed to play a key role in explaining the relationships among stress/arousal and mentalizing in different interpersonal contexts. They influence (a) the threshold at which the switch from controlled to automatic mentalizing occurs, (b) the strength of the relationship between the severity of stress/arousal and the activation of neural circuits involved in controlled versus automatic mentalizing, and (c) the time to recovery when controlled mentalizing is lost under stress/arousal

(Luyten, Campbell, Allison, & Fonagy, 2020). Noteworthy, disorganized/unresolved attachment is associated with increased amygdala activation when attachment is experimentally activated in all adults. But those with no diagnosis of BPD also show activation in the right dorsolateral prefrontal cortex (DLPFC) and the rostral cingulate zone (RCZ), which can be interpreted as the neural signature of BPD patients' inability to exert top-down control under conditions of attachment distress (Buchheim et al., 2016).

Given that the neural circuits involved in mentalizing follow a similar pathway to those of executive functioning, the observed comorbidity between depression other disorders, especially BPD, seems to involve all the systems relevant to this chapter: (a) increasing distress and negative affect (the stress system); (b) impairments in incentive motivation (the reward system), leading to compensatory strategies (e.g., drug abuse, sexual promiscuity, risk-taking); (c) impairments in mentalizing (the mentalizing system), leading to compensatory efforts to deal with a perceived loss of status and/or rejection (e.g., violent behavior to increase status, made possible by a denial or justification of the subjective suffering of others); and (d) loss of cognitive control mechanisms (the cognitive system) (Krause-Utz, Niedtfeld, Knauber, & Schmahl, 2017; Winsper et al., 2016).

From a developmental point of view, the capacity for mentalizing is first acquired in the context of attachment relationships. In particular, the capacity for parental mentalizing, or parental reflective functioning, that is, the caregiver's capacity to reflect upon his/her own internal mental experiences as well as those of the child, plays a key role in this process (Luyten, Nijssens, Fonagy, & Mayes, 2017; Sharp & Fonagy, 2008), but it does not explain the full picture of mentalization development (Zeegers, Colonnesi, Stams, & Meins, 2017). New advances in the study of mentalizing show that the role of the social environment in the functioning of mentalizing capacities is not restricted to early attachment relationships. In fact, mentalizing is viewed as fundamentally interactive in that the capacity to mentalize develops in the context of interactions with others, and as a result it is assumed to be continually influenced by the mentalizing capacity of those others. Mentalizing is thus, at least to an extent, relationship and context dependent (Fonagy et al., 2017a, 2017b; Luyten et al., 2020).

In the case of BPD, prospective studies showing very high rates of trauma in BPD patients provide more convincing evidence for hypothesized associations between disruptions in the development of the attachment-behavioral system and BPD. A recent review found that exposure to different types of trauma, including emotional abuse, neglect, and physical and sexual abuse, was associated with increased risk of BPD, which provides support for formulations emphasizing the broader socioecological context in the etiology of BPD, as it is found that BPD patients typically are exposed to a broader adverse context characterized by parental psychopathology, lower socioeconomic status, and/or violence (Stepp, Lazarus, & Byrd, 2016).

Like the neural circuits involved in the stress and reward systems, those involved in mentalizing undergo major functional and structural reorganization as a result of synaptogenesis in adolescence, followed by synaptic pruning into early adulthood.

At the same time, humans are faced with major developmental tasks involving a redefinition of autonomy and relatedness, necessitating considerable mentalizing skills. The inability to successfully navigate these changes may lead either to excessive mentalizing (hypermentalizing) and/or the avoidance of mentalizing (hypomentalizing) as a defensive strategy to avoid thinking about the often-painful nature of these changing experiences. Both hypermentalizing and hypomentalizing may be implicated in the reward deficiency syndrome mentioned in the previous sections (Krach, Paulus, Bodden, & Kircher, 2010; Preston, 2017).

4.6.2 Genetics

Most contemporary approaches to the genetics of social cognition in depression focus either on biological systems that influence social cognition, such as the oxytocinergic, dopaminergic, and serotonergic systems, or on specific domains of social cognition, such as empathy or theory of mind. For instance, polymorphisms in 5-HTTLPR have been related to biases in facial emotion interpretation. In fact, several polymorphisms implicated in the stress and reward domains have been related to openness to environmental influences. We have seen that these findings have led to a shift from diathesis-stress models to differential social susceptibility models (Ellis et al., 2011). There is also some evidence for gene-culture coevolution in relation to these genes, although research in this area remains controversial (Laland, Odling-Smee, & Myles, 2010). In this same line, genetic factors implicated in cognitive systems also influence the development of mentalizing, as well as the reward system. Developmentally speaking, genetic influences in reward, stress and mentalizing, mediated by attachment, start being more noticeable in adolescence than in earlier stages of the human life cycle (Blakemore & Mills, 2014; Fearon et al., 2014).

Behavioral genetic studies have generally found little heritability specific to social cognition that was not accounted for by genetic influence over executive functions, particularly verbal ability (Hughes et al., 2005). Once again, evidence suggests that learning about mental states is strongly influenced by the social and wider cultural context (Luyten et al., 2020; Mayer & Träuble, 2013; Pyers & Senghas, 2009).

Nevertheless, preliminary genetic data has found two single-nucleotide polymorphisms of the opioid delta 1 receptor gene as associated to identity disturbance and alterations in opioid receptor genes, including the μ-opioid receptor (OPRM1), with affective instability and sensitivity to abandonment (Siever, 2009). The speculation follows that genetically mediated disturbances in opioid neurotransmission may be related to difficulties of BPD patients in forming stable social bonds or coping with interpersonal distress (Bandelow et al., 2010). More research is needed, particularly to clarify the role of genetic variability on affective stability, attachment, and coherence of self-concept.

Both in animals and humans, the modulating role of neuropeptides, particularly oxytocin and vasopressin, has obtained slightly more consistent results. Genetic precursors of both of these neuropeptides have been found to modulate social behavior, specifically prosocial or altruistic decision making, pair bonding, and onset of sexual behavior (Ebstein et al., 2009; Israel et al., 2009; Walum et al., 2008). However, as stated above, these disturbances seem to be more related to the salience of social stimuli and reduced expectation of reward in BPD patients, and genetic studies referring to the capacity for human cognition and interaction are at best preliminary and have been difficult to replicate (Liu et al., 2012; Lubke et al., 2014; Luyten et al., 2020).

4.6.3 Behavioral Level

The most widespread theories about depression tended to focus on distortions in the content of beliefs and assumptions about the self and others. But more contemporary theories, chiefly those based on mindfulness, cognitive, and mentalizing approaches, focus on distortions of the process of mentalizing or metacognition itself (Luyten et al., 2013; Luyten et al., 2020; Watkins & Teasdale, 2004). Specifically, mood-congruent mentalizing impairments in depression have been identified in several areas, from facial emotion recognition and theory of mind to more complex social understanding.

Social-cognitive impairments have been related not only to the risk for depression but also to relapse. In fact, these impairments have been shown to persist during remission (Billeke, Boardman, & Doraiswamy, 2013; Bistricky, Ingram, & Atchley, 2011; Weightman, Air, & Baune, 2014). Conversely, both severity and duration of depressive episodes seem in turn to increase impairment of mentalizing, which suggests the existence of a vicious cycle between depression and mentalizing impairments (Bistricky et al., 2011; Fischer-Kern & Tmej, 2019; Weightman et al., 2014). Indeed, studies of clinical and subclinical depression in adults have consistently found depression to be associated with high empathic distress, suggesting poor self-other differentiation and high sensitivity to the mental states of others (Schreiter, Pijnenborg, & Aan Het Rot, 2013). Individual differences in the use of secondary attachment strategies again might explain some conflicting findings of studies in this area (Manstead, Dosmukhambetova, Shearn, & Clifton, 2013). Insecure attachment has also been associated with impairments (often severe) in mentalizing that are typical of BPD patients. There is evidence to suggest that depressed patients who predominantly use attachment hyperactivating strategies might be highly attuned to the mental states of others, whereas those who predominantly use attachment deactivating strategies might show severe deficits in this capacity (Luyten et al., 2012). Impairments in mentalizing thus present an important target in treatments for depression, regardless of the theoretical orientation of specific treatments. And as stated above, both cognitive behavioral and psychodynamic approaches have shifted from treatments focusing on the content of psychological dynamics in depression (e.g., schemas or attachment representations) to treatments that also include a focus on the process of mentalizing or metacognition, particularly in patients with more chronic presentations of depression (Luyten et al., 2013; Luyten et al., 2020).

Impairments in mentalizing are typical of patients with BPD. These tend to take the form of overly simplistic or overly analytic accounts of their own mental states and those of others (Fonagy & Luyten, 2009). However, research and clinical accounts have during decades reported what seems to be superior mentalizing capacities in BPD patients compared with normal controls, the so-called empathy paradox (Carter & Rinsley, 1977; Dinsdale & Crespi, 2013; Krohn, 1974). But these apparently conflicting findings regarding BPD make sense when we observe the characteristic pattern of mentalizing impairments of BPD patients. It implies a rapid loss of controlled mentalizing and overreliance on fast, automatic mentalizing, favoring affectively dominated and highly externally based mentalizing at the expense of mentalizing that is directly focused on mental interiors and cognitive in nature. This is accompanied by the tendency to conflate mental states of the self and others (so-called identity diffusion, typical of BPD), leading to increased susceptibility to emotional contagion. In conclusion, this "superiority" of mentalizing of BPD patients in certain circumstances appears to be largely based on a tendency toward hypermentalizing – an attempt to make sense of others' external cues (such as their facial expressions or posture) based on fast, automatic processing of such information. Besides the risk implied in jumping to rushed conclusions about the other's mental states (which might be at times accurate), if we consider the negativity bias present in BPD (that we reviewed in the section about reward, and the negative expectation of these patients) which, for example, is demonstrated by these patients when interpreting neutral faces as showing negative affect, or neutral social situations as negative and more aggressive when presented with video clips (Barnow et al., 2009; Herpertz & Bertsch, 2015), then we can not only explain the seemingly better capacity for empathy in BPD but also why that capacity does not lead to more fulfilling and deeper interpersonal relationships for these patients.

We have been insisting throughout this chapter both on the importance of attachment in the functioning of the neural systems described and their contribution to psychopathology, and at the same time, trying to highlight that the explanatory power of attachment theory, while important, it is not the sole contributor to the development of the stress, reward, and mentalizing systems. In fact, recent research provides five major challenges for contemporary attachment theory. First, the relationship between attachment in childhood and later outcomes is not as strong as may be expected from some traditional assumptions within attachment theory (Fearon, Bakermans-Kranenburg, Van IJzendoorn, Lapsley, & Roisman, 2010; Groh, Roisman, van IJzendoorn, Bakermans-Kranenburg, & Fearon, 2012; Madigan, Atkinson, Laurin, & Benoit, 2013). Second, meta-analytic investigations show only moderate stability of attachment styles across the life span (Fraley, 2002; Pinquart, Feußner, & Ahnert, 2013). The stability of attachment is greater in adolescence and adulthood than in childhood (Fraley & Roberts, 2005; Jones et al., 2018), but it is actually risk status (e.g., family conflict, parental separation, minority ethnic status, male gender) which has repeatedly been associated with lower stability in meta-analyses (see Verhage et al., 2018). Thus, the stability of attachment is largely a function of the stability of the environment (Fraley & Roberts, 2005). Third, historical, sociocultural, and environmental factors do determine the function of the attachment system, challenging Bowlby's original formulations of attachment as an innate, universal behavioral system (Bowlby, 1988). Fourth, parental sensitivity and parental mentalizing, which are considered key in the intergenerational transmission of attachment, explain only a fraction of the variance in the association between parent and infant attachment. The fifth challenge to attachment theory is the increasing evidence for genetic factors in determining the course of attachment (Fearon et al., 2014).

Faced with these inconsistencies, we have proposed a new way of understanding the development of psychopathology, particularly BPD, based on novel evolutionary developmental neurobiology findings (Fonagy et al., 2017a, 2017b; Luyten et al., 2020). This new theoretical understanding, the theory of epistemic trust, posits that humans have a unique capacity for the efficient intergenerational transmission of cultural knowledge. In this context, the capacity for epistemic trust is more fundamental than the capacity of mentalizing. The capacity for epistemic trust allows for identifying knowledge conveyed by others as personally relevant and generalizable to other contexts. This capacity is an important evolutionary advantage which bypasses having to work out cultural knowledge oneself (very time-consuming, difficult, and often impossible), but allows the recipient of information (e.g., a young child) to rely on the authority and perceived trustworthiness of the person communicating that information (e.g., a caregiver or teacher; Coan & Sbarra, 2015; Gergely, 2013; Konner, 2010; Sperber et al., 2010; Tomasello, 2010). The default mode of functioning of humans is not epistemic trust, but epistemic vigilance or the ability to identify and filter out information conveyed by others that is perceived to be misleading, inaccurate, or deceitful. Therefore, in order to overcome this vigilant state and be able to learn from the social environment, the caregiver must be able to trigger trust in the developing human through ostensive cues, which prime and highlight to him/her that forthcoming communications are significant. These ostensive cues lead the recipient to feel recognized as a subjective, agentive self (Gergely, 2013). This feeling of being recognized opens up the channel for the fast transmission of knowledge and, in turn, the pathway for benefiting from positive influences in one's environment. It is here that early attachment plays a crucial role. It is primarily in the context of (early) attachment relationships that children learn to recognize who is trustworthy, authoritative, and knowledgeable (Corriveau et al., 2009). In turn, mentalizing is an essential competence for caregivers, who must have a genuine interest in the child's mind (i.e., high levels of mentalizing), thus providing the most consistent ostensive cueing and, in turn, the most fertile ground in which the child can develop epistemic trust and generalize it to new relationships and contexts. Yet, this process goes beyond the attachment context. Other social contextual factors and learning processes also influence the development of epistemic trust. Peers, people in the community, and sociocultural influences more generally (like those transmitted through social media) may further foster or inhibit the development of epistemic trust. To date, only indirect evidence has shown the role of epistemic trust in BPD, showing, for example, that BPD patients are more distrustful. As we have seen, they show a negative bias of social interaction, expect to be hurt or abandoned, and perceive others as more hostile and untrustworthy (Bartz et al., 2011; Fertuck et al., 2018).

Nevertheless, this broader view of psychopathology as not only determined by the private relationship between the individual and early caregivers but also influenced by the extended cultural environment has important implications for the conception of psychopathology and, more importantly, for the conceptualization and design of therapeutic interventions. While the stress regulation system, the reward system, and the social-cognitive mentalizing system are doubtlessly important in the individual development of depression and BPD, the regulation of the relationship between oneself and others has to be conceived from a sociocultural point of view.

4.7 Conclusions

This chapter presented an integrative, evolutionary-based developmental framework for depression and BPD rooted in the RDoC approach. It argues that depression and BPD result from interacting impairments in stress systems, leading to problems with reward, particularly in the areas of attachment and agency/autonomy, and to problems with mentalizing, understood within a broader evolutionary sociocultural perspective. The implication of the three RDoC systems reviewed above as the individual backbones of the relationship between self and others, the effects of this relationship in the development of psychopathology, and the sociocultural context in which these systems must be placed have important consequences in the understanding of psychopathology deficits and presentations and in the design of treatments.

Indeed, for example, the high comorbidity of depression and BPD with other disorders follows from the fact that both depression and BPD involve impairments in these three basic biobehavioral systems. This is in line with the developmental psychopathology principles of equifinality and multifinality (Cicchetti & Rogosch, 1996). These principles hold that different etiological factors (e.g., childhood trauma, current stress, and impaired social functioning) are implicated in developmental pathways toward psychopathology (equifinality), while the same etiological factors that are implicated in one disorder may also play a role in the etiology of other disorders (multifinality). Because of its focus on more basic biobehavioral systems or domains implicated in depression and BPD, the RDoC framework provides a promising avenue for further research in this respect, particularly given the great heterogeneity in the clinical presentations of depression and BPD. Looking at the basic systems underlying these (very) heterogeneous diagnoses might help to explain their variations and to understand the particular deficits and advantages of various individual presentations, as they are usually encountered in clinical practice. The elementary, developmentally based and piecemeal conceptualization of both depression and BPD presented in this chapter does not necessarily replace the classifications of the ICD or DSM, but enriches them by offering a strategy for subtyping these current diagnostic entities. Moreover, given the focus on the neurobiological basis of disease, the RDoC framework implies a departure from the focus on single diagnoses, such as depression and BPD, in both research and clinical practice. This basis calls for an examination of psychopathology from a dimensional and developmental structure, rather than a categorical one.

In terms of treatment implications of these ideas, we conceive the change resulting from therapeutic interventions as the outcome of particular forms of social learning from the patients' environment. Effective treatments are a form of social relearning, which implies the lowering of epistemic vigilance, the rekindling of mechanisms for social learning, and the reengagement with the social world (Fonagy et al., 2017a, 2017b). This means that effective treatments are able to covey a model of the patient's mind to the patient, that is to say, they are able to show to the patients that they are being mentalized by the therapist. When the patient sees themselves mentalized through the therapist's use of ostensive cues, they feel recognized as an independent agent and epistemic vigilance gives way to trust, which ideally activates social learning in the patient. The therapist must be able to tailor interventions to the specific patient, demonstrating his/her ability to see the patient's problems from his/her perspective, and the patient needs to be able to recognize that the therapist is able to consider the patient's perspective, in a mutually mentalizing process. The achievement of epistemic trust in turn reactivates the patient's mentalizing capacity through modelling by the therapist, which in turn facilitates more epistemic trust. This helps the patient to benefit from the communication with the therapist, learn new skills, acquire self-knowledge, and/or restructure internal working models. More importantly, therapies that reopen epistemic trust through mentalizing enable a wider virtuous cycle of salutogenesis not restricted only to the psychotherapeutic situation, but enhancing the capacity to benefit from further positive social influences outside the consulting room. This reengagement with the social world frees the patient from their state of social isolation, but it implies that, besides therapy, new positive social experiences will be sought or existing relationships will be recalibrated to become more positive and enriching. A further implication is, of course, that psychological interventions may need to also intervene at the level of the social environment when needed or appropriate: psychological interventions do not act in a social void, but are intimately dependent on the social and cultural context that surrounds them.

References

Adolphs, R. (2015). The unsolved problems of neuroscience. *Trends in Cognitive Sciences, 19*, 173–175.

Afifi, T. O., Enns, M. W., Cox, B. J., Asmundson, G. J., Stein, M. B., & Sareen, J. (2008). Population attributable fractions of psychiatric disorders and suicide ideation and attempts associated with adverse childhood experiences. *American Journal of Public Health, 98*, 946–952.

Agerup, T., Lydersen, S., Wallander, J., & Sund, A. M. (2015). Associations between parental attachment and course of depression between adolescence and young adulthood. *Child Psychiatry & Human Development, 46*, 632–642.
Amad, A., Ramoz, N., Thomas, P., & Gorwood, P. (2016). The age-dependent plasticity highlights the conceptual interface between borderline personality disorder and PTSD. *European Archives of Psychiatry and Clinical Neuroscience, 266*, 373–375.
American Psychiatric Association. (2013). *Diagnostic and statistical manual of mental disorders (DSM-5®)*. Arlington, VA: American Psychiatric Publications.
Anda, R. F., Felitti, V. J., Bremner, J. D., Walker, J. D., Whitfield, C., Perry, B. D., … Giles, W. H. (2006). The enduring effects of abuse and related adverse experiences in childhood. *European Archives of Psychiatry and Clinical Neuroscience, 256*, 174–186.
Andersen, S. L., & Teicher, M. H. (2008). Stress, sensitive periods and maturational events in adolescent depression. *Trends in Neurosciences, 31*, 183–191.
Andreou, C., Kleinert, J., Steinmann, S., Fuger, U., Leicht, G., & Mulert, C. (2015). Oscillatory responses to reward processing in borderline personality disorder. *The World Journal of Biological Psychiatry, 16*, 575–586.
Angold, A., Erkanli, A., Silberg, J., Eaves, L., & Costello, E. J. (2002). Depression scale scores in 8–17-year-olds: Effects of age and gender. *Journal of Child Psychology and Psychiatry, 43*, 1052–1063.
Apter-Levi, Y., Zagoory-Sharon, O., & Feldman, R. (2014). Oxytocin and vasopressin support distinct configurations of social synchrony. *Brain Research, 1580*, 124–132.
Arce, E., & Santisteban, C. (2006). Impulsivity: A review. *Psicothema, 18*, 213–220.
Archer, T., Oscar-Berman, M., Blum, K., & Gold, M. (2012). Neurogenetics and epigenetics in impulsive behaviour: Impact on reward circuitry. *Journal of genetic syndrome & gene therapy, 3*, 1000115.
Arnsten, A. F. (1998). The biology of being frazzled. *Science, 280*, 1711–1712.
Arnsten, A. F. (2011). Prefrontal cortical network connections: Key site of vulnerability in stress and schizophrenia. *International Journal of Developmental Neuroscience, 29*, 215–223.
Aron, A., Fisher, H., Mashek, D. J., Strong, G., Li, H., & Brown, L. L. (2005). Reward, motivation, and emotion systems associated with early-stage intense romantic love. *Journal of Neurophysiology, 94*, 327–337.
Auerbach, R. P., Admon, R., & Pizzagalli, D. A. (2014). Adolescent depression: Stress and reward dysfunction. *Harvard Review of Psychiatry, 22*, 139.
Avenevoli, S., Swendsen, J., He, J.-P., Burstein, M., & Merikangas, K. R. (2015). Major depression in the national comorbidity survey–adolescent supplement: Prevalence, correlates, and treatment. *Journal of the American Academy of Child & Adolescent Psychiatry, 54*, 37–44. e32.
Bagot, R. C., Labonté, B., Peña, C. J., & Nestler, E. J. (2014). Epigenetic signaling in psychiatric disorders: Stress and depression. *Dialogues in Clinical Neuroscience, 16*, 281.
Bakusic, J., Schaufeli, W., Claes, S., & Godderis, L. (2017). Stress, burnout and depression: A systematic review on DNA methylation mechanisms. *Journal of Psychosomatic Research, 92*, 34–44.
Bandelow, B., Schmahl, C., Falkai, P., & Wedekind, D. (2010). Borderline personality disorder: A dysregulation of the endogenous opioid system? *Psychological Review, 117*, 623.
Barbano, M. F., & Cador, M. (2007). Opioids for hedonic experience and dopamine to get ready for it. *Psychopharmacology, 191*, 497–506.
Barker, V., Romaniuk, L., Cardinal, R., Pope, M., Nicol, K., & Hall, J. (2015). Impulsivity in borderline personality disorder. *Psychological Medicine, 45*, 1955–1964.
Barnow, S., Stopsack, M., Grabe, H. J., Meinke, C., Spitzer, C., Kronmüller, K., & Sieswerda, S. (2009). Interpersonal evaluation bias in borderline personality disorder. *Behaviour Research and Therapy, 47*, 359–365.
Barr, C. S., Schwandt, M. L., Lindell, S. G., Higley, J. D., Maestripieri, D., Goldman, D., … Heilig, M. (2008). Variation at the mu-opioid receptor gene (OPRM1) influences attachment behavior in infant primates. *Proceedings of the National Academy of Sciences, 105*, 5277–5281.

Bartz, J. A., Zaki, J., Bolger, N., & Ochsner, K. N. (2011). Social effects of oxytocin in humans: Context and person matter. *Trends in Cognitive Sciences, 15*, 301–309.
Beck, A. T. (2009). Cognitive aspects of personality disorders and their relation to syndromal disorders: A psychoevolutionary approach. In C. R. Cloninger (Ed.), *Personality and psychopathology* (pp. 411–429). Washington, DC: American Psychiatric Press.
Berenson, K. R., Gregory, W. E., Glaser, E., Romirowsky, A., Rafaeli, E., Yang, X., & Downey, G. (2016). Impulsivity, rejection sensitivity, and reactions to stressors in borderline personality disorder. *Cognitive Therapy and Research, 40*, 510–521.
Berg, J. M., Latzman, R. D., Bliwise, N. G., & Lilienfeld, S. O. (2015). Parsing the heterogeneity of impulsivity: A meta-analytic review of the behavioral implications of the UPPS for psychopathology. *Psychological Assessment, 27*, 1129.
Bertsch, K., Gamer, M., Schmidt, B., Schmidinger, I., Walther, S., Kästel, T., … Herpertz, S. C. (2013). Oxytocin and reduction of social threat hypersensitivity in women with borderline personality disorder. *American Journal of Psychiatry, 170*, 1169–1177.
Bifulco, A., Kwon, J., Jacobs, C., Moran, P. M., Bunn, A., & Beer, N. (2006). Adult attachment style as mediator between childhood neglect/abuse and adult depression and anxiety. *Social Psychiatry and Psychiatric Epidemiology, 41*, 796–805.
Billeke, P., Boardman, S., & Doraiswamy, P. (2013). Social cognition in major depressive disorder: A new paradigm? *Translational Neuroscience, 4*, 437–447.
Birmaher, B., Brent, D., & Issues, A. W. (2007). Practice parameter for the assessment and treatment of children and adolescents with depressive disorders. *Journal of the American Academy of Child & Adolescent Psychiatry, 46*, 1503–1526.
Birmaher, B., Ryan, N. D., Williamson, D. E., Brent, D. A., & Kaufman, J. (1996). Childhood and adolescent depression: A review of the past 10 years. Part II. *Journal of the American Academy of Child & Adolescent Psychiatry, 35*, 1575–1583.
Bistricky, S. L., Ingram, R. E., & Atchley, R. A. (2011). Facial affect processing and depression susceptibility: Cognitive biases and cognitive neuroscience. *Psychological Bulletin, 137*, 998.
Blakemore, S.-J., & Mills, K. L. (2014). Is adolescence a sensitive period for sociocultural processing? *Annual Review of Psychology, 65*, 187–207.
Blatt, S. J. (2008). *Polarities of experience: Relatedness and self-definition in personality development, psychopathology, and the therapeutic process*. Washington, DC: American Psychological Association.
Blatt, S. J., Zuroff, D. C., Hawley, L. L., & Auerbach, J. S. (2010). Predictors of sustained therapeutic change. *Psychotherapy Research, 20*, 37–54.
Bøen, E., Westlye, L. T., Elvsåshagen, T., Hummelen, B., Hol, P. K., Boye, B., … Malt, U. F. (2014). Smaller stress-sensitive hippocampal subfields in women with borderline personality disorder without posttraumatic stress disorder. *Journal of Psychiatry & Neuroscience: JPN, 39*, 127.
Bogdan, R., Nikolova, Y. S., & Pizzagalli, D. A. (2013). Neurogenetics of depression: A focus on reward processing and stress sensitivity. *Neurobiology of Disease, 52*, 12–23.
Bokhorst, C. L., Bakermans-kranenburg, M. J., Pasco Fearon, R., Van Ijzendoorn, M. H., Fonagy, P., & Schuengel, C. (2003). The importance of shared environment in mother–infant attachment security: A behavioral genetic study. *Child Development, 74*, 1769–1782.
Bolton, E. E., Mueser, K. T., & Rosenberg, S. D. (2006). Symptom correlates of posttraumatic stress disorder in clients with borderline personality disorder. *Comprehensive Psychiatry, 47*, 357–361.
Bornovalova, M. A., Verhulst, B., Webber, T., McGue, M., Iacono, W. G., & Hicks, B. M. (2018). Genetic and environmental influences on the codevelopment among borderline personality disorder traits, major depression symptoms, and substance use disorder symptoms from adolescence to young adulthood. *Development and Psychopathology, 30*, 49–65.
Bourvis, N., Aouidad, A., Cabelguen, C., Cohen, D., & Xavier, J. (2017). How do stress exposure and stress regulation relate to borderline personality disorder? *Frontiers in Psychology, 8*, 2054.
Bowlby, J. (1988). *A secure base: Parent-child attachment and healthy human development*. New York, NY: Basic Books.

Bresin, K., & Gordon, K. H. (2013). Endogenous opioids and nonsuicidal self-injury: A mechanism of affect regulation. *Neuroscience & Biobehavioral Reviews, 37*, 374–383.
Bress, J. N., Smith, E., Foti, D., Klein, D. N., & Hajcak, G. (2012). Neural response to reward and depressive symptoms in late childhood to early adolescence. *Biological Psychology, 89*, 156–162.
Buchheim, A., Erk, S., George, C., Kächele, H., Martius, P., Pokorny, D., … Walter, H. (2016). Neural response during the activation of the attachment system in patients with borderline personality disorder: An fMRI study. *Frontiers in Human Neuroscience, 10*, 389.
Calati, R., Gressier, F., Balestri, M., & Serretti, A. (2013). Genetic modulation of borderline personality disorder: Systematic review and meta-analysis. *Journal of Psychiatric Research, 47*, 1275–1287.
Carlson, E. A., Egeland, B., & Sroufe, L. A. (2009). A prospective investigation of the development of borderline personality symptoms. *Development and Psychopathology, 21*, 1311–1334.
Carragher, N., Teesson, M., Sunderland, M., Newton, N., Krueger, R., Conrod, P., … Slade, T. (2016). The structure of adolescent psychopathology: A symptom-level analysis. *Psychological Medicine, 46*, 981–994.
Carter, L., & Rinsley, D. B. (1977). Vicissitudes of 'empathy' in a borderline adolescent. *International Review of Psycho-Analysis, 4*, 317–326.
Carvalho Fernando, S., Beblo, T., Schlosser, N., Terfehr, K., Otte, C., Löwe, B., … Wingenfeld, K. (2012). Associations of childhood trauma with hypothalamic-pituitary-adrenal function in borderline personality disorder and major depression. *Psychoneuroendocrinology, 37*, 1659–1668.
Carvalho Fernando, S., Beblo, T., Schlosser, N., Terfehr, K., Otte, C., Löwe, B., … Wingenfeld, K. (2014). The impact of self-reported childhood trauma on emotion regulation in borderline personality disorder and major depression. *Journal of Trauma & Dissociation, 15*, 384–401.
Caspi, A., Hariri, A. R., Holmes, A., Uher, R., & Moffitt, T. E. (2010). Genetic sensitivity to the environment: The case of the serotonin transporter gene and its implications for studying complex diseases and traits. *American Journal of Psychiatry, 167*, 509–527.
Caspi, A., Houts, R. M., Belsky, D. W., Goldman-Mellor, S. J., Harrington, H., Israel, S., … Poulton, R. (2014). The p factor: One general psychopathology factor in the structure of psychiatric disorders? *Clinical Psychological Science, 2*, 119–137.
Cattane, N., Rossi, R., Lanfredi, M., & Cattaneo, A. (2017). Borderline personality disorder and childhood trauma: Exploring the affected biological systems and mechanisms. *BMC Psychiatry, 17*, 221.
Champagne, F. A., & Curley, J. P. (2009). Epigenetic mechanisms mediating the long-term effects of maternal care on development. *Neuroscience & Biobehavioral Reviews, 33*, 593–600.
Chanen, A. M., & Kaess, M. (2012). Developmental pathways to borderline personality disorder. *Current Psychiatry Reports, 14*, 45–53.
Chanen, A. M., Velakoulis, D., Carison, K., Gaunson, K., Wood, S. J., Yuen, H. P., … Pantelis, C. (2008). Orbitofrontal, amygdala and hippocampal volumes in teenagers with first-presentation borderline personality disorder. *Psychiatry Research: Neuroimaging, 163*, 116–125.
Charoensook, J. (2017). Is epigenetic stress the link between childhood maltreatment and borderline personality disorder? *American Journal of Psychiatry Residents' Journal, 12*, 2–4.
Cicchetti, D., & Rogosch, F. A. (1996). Equifinality and multifinality in developmental psychopathology. *Development and Psychopathology, 8*, 597–600.
Cicchetti, D., & Toth, S. L. (2005). Child maltreatment. *Annual Review of Clinical Psychology, 1*, 409–438.
Clark, L. A., Nuzum, H., & Ro, E. (2018). Manifestations of personality impairment severity: Comorbidity, course/prognosis, psychosocial dysfunction, and 'borderline' personality features. *Current Opinion in Psychology, 21*, 117–121.

Clarke, S. B., Rizvi, S. L., & Resick, P. A. (2008). Borderline personality characteristics and treatment outcome in cognitive-behavioral treatments for PTSD in female rape victims. *Behavior Therapy, 39*, 72–78.
Coan, J. A., & Sbarra, D. A. (2015). Social baseline theory: The social regulation of risk and effort. *Current Opinion in Psychology, 1*, 87–91.
Collins, P. Y., Patel, V., Joestl, S. S., March, D., Insel, T. R., Daar, A. S., ... Fairburn, C. (2011). Grand challenges in global mental health. *Nature, 475*, 27.
Comings, D. E., & Blum, K. (2000). Reward deficiency syndrome: Genetic aspects of behavioral disorders. In *Progress in brain research* (Vol. 126, pp. 325–341). Amsterdam, The Netherlands: Elsevier.
Corriveau, K. H., Harris, P. L., Meins, E., Fernyhough, C., Arnott, B., Elliott, L., ... De Rosnay, M. (2009). Young children's trust in their mother's claims: Longitudinal links with attachment security in infancy. *Child Development, 80*, 750–761.
Costa, B., Pini, S., Gabelloni, P., Abelli, M., Lari, L., Cardini, A., ... Galderisi, S. (2009). Oxytocin receptor polymorphisms and adult attachment style in patients with depression. *Psychoneuroendocrinology, 34*, 1506–1514.
Costello, J. E., Erkanli, A., & Angold, A. (2006). Is there an epidemic of child or adolescent depression? *Journal of Child Psychology and Psychiatry, 47*, 1263–1271.
Crone, E. A., & Dahl, R. E. (2012). Understanding adolescence as a period of social–affective engagement and goal flexibility. *Nature Reviews Neuroscience, 13*, 636–650.
Cusi, A. M., Nazarov, A., Holshausen, K., MacQueen, G. M., & McKinnon, M. C. (2012). Systematic review of the neural basis of social cognition in patients with mood disorders. *Journal of Psychiatry & Neuroscience, 37*(3), 154–169.
Cuthbert, B. N., & Insel, T. R. (2013). Toward the future of psychiatric diagnosis: The seven pillars of RDoC. *BMC Medicine, 11*, 126.
Cyranowski, J. M., Hofkens, T. L., Frank, E., Seltman, H., Cai, H.-M., & Amico, J. A. (2008). Evidence of dysregulated peripheral oxytocin release among depressed women. *Psychosomatic Medicine, 70*, 967.
Dammann, G., Teschler, S., Haag, T., Altmüller, F., Tuczek, F., & Dammann, R. H. (2011). Increased DNA methylation of neuropsychiatric genes occurs in borderline personality disorder. *Epigenetics, 6*, 1454–1462.
Davey, C. G., Yücel, M., & Allen, N. B. (2008). The emergence of depression in adolescence: Development of the prefrontal cortex and the representation of reward. *Neuroscience & Biobehavioral Reviews, 32*, 1–19.
Deckers, J. W., Lobbestael, J., Van Wingen, G. A., Kessels, R. P., Arntz, A., & Egger, J. I. (2015). The influence of stress on social cognition in patients with borderline personality disorder. *Psychoneuroendocrinology, 52*, 119–129.
Dick, D. M., Agrawal, A., Keller, M. C., Adkins, A., Aliev, F., Monroe, S., ... Sher, K. J. (2015). Candidate gene–environment interaction research: Reflections and recommendations. *Perspectives on Psychological Science, 10*, 37–59.
Dillon, D. G., Rosso, I. M., Pechtel, P., Killgore, W. D., Rauch, S. L., & Pizzagalli, D. A. (2014). Peril and pleasure: An RDOC-inspired examination of threat responses and reward processing in anxiety and depression. *Depression and Anxiety, 31*, 233–249.
Dinsdale, N., & Crespi, B. J. (2013). The borderline empathy paradox: Evidence and conceptual models for empathic enhancements in borderline personality disorder. *Journal of Personality Disorders, 27*, 172–195.
Distel, M. A., Rebollo-Mesa, I., Willemsen, G., Derom, C. A., Trull, T. J., Martin, N. G., & Boomsma, D. I. (2009). Familial resemblance of borderline personality disorder features: Genetic or cultural transmission? *PLoS One, 4*, e5334.
Distel, M. A., Trull, T. J., Willemsen, G., Vink, J. M., Derom, C. A., Lynskey, M., ... Boomsma, D. I. (2009). The five-factor model of personality and borderline personality disorder: A genetic analysis of comorbidity. *Biological Psychiatry, 66*, 1131–1138.

Distel, M. A., Willemsen, G., Ligthart, L., Derom, C. A., Martin, N. G., Neale, M. C., ... Boomsma, D. I. (2010). Genetic covariance structure of the four main features of borderline personality disorder. *Journal of Personality Disorders, 24*, 427–444.

Dixon-Gordon, K. L., Gratz, K. L., & Tull, M. T. (2013). Multimodal assessment of emotional reactivity in borderline personality pathology: The moderating role of posttraumatic stress disorder symptoms. *Comprehensive Psychiatry, 54*, 639–648.

Dölen, G., Darvishzadeh, A., Huang, K. W., & Malenka, R. C. (2013). Social reward requires coordinated activity of nucleus accumbens oxytocin and serotonin. *Nature, 501*, 179–184.

Drevets, W. C., Price, J. L., & Furey, M. L. (2008). Brain structural and functional abnormalities in mood disorders: Implications for neurocircuitry models of depression. *Brain Structure and Function, 213*, 93–118.

Dube, S. R., Anda, R. F., Felitti, V. J., Chapman, D. P., Williamson, D. F., & Giles, W. H. (2001). Childhood abuse, household dysfunction, and the risk of attempted suicide throughout the life span: Findings from the adverse childhood experiences study. *JAMA, 286*, 3089–3096.

Ebstein, R. P., Israel, S., Lerer, E., Uzefovsky, F., Shalev, I., Gritsenko, I., ... Yirmiya, N. (2009). Arginine vasopressin and oxytocin modulate human social behavior. *Annals of the New York Academy of Sciences, 1167*, 87–102.

Ehrenthal, J. C., Levy, K. N., Scott, L. N., & Granger, D. A. (2018). Attachment-related regulatory processes moderate the impact of adverse childhood experiences on stress reaction in borderline personality disorder. *Journal of Personality Disorders, 32*, 93–114.

Eiland, L., & Romeo, R. D. (2013). Stress and the developing adolescent brain. *Neuroscience, 249*, 162–171.

Ein-Dor, T., Mikulincer, M., Doron, G., & Shaver, P. R. (2010). The attachment paradox: How can so many of us (the insecure ones) have no adaptive advantages? *Perspectives on Psychological Science, 5*, 123–141.

Ellis, B. J., Boyce, W. T., Belsky, J., Bakermans-Kranenburg, M. J., & Van IJzendoorn, M. H. (2011). Differential susceptibility to the environment: An evolutionary–neurodevelopmental theory. *Development and Psychopathology, 23*, 7–28.

Enzi, B., Doering, S., Faber, C., Hinrichs, J., Bahmer, J., & Northoff, G. (2013). Reduced deactivation in reward circuitry and midline structures during emotion processing in borderline personality disorder. *The World Journal of Biological Psychiatry, 14*, 45–56.

Essex, M. J., Thomas Boyce, W., Hertzman, C., Lam, L. L., Armstrong, J. M., Neumann, S. M., & Kobor, M. S. (2013). Epigenetic vestiges of early developmental adversity: Childhood stress exposure and DNA methylation in adolescence. *Child Development, 84*, 58–75.

Fearon, P., Shmueli-Goetz, Y., Viding, E., Fonagy, P., & Plomin, R. (2014). Genetic and environmental influences on adolescent attachment. *Journal of Child Psychology and Psychiatry, 55*, 1033–1041.

Fearon, R. P., Bakermans-Kranenburg, M. J., Van IJzendoorn, M. H., Lapsley, A. M., & Roisman, G. I. (2010). The significance of insecure attachment and disorganization in the development of children's externalizing behavior: A meta-analytic study. *Child Development, 81*, 435–456.

Feldman, R., Vengrober, A., & Ebstein, R. (2014). Affiliation buffers stress: Cumulative genetic risk in oxytocin–vasopressin genes combines with early caregiving to predict PTSD in war-exposed young children. *Translational Psychiatry, 4*, e370–e370.

Fertuck, E. A., Fischer, S., & Beeney, J. (2018). Social cognition and borderline personality disorder: Splitting and trust impairment findings. *Psychiatric Clinics, 41*, 613–632.

Fertuck, E. A., Lenzenweger, M. F., Clarkin, J. F., Hoermann, S., & Stanley, B. (2006). Executive neurocognition, memory systems, and borderline personality disorder. *Clinical Psychology Review, 26*, 346–375.

Fineberg, S. K., Leavitt, J., Stahl, D. S., Kronemer, S., Landry, C. D., Alexander-Bloch, A., ... Corlett, P. R. (2018). Differential valuation and learning from social and nonsocial cues in borderline personality disorder. *Biological Psychiatry, 84*, 838–845.

Fischer-Kern, M., & Tmej, A. (2019). Mentalization and depression: Theoretical concepts, treatment approaches and empirical studies – An overview. *Zeitschrift für Psychosomatische Medizin und Psychotherapie, 65*, 162–177.
Fonagy, P. (2000). Attachment and borderline personality disorder. *Journal of the American Psychoanalytic Association, 48*, 1129–1146.
Fonagy, P., & Bateman, A. W. (2016). Adversity, attachment, and mentalizing. *Comprehensive Psychiatry, 64*, 59–66.
Fonagy, P., Bateman, A. W., Lorenzini, N., Luyten, P., & Campbell, C. (2021). Development, attachment and childhood experiences. In J. Oldham & A. Skodol (Eds.), *American Psychiatric Association Publishing textbook of personality disorders, 3rd edn*. Washington, DC: American Psychiatric Association Publishing.
Fonagy, P., & Campbell, C. (2015). Bad blood revisited: Attachment and psychoanalysis, 2015. *British Journal of Psychotherapy, 31*, 229–250.
Fonagy, P., Leigh, T., Steele, M., Steele, H., Kennedy, R., Mattoon, G., … Gerber, A. (1996). The relation of attachment status, psychiatric classification, and response to psychotherapy. *Journal of Consulting and Clinical Psychology, 64*, 22.
Fonagy, P., Lorenzini, N., & Campbell, C. (2014). Why are we interested in attachments? In *The Routledge handbook of attachment: Theory* (pp. 45–62). New York, NY: Routledge.
Fonagy, P., & Luyten, P. (2009). A developmental, mentalization-based approach to the understanding and treatment of borderline personality disorder. *Development and Psychopathology, 21*, 1355–1381.
Fonagy, P., & Luyten, P. (2016). A multilevel perspective on the development of borderline personality disorder. *Development and Psychopathology, 3*, 1–67.
Fonagy, P., Luyten, P., & Allison, E. (2015). Epistemic petrification and the restoration of epistemic trust: A new conceptualization of borderline personality disorder and its psychosocial treatment. *Journal of Personality Disorders, 29*, 575–609.
Fonagy, P., Luyten, P., Allison, E., & Campbell, C. (2017a). What we have changed our minds about: Part 1. Borderline personality disorder as a limitation of resilience. *Borderline Personality Disorder and Emotion Dysregulation, 4*, 11.
Fonagy, P., Luyten, P., Allison, E., & Campbell, C. (2017b). What we have changed our minds about: Part 2. Borderline personality disorder, epistemic trust and the developmental significance of social communication. *Borderline Personality Disorder and Emotion Dysregulation, 4*, 9.
Fonagy, P., Target, M., & Gergely, G. (2000). Attachment and borderline personality disorder: A theory and some evidence. *Psychiatric Clinics, 23*, 103–122.
Forbes, E., Brown, S., Kimak, M., Ferrell, R., Manuck, S., & Hariri, A. (2009). Genetic variation in components of dopamine neurotransmission impacts ventral striatal reactivity associated with impulsivity. *Molecular Psychiatry, 14*, 60–70.
Forbes, E. E. (2009). Where's the fun in that? Broadening the focus on reward function in depression. *Biological Psychiatry, 66*, 199.
Forbes, E. E., & Dahl, R. E. (2012). Research review: Altered reward function in adolescent depression: What, when and how? *Journal of Child Psychology and Psychiatry, 53*, 3–15.
Fraley, C. R. (2002). Attachment stability from infancy to adulthood: Meta-analysis and dynamic modeling of developmental mechanisms. *Personality and Social Psychology Review, 6*, 123–151.
Fraley, R. C., & Roberts, B. W. (2005). Patterns of continuity: A dynamic model for conceptualizing the stability of individual differences in psychological constructs across the life course. *Psychological Review, 112*, 60.
Fredrickson, B. L. (2001). The role of positive emotions in positive psychology: The broaden-and-build theory of positive emotions. *American Psychologist, 56*, 218.
Frith, C. D., & Frith, U. (2006). The neural basis of mentalizing. *Neuron, 50*, 531–534.
Gagnon, J. (2017). Defining borderline personality disorder impulsivity: Review of neuropsychological data and challenges that face researchers. *Journal of Psychiatry and Psychiatric Disorders, 1*, 154–176.

Gergely, G. (2013). Ostensive communication and cultural learning: The natural pedagogy hypothesis. In J. Metcalfe & H. S. Terrace (Eds.), *Agency and joint attention* (pp. 139–151). Oxford, UK: Oxford University Press.
Giedd, J. N., Lalonde, F. M., Celano, M. J., White, S. L., Wallace, G. L., Lee, N. R., & Lenroot, R. K. (2009). Anatomical brain magnetic resonance imaging of typically developing children and adolescents. *Journal of the American Academy of Child and Adolescent Psychiatry, 48*, 465.
Gilbert, P. (2006). Evolution and depression: Issues and implications. *Psychological Medicine, 36*, 287–297.
Gluckman, P. D., Hanson, M. A., Bateson, P., Beedle, A. S., Law, C. M., Bhutta, Z. A., … Dasgupta, P. (2009). Towards a new developmental synthesis: Adaptive developmental plasticity and human disease. *The Lancet, 373*, 1654–1657.
Gold, P. W., Machado-Vieira, R., & Pavlatou, M. G. (2015). Clinical and biochemical manifestations of depression: Relation to the neurobiology of stress. *Neural Plasticity, 2015*, 581976.
Golden, S. A., Christoffel, D. J., Heshmati, M., Hodes, G. E., Magida, J., Davis, K., … Russo, S. J. (2013). Epigenetic regulation of RAC1 induces synaptic remodeling in stress disorders and depression. *Nature Medicine, 19*, 337–344.
Golier, J. A., Yehuda, R., Bierer, L. M., Mitropoulou, V., New, A. S., Schmeidler, J., … Siever, L. J. (2003). The relationship of borderline personality disorder to posttraumatic stress disorder and traumatic events. *American Journal of Psychiatry, 160*, 2018–2024.
Gotlib, I. H., Hamilton, J. P., Cooney, R. E., Singh, M. K., Henry, M. L., & Joormann, J. (2010). Neural processing of reward and loss in girls at risk for major depression. *Archives of General Psychiatry, 67*, 380–387.
Grassetti, S. N. (2011). *Borderline features and attachment in adolescents whose mothers have borderline personality disorder* [Maters Thesis. University of Tennessee, Knoxville]. Retreived from https://trace.tennessee.edu/utk_gradthes/973/
Groh, A. M., Roisman, G. I., van IJzendoorn, M. H., Bakermans-Kranenburg, M. J., & Fearon, R. P. (2012). The significance of insecure and disorganized attachment for children's internalizing symptoms: A meta-analytic study. *Child Development, 83*, 591–610.
Grunebaum, M. F., Galfalvy, H. C., Mortenson, L. Y., Burke, A. K., Oquendo, M. A., & Mann, J. J. (2010). Attachment and social adjustment: Relationships to suicide attempt and major depressive episode in a prospective study. *Journal of Affective Disorders, 123*, 123–130.
Guilé, J. M., Boissel, L., Alaux-Cantin, S., & de La Rivière, S. G. (2018). Borderline personality disorder in adolescents: Prevalence, diagnosis, and treatment strategies. *Adolescent Health, Medicine and Therapeutics, 9*, 199.
Gunderson, J. G., & Sabo, A. N. (1993). The phenomenological and conceptual interface between borderline personality disorder and PTSD. *The American Journal of Psychiatry, 150*, 19–27.
Gunnar, M., & Quevedo, K. (2007). The neurobiology of stress and development. *Annual Review of Psychology, 58*, 145–173.
Hammen, C. (2005). Stress and depression. *Annual Review of Clinical Psychology, 1*, 293–319.
Hammen, C., Bower, J. E., & Cole, S. W. (2015). Oxytocin receptor gene variation and differential susceptibility to family environment in predicting youth borderline symptoms. *Journal of Personality Disorders, 29*, 177–192.
Han, B., Compton, W. M., Gfroerer, J., & McKeon, R. (2015). Prevalence and correlates of past 12-month suicide attempt among adults with past-year suicidal ideation in the United States. *The Journal of Clinical Psychiatry, 76*, 295–302.
Hastings, R. S., Parsey, R. V., Oquendo, M. A., Arango, V., & Mann, J. J. (2004). Volumetric analysis of the prefrontal cortex, amygdala, and hippocampus in major depression. *Neuropsychopharmacology, 29*, 952–959.
Hazlett, E. A., Zhang, J., New, A. S., Zelmanova, Y., Goldstein, K. E., Haznedar, M. M., … Chu, K.-W. (2012). Potentiated amygdala response to repeated emotional pictures in borderline personality disorder. *Biological Psychiatry, 72*, 448–456.
Heffernan, K., & Cloitre, M. (2000). A comparison of posttraumatic stress disorder with and without borderline personality disorder among women with a history of childhood sexual abuse:

Etiological and clinical characteristics. *The Journal of Nervous and Mental Disease, 188*, 589–595.
Heim, C., & Binder, E. B. (2012). Current research trends in early life stress and depression: Review of human studies on sensitive periods, gene–environment interactions, and epigenetics. *Experimental Neurology, 233*, 102–111.
Heim, C., Newport, D. J., Mletzko, T., Miller, A. H., & Nemeroff, C. B. (2008). The link between childhood trauma and depression: Insights from HPA axis studies in humans. *Psychoneuroendocrinology, 33*, 693–710.
Herbort, M. C., Soch, J., Wüstenberg, T., Krauel, K., Pujara, M., Koenigs, M., … Schott, B. H. (2016). A negative relationship between ventral striatal loss anticipation response and impulsivity in borderline personality disorder. *NeuroImage: Clinical, 12*, 724–736.
Herpertz, S. C., & Bertsch, K. (2015). A new perspective on the pathophysiology of borderline personality disorder: A model of the role of oxytocin. *American Journal of Psychiatry, 172*, 840–851.
Heshmati, M., & Russo, S. J. (2015). Anhedonia and the brain reward circuitry in depression. *Current Behavioral Neuroscience Reports, 2*, 146–153.
Hostinar, C. E., Sullivan, R. M., & Gunnar, M. R. (2014). Psychobiological mechanisms underlying the social buffering of the hypothalamic–pituitary–adrenocortical axis: A review of animal models and human studies across development. *Psychological Bulletin, 140*, 256.
Hsu, D. T., Sanford, B. J., Meyers, K. K., Love, T. M., Hazlett, K. E., Walker, S. J., … Zubieta, J.-K. (2015). It still hurts: Altered endogenous opioid activity in the brain during social rejection and acceptance in major depressive disorder. *Molecular Psychiatry, 20*, 193–200.
Hughes, C., Jaffee, S. R., Happé, F., Taylor, A., Caspi, A., & Moffitt, T. E. (2005). Origins of individual differences in theory of mind: From nature to nurture? *Child Development, 76*, 356–370.
Hulvershorn, L. A., Cullen, K., & Anand, A. (2011). Toward dysfunctional connectivity: A review of neuroimaging findings in pediatric major depressive disorder. *Brain Imaging and Behavior, 5*, 307–328.
Humphrey, N. K. (1976). The social function of intellect. In *Growing points in ethology* (pp. 303–317). Cambridge, UK: Cambridge University Press.
Hüpen, P., Wagels, L., Weidler, C., Kable, J. W., Schneider, F., & Habel, U. (2020). Altered psychophysiological correlates of risk-taking in borderline personality disorder. *Psychophysiology, 57*, e13540.
Ibrahim, A. K., Kelly, S. J., Adams, C. E., & Glazebrook, C. (2013). A systematic review of studies of depression prevalence in university students. *Journal of Psychiatric Research, 47*, 391–400.
Ibrahim, J., Cosgrave, N., & Woolgar, M. (2018). Childhood maltreatment and its link to borderline personality disorder features in children: A systematic review approach. *Clinical Child Psychology and Psychiatry, 23*, 57–76.
Insel, T., Cuthbert, B., Garvey, M., Heinssen, R., Pine, D. S., Quinn, K., … Wang, P. (2010). Research domain criteria (RDoC): Toward a new classification framework for research on mental disorders. *American Journal of Psychiatry, 167*(7), 748–751.
Insel, T. R., & Young, L. J. (2001). The neurobiology of attachment. *Nature Reviews Neuroscience, 2*, 129–136.
Israel, S., Lerer, E., Shalev, I., Uzefovsky, F., Riebold, M., Laiba, E., … Knafo, A. (2009). The oxytocin receptor (OXTR) contributes to prosocial fund allocations in the dictator game and the social value orientations task. *PLoS One, 4*, e5535.
Jin, X., Zhong, M., Yao, S., Cao, X., Tan, C., Gan, J., … Yi, J. (2016). A voxel-based morphometric MRI study in young adults with borderline personality disorder. *PloS One, 11*, e0147938.
Jones, J. D., Fraley, R. C., Ehrlich, K. B., Stern, J. A., Lejuez, C., Shaver, P. R., & Cassidy, J. (2018). Stability of attachment style in adolescence: An empirical test of alternative developmental processes. *Child Development, 89*, 871–880.
Joyce, P. R., McHugh, P. C., McKenzie, J. M., Sullivan, P. F., Mulder, R. T., Luty, S. E., … Miller, A. M. (2006). A dopamine transporter polymorphism is a risk factor for borderline personality disorder in depressed patients. *Psychological Medicine, 36*, 807–813.

Kaplan, C., Tarlow, N., Stewart, J. G., Aguirre, B., Galen, G., & Auerbach, R. P. (2016). Borderline personality disorder in youth: The prospective impact of child abuse on non-suicidal self-injury and suicidality. *Comprehensive Psychiatry, 71*, 86–94.
Kendler, K., Myers, J., & Reichborn-Kjennerud, T. (2011). Borderline personality disorder traits and their relationship with dimensions of normative personality: A web-based cohort and twin study. *Acta Psychiatrica Scandinavica, 123*, 349–359.
Kendler, K. S., & Gardner, C. O. (2014). Sex differences in the pathways to major depression: A study of opposite-sex twin pairs. *American Journal of Psychiatry, 171*, 426–435.
Kendler, K. S., Kuhn, J., & Prescott, C. A. (2004). The interrelationship of neuroticism, sex, and stressful life events in the prediction of episodes of major depression. *American Journal of Psychiatry, 161*, 631–636.
Kerestes, R., Davey, C. G., Stephanou, K., Whittle, S., & Harrison, B. J. (2014). Functional brain imaging studies of youth depression: A systematic review. *NeuroImage: Clinical, 4*, 209–231.
Kessler, R. C., Berglund, P., Demler, O., Jin, R., Koretz, D., Merikangas, K. R., … Wang, P. S. (2003). The epidemiology of major depressive disorder: Results from the National Comorbidity Survey Replication (NCS-R). *JAMA, 289*, 3095–3105.
Kessler, R. C., Berglund, P., Demler, O., Jin, R., Merikangas, K. R., & Walters, E. E. (2005). Lifetime prevalence and age-of-onset distributions of DSM-IV disorders in the National Comorbidity Survey Replication. *Archives of General Psychiatry, 62*, 593–602.
Kim, S., Fonagy, P., Koos, O., Dorsett, K., & Strathearn, L. (2014). Maternal oxytocin response predicts mother-to-infant gaze. *Brain Research, 1580*, 133–142.
Kluetsch, R. C., Schmahl, C., Niedtfeld, I., Densmore, M., Calhoun, V. D., Daniels, J., … Lanius, R. A. (2012). Alterations in default mode network connectivity during pain processing in borderline personality disorder. *Archives of General Psychiatry, 69*, 993–1002.
Koenig, J., Kemp, A. H., Feeling, N. R., Thayer, J. F., & Kaess, M. (2016). Resting state vagal tone in borderline personality disorder: A meta-analysis. *Progress in Neuro-Psychopharmacology and Biological Psychiatry, 64*, 18–26.
Koenigsberg, H. W., Siever, L. J., Lee, H., Pizzarello, S., New, A. S., Goodman, M., … Prohovnik, I. (2009). Neural correlates of emotion processing in borderline personality disorder. *Psychiatry Research: Neuroimaging, 172*, 192–199.
Konner, M. (2010). *The evolution of childhood: Relationships, emotion, mind*. Cambridge, MA: Harvard University Press.
Krach, S., Paulus, F. M., Bodden, M., & Kircher, T. (2010). The rewarding nature of social interactions. *Frontiers in Behavioral Neuroscience, 4*, 22.
Krause-Utz, A., Cackowski, S., Daffner, S., Sobanski, E., Plichta, M. M., Bohus, M., … Schmahl, C. (2016). Delay discounting and response disinhibition under acute experimental stress in women with borderline personality disorder and adult attention deficit hyperactivity disorder. *Psychological Medicine, 46*, 3137–3149.
Krause-Utz, A., Niedtfeld, I., Knauber, J., & Schmahl, C. (2017). Neurobiology in borderline personality disorder. In B. Stanley & A. New (Eds.), *Primer on borderline personality disorder* (pp. 83–111). New York, NY: Oxford University Press.
Krause-Utz, A., Winter, D., Niedtfeld, I., & Schmahl, C. (2014). The latest neuroimaging findings in borderline personality disorder. *Current Psychiatry Reports, 16*, 438.
Krohn, A. (1974). Borderline "empathy" and differentiation of object representations: A contribution to the psychology of object relations. *International Journal of Psychoanalytic Psychotherapy, 3*, 142.
Kuhlmann, A., Bertsch, K., Schmidinger, I., Thomann, P. A., & Herpertz, S. C. (2013). Morphometric differences in central stress-regulating structures between women with and without borderline personality disorder. *Journal of psychiatry & neuroscience: JPN, 38*, 129.
Kulacaoglu, F., & Kose, S. (2018). Borderline Personality Disorder (BPD): In the midst of vulnerability, Chaos, and Awe. *Brain Sciences, 8*, 201.
Kuo, J. R., Fitzpatrick, S., Metcalfe, R. K., & McMain, S. (2016). A multi-method laboratory investigation of emotional reactivity and emotion regulation abilities in borderline personality disorder. *Journal of Behavior Therapy and Experimental Psychiatry, 50*, 52–60.

Laceulle, O. M., Vollebergh, W. A., & Ormel, J. (2015). The structure of psychopathology in adolescence: Replication of a general psychopathology factor in the TRAILS study. *Clinical Psychological Science, 3*, 850–860.
Lahey, B. B., Rathouz, P. J., Keenan, K., Stepp, S. D., Loeber, R., & Hipwell, A. E. (2015). Criterion validity of the general factor of psychopathology in a prospective study of girls. *Journal of Child Psychology and Psychiatry, 56*, 415–422.
Laland, K. N., Odling-Smee, J., & Myles, S. (2010). How culture shaped the human genome: Bringing genetics and the human sciences together. *Nature Reviews Genetics, 11*, 137–148.
Lawrence, K. A., Allen, J. S., & Chanen, A. M. (2010). Impulsivity in borderline personality disorder: Reward-based decision-making and its relationship to emotional distress. *Journal of Personality Disorders, 24*, 785–799.
Leckman, J. F., Carter, C. S., Hennessy, M. B., Hrdy, S. B., Keverne, E. B., Klann-Delius, G., ... von Holst, D. (2005). Biobehavioral processes in attachment and bonding. In C. S. Carter, L. Ahnert, K. E. Grossman, S. B. Hrdy, M. E. Lamb, S. W. Porges, & N. Sachser (Eds.), *Attachment and bonding: A new synthesis* (pp. 1011–1021). Boston, MA: MIT Press.
Lecompte, V., Moss, E., Cyr, C., & Pascuzzo, K. (2014). Preschool attachment, self-esteem and the development of preadolescent anxiety and depressive symptoms. *Attachment & Human Development, 16*, 242–260.
Lee, A., & Hankin, B. L. (2009). Insecure attachment, dysfunctional attitudes, and low self-esteem predicting prospective symptoms of depression and anxiety during adolescence. *Journal of Clinical Child & Adolescent Psychology, 38*, 219–231.
Lee, E. J., & Stone, S. I. (2012). Co-occurring internalizing and externalizing behavioral problems: The mediating effect of negative self-concept. *Journal of Youth and Adolescence, 41*, 717–731.
Lee Raby, K., Cicchetti, D., Carlson, E. A., Egeland, B., & Andrew Collins, W. (2013). Genetic contributions to continuity and change in attachment security: A prospective, longitudinal investigation from infancy to young adulthood. *Journal of Child Psychology and Psychiatry, 54*, 1223–1230.
Leichsenring, F., Leibing, E., Kruse, J., New, A. S., & Leweke, F. (2011). Borderline personality disorder. *The Lancet, 377*, 74–84.
Lereya, S. T., Winsper, C., Tang, N. K., & Wolke, D. (2017). Sleep problems in childhood and borderline personality disorder symptoms in early adolescence. *Journal of Abnormal Child Psychology, 45*, 193–206.
Lewis, K. L., & Grenyer, B. F. (2009). Borderline personality or complex posttraumatic stress disorder? An update on the controversy. *Harvard Review of Psychiatry, 17*, 322–328.
Lieb, K., Zanarini, M. C., Schmahl, C., Linehan, M. M., & Bohus, M. (2004). Borderline personality disorder. *The Lancet, 364*, 453–461.
Lieberman, M. D. (2007). Social cognitive neuroscience: A review of core processes. *Annual Review of Psychology, 58*, 259–289.
Liu, J., Dietz, K., DeLoyht, J. M., Pedre, X., Kelkar, D., Kaur, J., ... Nestler, E. J. (2012). Impaired adult myelination in the prefrontal cortex of socially isolated mice. *Nature Neuroscience, 15*, 1621–1623.
Lorenzini, N., & Fonagy, P. (2013). Attachment and personality disorders: A short review. *Focus, 11*, 155–166.
Lubke, G., Laurin, C., Amin, N., Hottenga, J. J., Willemsen, G., van Grootheest, G., ... Van Duijn, C. (2014). Genome-wide analyses of borderline personality features. *Molecular Psychiatry, 19*, 923–929.
Luciana, M. (2013). Adolescent brain development in normality and psychopathology. *Development and Psychopathology, 25*, 1325–1345.
Lupien, S. J., McEwen, B. S., Gunnar, M. R., & Heim, C. (2009). Effects of stress throughout the lifespan on the brain, behaviour and cognition. *Nature Reviews Neuroscience, 10*, 434–445.
Luyten, P., & Blatt, S. J. (2013). Interpersonal relatedness and self-definition in normal and disrupted personality development: Retrospect and prospect. *American Psychologist, 68*, 172.

Luyten, P., Blatt, S. J., & Fonagy, P. (2013). Impairments in self structures in depression and suicide in psychodynamic and cognitive behavioral approaches: Implications for clinical practice and research. *International Journal of Cognitive Therapy, 6*, 265–279.

Luyten, P., Blatt, S. J., Van Houdenhove, B., & Corveleyn, J. (2006). Depression research and treatment: Are we skating to where the puck is going to be? *Clinical Psychology Review, 26*, 985–999.

Luyten, P., Campbell, C., Allison, E., & Fonagy, P. (2020). The mentalizing approach to psychopathology: State of the art and future directions. *Annual Review of Clinical Psychology, 16*, 297–325.

Luyten, P., & Fonagy, P. (2015a). The neurobiology of mentalizing. *Personality Disorders: Theory, Research, and Treatment, 6*, 366.

Luyten, P., & Fonagy, P. (2015b). Psychodynamic treatment for borderline personality disorder and mood disorders: A mentalizing perspective. In *Borderline personality and mood disorders* (pp. 223–251). New York, NY: Springer.

Luyten, P., Fonagy, P., Lemma, A., & Target, M. (2012). Depression. In A. W. Bateman & P. Fonagy (Eds.), *Handbook of mentalizing in mental health practice* (pp. 385–417). Washington, DC: American Psychiatric Association.

Luyten, P., Nijssens, L., Fonagy, P., & Mayes, L. C. (2017). Parental reflective functioning: Theory, research, and clinical applications. *The Psychoanalytic Study of the Child, 70*, 174–199.

MacGregor, E. K., Grunebaum, M. F., Galfalvy, H. C., Melhem, N., Burke, A. K., Brent, D. A., ... Mann, J. J. (2014). Depressed parents' attachment: Effects on offspring suicidal behavior in a longitudinal, family study. *The Journal of Clinical Psychiatry, 75*, 879.

Machizawa-Summers, S. (2007). Childhood trauma and parental bonding among Japanese female patients with borderline personality disorder. *International Journal of Psychology, 42*, 265–273.

MacIntosh, H. B., Godbout, N., & Dubash, N. (2015). Borderline personality disorder: Disorder of trauma or personality, a review of the empirical literature. *Canadian Psychology/Psychologie Canadienne, 56*, 227.

MacKillop, J., Gray, J. C., Weafer, J., Sanchez-Roige, S., Palmer, A. A., & de Wit, H. (2019). Genetic influences on delayed reward discounting: A genome-wide prioritized subset approach. *Experimental and Clinical Psychopharmacology, 27*, 29.

Madigan, S., Atkinson, L., Laurin, K., & Benoit, D. (2013). Attachment and internalizing behavior in early childhood: A meta-analysis. *Developmental Psychology, 49*, 672.

Manstead, A. S., Dosmukhambetova, D., Shearn, J., & Clifton, A. (2013). The influence of dysphoria and depression on mental state decoding. *Journal of Social and Clinical Psychology, 32*, 116–133.

Martel, M. M., Pan, P. M., Hoffmann, M. S., Gadelha, A., do Rosário, M. C., Mari, J. J., ... Bressan, R. A. (2017). A general psychopathology factor (P factor) in children: Structural model analysis and external validation through familial risk and child global executive function. *Journal of Abnormal Psychology, 126*, 137.

Martin, L. E., & Potts, G. F. (2004). Reward sensitivity in impulsivity. *Neuroreport, 15*, 1519–1522.

Martín-Blanco, A., Ferrer, M., Soler, J., Arranz, M. J., Vega, D., Bauzà, J., ... García-Martinez, I. (2015). An exploratory association study of the influence of noradrenergic genes and childhood trauma in borderline personality disorder. *Psychiatry Research, 229*, 589–592.

Martín-Blanco, A., Ferrer, M., Soler, J., Arranz, M. J., Vega, D., Calvo, N., ... Salazar, J. (2016). The role of hypothalamus–pituitary–adrenal genes and childhood trauma in borderline personality disorder. *European Archives of Psychiatry and Clinical Neuroscience, 266*, 307–316.

Matthews, K., & Robbins, T. W. (2003). Early experience as a determinant of adult behavioural responses to reward: The effects of repeated maternal separation in the rat. *Neuroscience & Biobehavioral Reviews, 27*, 45–55.

Mayer, A., & Träuble, B. E. (2013). Synchrony in the onset of mental state understanding across cultures? A study among children in Samoa. *International Journal of Behavioral Development, 37*, 21–28.

Mayes, L. C. (2000). *A developmental perspective on the regulation of arousal states.* Paper presented at the Seminars in perinatology.
Mazure, C. M. (1998). Life stressors as risk factors in depression. *Clinical Psychology: Science and Practice, 5*, 291–313.
McCloskey, M. S., New, A. S., Siever, L. J., Goodman, M., Koenigsberg, H. W., Flory, J. D., & Coccaro, E. F. (2009). Evaluation of behavioral impulsivity and aggression tasks as endophenotypes for borderline personality disorder. *Journal of Psychiatric Research, 43*, 1036–1048.
McCrory, E., De Brito, S. A., & Viding, E. (2012). The link between child abuse and psychopathology: A review of neurobiological and genetic research. *Journal of the Royal Society of Medicine, 105*, 151–156.
McEwen, B. S. (2006). Sleep deprivation as a neurobiologic and physiologic stressor: Allostasis and allostatic load. *Metabolism, 55*, S20–S23.
McEwen, B. S. (2007). Physiology and neurobiology of stress and adaptation: Central role of the brain. *Physiological Reviews, 87*, 873–904.
McLaughlin, K. A., Green, J. G., Gruber, M. J., Sampson, N. A., Zaslavsky, A. M., & Kessler, R. C. (2010). Childhood adversities and adult psychiatric disorders in the national comorbidity survey replication II: Associations with persistence of DSM-IV disorders. *Archives of General Psychiatry, 67*, 124–132.
McLean, L. M., & Gallop, R. (2003). Implications of childhood sexual abuse for adult borderline personality disorder and complex posttraumatic stress disorder. *American Journal of Psychiatry, 160*, 369–371.
McQuaid, R. J., McInnis, O. A., Abizaid, A., & Anisman, H. (2014). Making room for oxytocin in understanding depression. *Neuroscience & Biobehavioral Reviews, 45*, 305–322.
Meaney, R., Hasking, P., & Reupert, A. (2016). Prevalence of borderline personality disorder in university samples: Systematic review, meta-analysis and meta-regression. *PLoS One, 11*, e0155439.
Mikulincer, M., & Shaver, P. R. (2007). *Attachment in adulthood: Structure, dynamics, and change*. New York, NY: Guilford Press.
Miller, G. E., Chen, E., & Zhou, E. S. (2007). If it goes up, must it come down? Chronic stress and the hypothalamic-pituitary-adrenocortical axis in humans. *Psychological Bulletin, 133*, 25.
Minzenberg, M. J., Fan, J., New, A. S., Tang, C. Y., & Siever, L. J. (2007). Fronto-limbic dysfunction in response to facial emotion in borderline personality disorder: An event-related fMRI study. *Psychiatry Research: Neuroimaging, 155*, 231–243.
Mojtabai, R., Olfson, M., & Han, B. (2016). National trends in the prevalence and treatment of depression in adolescents and young adults. *Pediatrics, 138*, e20161878.
Monroe, S. M., Anderson, S. F., & Harkness, K. L. (2019). Life stress and major depression: The mysteries of recurrences. *Psychological Review, 126*, 791–816.
Monroe, S. M., & Harkness, K. L. (2005). Life stress, the "kindling" hypothesis, and the recurrence of depression: Considerations from a life stress perspective. *Psychological Review, 112*, 417.
Morrissey, H., Ball, P., & Pandal, G. (2020). *The association between lifestyle and social factors with onset of depression, anxiety and stress.*
Moutsiana, C., Fearon, P., Murray, L., Cooper, P., Goodyer, I., Johnstone, T., & Halligan, S. (2014). Making an effort to feel positive: Insecure attachment in infancy predicts the neural underpinnings of emotion regulation in adulthood. *Journal of Child Psychology and Psychiatry, 55*, 999–1008.
Moutsiana, C., Johnstone, T., Murray, L., Fearon, P., Cooper, P. J., Pliatsikas, C., … Halligan, S. L. (2015). Insecure attachment during infancy predicts greater amygdala volumes in early adulthood. *Journal of Child Psychology and Psychiatry, 56*, 540–548.
Murayama, K., Matsumoto, M., Izuma, K., & Matsumoto, K. (2010). Neural basis of the undermining effect of monetary reward on intrinsic motivation. *Proceedings of the National Academy of Sciences, 107*, 20911–20916.

Murray, L., Arteche, A., Fearon, P., Halligan, S., Goodyer, I., & Cooper, P. (2011). Maternal postnatal depression and the development of depression in offspring up to 16 years of age. *Journal of the American Academy of Child & Adolescent Psychiatry, 50*, 460–470.
Mutlu, A. K., Schneider, M., Debbané, M., Badoud, D., Eliez, S., & Schaer, M. (2013). Sex differences in thickness, and folding developments throughout the cortex. *NeuroImage, 82*, 200–207.
Naoum, J., Reitz, S., Krause-Utz, A., Kleindienst, N., Willis, F., Kuniss, S., … Schmahl, C. (2016). The role of seeing blood in non-suicidal self-injury in female patients with borderline personality disorder. *Psychiatry Research, 246*, 676–682.
Naranjo, C. A., Tremblay, L. K., & Busto, U. E. (2001). The role of the brain reward system in depression. *Progress in Neuro-Psychopharmacology and Biological Psychiatry, 25*, 781–823.
Nater, U. M., Bohus, M., Abbruzzese, E., Ditzen, B., Gaab, J., Kleindienst, N., … Ehlert, U. (2010). Increased psychological and attenuated cortisol and alpha-amylase responses to acute psychosocial stress in female patients with borderline personality disorder. *Psychoneuroendocrinology, 35*, 1565–1572.
Nemoda, Z., Lyons-Ruth, K., Szekely, A., Bertha, E., Faludi, G., & Sasvari-Szekely, M. (2010). Association between dopaminergic polymorphisms and borderline personality traits among at-risk young adults and psychiatric inpatients. *Behavioral and Brain Functions, 6*, 4.
Nestler, E. J., & Carlezon, W. A., Jr. (2006). The mesolimbic dopamine reward circuit in depression. *Biological Psychiatry, 59*, 1151–1159.
Neumann, I. D. (2008). Brain oxytocin: A key regulator of emotional and social behaviours in both females and males. *Journal of Neuroendocrinology, 20*, 858–865.
New, A. S., Perez-Rodriguez, M. M., & Ripoll, L. H. (2012). Neuroimaging and borderline personality disorder. *Psychiatric Annals, 42*, 65–71.
Newnham, E. A., & Janca, A. (2014). Childhood adversity and borderline personality disorder: A focus on adolescence. *Current Opinion in Psychiatry, 27*, 68–72.
Nicol, K., Pope, M., Romaniuk, L., & Hall, J. (2015). Childhood trauma, midbrain activation and psychotic symptoms in borderline personality disorder. *Translational Psychiatry, 5*, e559–e559.
Niedtfeld, I., Schulze, L., Krause-Utz, A., Demirakca, T., Bohus, M., & Schmahl, C. (2013). Voxel-based morphometry in women with borderline personality disorder with and without comorbid posttraumatic stress disorder. *PloS One, 8*, e65824.
Nock, M. K., Green, J. G., Hwang, I., McLaughlin, K. A., Sampson, N. A., Zaslavsky, A. M., & Kessler, R. C. (2013). Prevalence, correlates, and treatment of lifetime suicidal behavior among adolescents: Results from the National Comorbidity Survey Replication Adolescent Supplement. *JAMA Psychiatry, 70*, 300–310.
Pagura, J., Stein, M. B., Bolton, J. M., Cox, B. J., Grant, B., & Sareen, J. (2010). Comorbidity of borderline personality disorder and posttraumatic stress disorder in the US population. *Journal of Psychiatric Research, 44*, 1190–1198.
Panksepp, J., Herman, B., Conner, R., Bishop, P., & Scott, J. (1978). The biology of social attachments: Opiates alleviate separation distress. *Biological Psychiatry, 13*, 607–618.
Panksepp, J., & Watt, D. (2011). Why does depression hurt? Ancestral primary-process separation-distress (PANIC/GRIEF) and diminished brain reward (SEEKING) processes in the genesis of depressive affect. *Psychiatry: Interpersonal & Biological Processes, 74*, 5–13.
Patalay, P., Fonagy, P., Deighton, J., Belsky, J., Vostanis, P., & Wolpert, M. (2015). A general psychopathology factor in early adolescence. *The British Journal of Psychiatry, 207*, 15–22.
Pervanidou, P., & Chrousos, G. P. (2012). Metabolic consequences of stress during childhood and adolescence. *Metabolism, 61*, 611–619.
Pinquart, M., Feußner, C., & Ahnert, L. (2013). Meta-analytic evidence for stability in attachments from infancy to early adulthood. *Attachment & Human Development, 15*, 189–218.
Pizzagalli, D. A. (2014). Depression, stress, and anhedonia: Toward a synthesis and integrated model. *Annual Review of Clinical Psychology, 10*, 393–423.
Porter, C., Palmier-Claus, J., Branitsky, A., Mansell, W., Warwick, H., & Varese, F. (2019). Childhood adversity and borderline personality disorder: A meta-analysis. *Acta Psychiatrica Scandinavica, 141*, 6–20.

Preston, S. D. (2017). The rewarding nature of social contact. *Science, 357*, 1353–1354.
Pyers, J. E., & Senghas, A. (2009). Language promotes false-belief understanding: Evidence from learners of a new sign language. *Psychological Science, 20*, 805–812.
Raabe, F. J., & Spengler, D. (2013). Epigenetic risk factors in PTSD and depression. *Frontiers in Psychiatry, 4*, 80.
Reich, R. B., Vera, S. C., Marino, M. F., Levin, A., Yong, L., & Frankenburg, F. R. (1997). Reported pathological childhood experiences associated with the development of borderline personality disorder. *American Journal of Psychiatry, 154*, 11011106.
Reichborn-Kjennerud, T., Ystrom, E., Neale, M. C., Aggen, S. H., Mazzeo, S. E., Knudsen, G. P., ... Kendler, K. S. (2013). Structure of genetic and environmental risk factors for symptoms of DSM-IV borderline personality disorder. *JAMA Psychiatry, 70*, 1206–1214.
Reitz, S., Kluetsch, R., Niedtfeld, I., Knorz, T., Lis, S., Paret, C., ... Baumgärtner, U. (2015). Incision and stress regulation in borderline personality disorder: Neurobiological mechanisms of self-injurious behaviour. *The British Journal of Psychiatry, 207*, 165–172.
Repetti, R. L., Taylor, S. E., & Seeman, T. E. (2002). Risky families: Family social environments and the mental and physical health of offspring. *Psychological Bulletin, 128*, 330.
Retz, W., Reif, A., Freitag, C. M., Retz-Junginger, P., & Rösler, M. (2010). Association of a functional variant of neuronal nitric oxide synthase gene with self-reported impulsiveness, venturesomeness and empathy in male offenders. *Journal of Neural Transmission, 117*, 321–324.
Rogosch, F. A., & Cicchetti, D. (2005). Child maltreatment, attention networks, and potential precursors to borderline personality disorder. *Development and Psychopathology, 17*, 1071–1089.
Roseboom, T. J., Painter, R. C., van Abeelen, A. F., Veenendaal, M. V., & de Rooij, S. R. (2011). Hungry in the womb: What are the consequences? Lessons from the Dutch famine. *Maturitas, 70*, 141–145.
Rung, J. M., & Madden, G. J. (2018). Experimental reductions of delay discounting and impulsive choice: A systematic review and meta-analysis. *Journal of Experimental Psychology: General, 147*, 1349.
Russ, M. J. (1992). Self-injurious behavior in patients with borderline personality disorder: Biological perspectives. *Journal of Personality Disorders, 6*, 64–81.
Russo, S. J., & Nestler, E. J. (2013). The brain reward circuitry in mood disorders. *Nature Reviews Neuroscience, 14*, 609–625.
Rutherford, H., Williams, S., Moy, S., Mayes, L., & Johns, J. (2011). Disruption of maternal parenting circuitry by addictive process: Rewiring of reward and stress systems. *Frontiers in Psychiatry, 2*, 37.
Ryan, R. M., Deci, E. L., & Vansteenkiste, M. (2016). Autonomy and autonomy disturbances in self-development and psychopathology: Research on motivation, attachment, and clinical process. In Cicchetti, D. (Ed.) *Development and Psychopathology, Volume I.* pp.1–54.
Sarkheil, P., Ibrahim, C. N., Schneider, F., Mathiak, K., & Klasen, M. (2019). Aberrant functional connectivity profiles of brain regions associated with salience and reward processing in female patients with borderline personality disorder. *Brain Imaging and Behavior, 14*(2), 1–11.
Sato, S., & Sassone-Corsi, P. (2019). Circadian and epigenetic control of depression-like behaviors. *Current Opinion in Behavioral Sciences, 25*, 15–22.
Satpute, A. B., & Lieberman, M. D. (2006). Integrating automatic and controlled processes into neurocognitive models of social cognition. *Brain Research, 1079*, 86–97.
Schauer, P. A., Rauh, J., Leicht, G., Andreou, C., & Mulert, C. (2019). Altered oscillatory responses to feedback in borderline personality disorder are linked to symptom severity. *Brain Topography, 32*, 482–491.
Schmahl, C., & Bremner, J. D. (2006). Neuroimaging in borderline personality disorder. *Journal of Psychiatric Research, 40*, 419–427.
Schreiter, S., Pijnenborg, G., & Aan Het Rot, M. (2013). Empathy in adults with clinical or subclinical depressive symptoms. *Journal of Affective Disorders, 150*, 1–16.

Schulze, L., Domes, G., Krüger, A., Berger, C., Fleischer, M., Prehn, K., … Herpertz, S. C. (2011). Neuronal correlates of cognitive reappraisal in borderline patients with affective instability. *Biological Psychiatry, 69*, 564–573.

Schulze, L., Schmahl, C., & Niedtfeld, I. (2016). Neural correlates of disturbed emotion processing in borderline personality disorder: A multimodal meta-analysis. *Biological Psychiatry, 79*, 97–106.

Scott, L. N., Levy, K. N., & Granger, D. A. (2013). Biobehavioral reactivity to social evaluative stress in women with borderline personality disorder. *Personality Disorders: Theory, Research, and Treatment, 4*, 91.

Seres, I., Unoka, Z., & Keri, S. (2009). The broken trust and cooperation in borderline personality disorder. *Neuroreport, 20*, 388–392.

Shahar, G. (2006). Clinical action: Introduction to the special section on the action perspective in clinical psychology. *Journal of Clinical Psychology, 62*, 1053–1064.

Shahar, G. (2015). *Erosion: The psychopathology of self-criticism*. New York, NY: Oxford University Press.

Sharp, C. (2020). Adolescent personality pathology and the alternative model for personality disorders: Self development as nexus. *Psychopathology, 53*, 1–7.

Sharp, C., & Fonagy, P. (2008). The parent's capacity to treat the child as a psychological agent: Constructs, measures and implications for developmental psychopathology. *Social Development, 17*, 737–754.

Sharp, C., Penner, F., & Ensink, K. (2019). Reflective function and borderline traits in adolescents. *Journal of Personality Disorders, 33*, 1–16.

Sharp, C., & Sieswerda, S. (2013). *The social-cognitive basis of borderline and antisocial personality disorder: Introduction*. New York, NY: Guilford Press.

Sharp, C., Vanwoerden, S., & Wall, K. (2018). Adolescence as a sensitive period for the development of personality disorder. *Psychiatric Clinics, 41*, 669–683.

Sharp, C., & Wall, K. (2018). Personality pathology grows up: Adolescence as a sensitive period. *Current Opinion in Psychology, 21*, 111–116.

Shaw, P., Kabani, N. J., Lerch, J. P., Eckstrand, K., Lenroot, R., Gogtay, N., … Rapoport, J. L. (2008). Neurodevelopmental trajectories of the human cerebral cortex. *Journal of Neuroscience, 28*, 3586–3594.

Shirley, R. (2017). *The role of childhood adversity in the development of psychotic experiences in borderline personality disorder*. London, UK: UCL (University College London).

Siegle, G. J., Konecky, R. O., Thase, M. E., & Carter, C. S. (2003). Relationships between amygdala volume and activity during emotional information processing tasks in depressed and never-depressed individuals: An fMRI investigation. *Annals of the New York Academy of Sciences, 985*, 481–484.

Siever, L. (2009). Opioid receptor and oxytocin genotypes in BPD. *Annual Meeting Syllabus and Proceedings Summary*.

Simeon, D., Bartz, J., Hamilton, H., Crystal, S., Braun, A., Ketay, S., & Hollander, E. (2011). Oxytocin administration attenuates stress reactivity in borderline personality disorder: A pilot study. *Psychoneuroendocrinology, 36*, 1418–1421.

Smith, T. B., & Silva, L. (2011). Ethnic identity and personal well-being of people of color: A meta-analysis. *Journal of Counseling Psychology, 58*, 42.

Spear, L. (2007). *The developing brain and adolescent-typical behavior patterns: An evolutionary approach*. New York, NY: Oxford Universuity Press.

Spear, L. P. (2000). The adolescent brain and age-related behavioral manifestations. *Neuroscience & Biobehavioral Reviews, 24*, 417–463.

Sperber, D., Clément, F., Heintz, C., Mascaro, O., Mercier, H., Origgi, G., & Wilson, D. (2010). Epistemic vigilance. *Mind & Language, 25*, 359–393.

Sroufe, L. A. (2005). Attachment and development: A prospective, longitudinal study from birth to adulthood. *Attachment & Human Development, 7*, 349–367.

Stepp, S. D., Lazarus, S. A., & Byrd, A. L. (2016). A systematic review of risk factors prospectively associated with borderline personality disorder: Taking stock and moving forward. *Personality Disorders: Theory, Research, and Treatment, 7*, 316.

Stewart, J. G., Singleton, P., Benau, E. M., Foti, D., Allchurch, H., Kaplan, C. S., ... Auerbach, R. P. (2019). Neurophysiological activity following rewards and losses among female adolescents and young adults with borderline personality disorder. *Journal of Abnormal Psychology, 128*, 610.

Stiglmayr, C., Ebner-Priemer, U., Bretz, J., Behm, R., Mohse, M., Lammers, C. H., ... Kleindienst, N. (2008). Dissociative symptoms are positively related to stress in borderline personality disorder. *Acta Psychiatrica Scandinavica, 117*, 139–147.

Strang, N. M., Pruessner, J., & Pollak, S. D. (2011). Developmental changes in adolescents' neural response to challenge. *Developmental Cognitive Neuroscience, 1*, 560–569.

Strathearn, L. (2011). Maternal neglect: Oxytocin, dopamine and the neurobiology of attachment. *Journal of Neuroendocrinology, 23*, 1054–1065.

Styron, T., & Janoff-Bulman, R. (1997). Childhood attachment and abuse: Long-term effects on adult attachment, depression, and conflict resolution. *Child Abuse & Neglect, 21*, 1015–1023.

Sullivan, P. F., Neale, M. C., & Kendler, K. S. (2000). Genetic epidemiology of major depression: Review and meta-analysis. *American Journal of Psychiatry, 157*, 1552–1562.

Swain, J. E., Kim, P., Spicer, J., Ho, S., Dayton, C. J., Elmadih, A., & Abel, K. (2014). Approaching the biology of human parental attachment: Brain imaging, oxytocin and coordinated assessments of mothers and fathers. *Brain Research, 1580*, 78–101.

Swain, J. E., Lorberbaum, J. P., Kose, S., & Strathearn, L. (2007). Brain basis of early parent–infant interactions: Psychology, physiology, and in vivo functional neuroimaging studies. *Journal of Child Psychology and Psychiatry, 48*, 262–287.

Temes, C. M., Magni, L. R., Fitzmaurice, G. M., Aguirre, B. A., Goodman, M., & Zanarini, M. C. (2017). Prevalence and severity of childhood adversity in adolescents with BPD, psychiatrically healthy adolescents, and adults with BPD. *Personality and Mental Health, 11*, 171–178.

Thompson, S. M., Hammen, C., Starr, L. R., & Najman, J. M. (2014). Oxytocin receptor gene polymorphism (rs53576) moderates the intergenerational transmission of depression. *Psychoneuroendocrinology, 43*, 11–19.

Tomasello, M. (2010). *Origins of human communication*. Cambridge, MA: MIT Press.

Tomko, R. L., Trull, T. J., Wood, P. K., & Sher, K. J. (2014). Characteristics of borderline personality disorder in a community sample: Comorbidity, treatment utilization, and general functioning. *Journal of Personality Disorders, 28*, 734–750.

Torgensen, S. (2014). Prevalence, sociodemographics and functional impairment. In J. M. Oldham, A. E. Skodol, & D. S. Bender (Eds.), *The American Psychiatric Publishing textbook of personality disorder* (2nd ed., pp. 109–130). Arlington, VA: American Psychiatric Publishing.

Tsuno, N., Besset, A., & Ritchie, K. (2005). Sleep and depression. *The Journal of Clinical Psychiatry, 66*, 1254–1269.

Uchida, S., Yamagata, H., Seki, T., & Watanabe, Y. (2018). Epigenetic mechanisms of major depression: Targeting neuronal plasticity. *Psychiatry and Clinical Neurosciences, 72*, 212–227.

Uddin, L. Q., Iacoboni, M., Lange, C., & Keenan, J. P. (2007). The self and social cognition: The role of cortical midline structures and mirror neurons. *Trends in Cognitive Sciences, 11*, 153–157.

Ullrich, S., & Coid, J. (2009). The age distribution of self-reported personality disorder traits in a household population. *Journal of Personality Disorders, 23*, 187–200.

Van Overwalle, F. (2009). Social cognition and the brain: A meta-analysis. *Human Brain Mapping, 30*, 829–858.

Van Overwalle, F. (2011). A dissociation between social mentalizing and general reasoning. *NeuroImage, 54*, 1589–1599.

van Zutphen, L., Siep, N., Jacob, G. A., Goebel, R., & Arntz, A. (2015). Emotional sensitivity, emotion regulation and impulsivity in borderline personality disorder: A critical review of fMRI studies. *Neuroscience & Biobehavioral Reviews, 51*, 64–76.
Vega, D., Ripollés, P., Soto, À., Torrubia, R., Ribas, J., Monreal, J. A., ... Rodríguez-Fornells, A. (2018). Orbitofrontal overactivation in reward processing in borderline personality disorder: The role of non-suicidal self-injury. *Brain Imaging and Behavior, 12*, 217–228.
Vega, D., Soto, À., Amengual, J. L., Ribas, J., Torrubia, R., Rodríguez-Fornells, A., & Marco-Pallarés, J. (2013). Negative reward expectations in borderline personality disorder patients: Neurophysiological evidence. *Biological Psychology, 94*, 388–396.
Verhage, M. L., Fearon, R. P., Schuengel, C., van IJzendoorn, M. H., Bakermans-Kranenburg, M. J., Madigan, S., ... Wong, M. S. (2018). Examining ecological constraints on the intergenerational transmission of attachment via individual participant data meta-analysis. *Child Development, 89*, 2023–2037.
Vogt, D., Waeldin, S., Hellhammer, D., & Meinlschmidt, G. (2016). The role of early adversity and recent life stress in depression severity in an outpatient sample. *Journal of Psychiatric Research, 83*, 61–70.
Völlm, B., Richardson, P., McKie, S., Elliott, R., Dolan, M., & Deakin, B. (2007). Neuronal correlates of reward and loss in cluster B personality disorders: A functional magnetic resonance imaging study. *Psychiatry Research: Neuroimaging, 156*, 151–167.
Vrticka, P., & Vuilleumier, P. (2012). Neuroscience of human social interactions and adult attachment style. *Frontiers in Human Neuroscience, 6*, 212.
Wagner, S., Baskaya, Ö., Anicker, N. J., Dahmen, N., Lieb, K., & Tadić, A. (2010). The catechol o-methyltransferase (COMT) val158met polymorphism modulates the association of serious life events (SLE) and impulsive aggression in female patients with borderline personality disorder (BPD). *Acta Psychiatrica Scandinavica, 122*, 110–117.
Wagner, S., Baskaya, Ö., Lieb, K., Dahmen, N., & Tadić, A. (2009). The 5-HTTLPR polymorphism modulates the association of serious life events (SLE) and impulsivity in patients with borderline personality disorder. *Journal of Psychiatric Research, 43*, 1067–1072.
Walum, H., Westberg, L., Henningsson, S., Neiderhiser, J. M., Reiss, D., Igl, W., ... Eriksson, E. (2008). Genetic variation in the vasopressin receptor 1a gene (AVPR1A) associates with pair-bonding behavior in humans. *Proceedings of the National Academy of Sciences, 105*, 14153–14156.
Watkins, E., & Teasdale, J. D. (2004). Adaptive and maladaptive self-focus in depression. *Journal of Affective Disorders, 82*, 1–8.
Weightman, M. J., Air, T. M., & Baune, B. T. (2014). A review of the role of social cognition in major depressive disorder. *Frontiers in Psychiatry, 5*, 179.
Weinberg, A., Klonsky, E. D., & Hajcak, G. (2009). Autonomic impairment in borderline personality disorder: A laboratory investigation. *Brain and Cognition, 71*, 279–286.
Widom, C. S., Czaja, S. J., & Paris, J. (2009). A prospective investigation of borderline personality disorder in abused and neglected children followed up into adulthood. *Journal of Personality Disorders, 23*, 433–446.
Wilkinson, P., Kelvin, R., Roberts, C., Dubicka, B., & Goodyer, I. (2011). Clinical and psychosocial predictors of suicide attempts and nonsuicidal self-injury in the Adolescent Depression Antidepressants and Psychotherapy Trial (ADAPT). *American Journal of Psychiatry, 168*, 495–501.
Willis, F., Kuniss, S., Kleindienst, N., Naoum, J., Reitz, S., Boll, S., ... Schmahl, C. (2017). The role of nociceptive input and tissue injury on stress regulation in borderline personality disorder. *Pain, 158*, 479–487.
Wingenfeld, K., Hill, A., Adam, B., & Driessen, M. (2007). Dexamethasone suppression test in borderline personality disorder: Impact of PTSD symptoms. *Psychiatry and Clinical Neurosciences, 61*, 681–683.

Wingenfeld, K., Spitzer, C., Rullkötter, N., & Löwe, B. (2010). Borderline personality disorder: Hypothalamus pituitary adrenal axis and findings from neuroimaging studies. *Psychoneuroendocrinology, 35*, 154–170.

Winsper, C., Marwaha, S., Lereya, S. T., Thompson, A., Eyden, J., & Singh, S. P. (2016). A systematic review of the neurobiological underpinnings of borderline personality disorder (BPD) in childhood and adolescence. *Reviews in the Neurosciences, 27*, 827–847.

Witt, S. H., Streit, F., Jungkunz, M., Frank, J., Awasthi, S., Reinbold, C., … Heilmann-Heimbach, S. (2017). Genome-wide association study of borderline personality disorder reveals genetic overlap with bipolar disorder, major depression and schizophrenia. *Translational Psychiatry, 7*, e1155–e1155.

Yurgelun-Todd, D. A., & Killgore, W. D. (2006). Fear-related activity in the prefrontal cortex increases with age during adolescence: A preliminary fMRI study. *Neuroscience Letters, 406*, 194–199.

Zanarini, M. C., Temes, C. M., Magni, L. R., Fitzmaurice, G. M., Aguirre, B. A., & Goodman, M. (2017). Prevalence rates of borderline symptoms reported by adolescent inpatients with BPD, psychiatrically healthy adolescents and adult inpatients with BPD. *Personality and Mental Health, 11*, 150–156.

Zanarini, M. C., Yong, L., Frankenburg, F. R., Hennen, J., Reich, D. B., Marino, M. F., & Vujanovic, A. A. (2002). Severity of reported childhood sexual abuse and its relationship to severity of borderline psychopathology and psychosocial impairment among borderline inpatients. *The Journal of Nervous and Mental Disease, 190*, 381–387.

Zeegers, M. A., Colonnesi, C., Stams, G.-J. J., & Meins, E. (2017). Mind matters: A meta-analysis on parental mentalization and sensitivity as predictors of infant–parent attachment. *Psychological Bulletin, 143*, 1245.

Zimmerman, D. J., & Choi-Kain, L. W. (2009). The hypothalamic-pituitary-adrenal axis in borderline personality disorder: A review. *Harvard Review of Psychiatry, 17*, 167–183.

Zlotnick, C., Franklin, C. L., & Zimmerman, M. (2002). Is comorbidity of posttraumatic stress disorder and borderline personality disorder related to greater pathology and impairment? *American Journal of Psychiatry, 159*, 1940–1943.

Chapter 5
The Domain of Social Dysfunction in Complex Depressive Disorders

Devika Duggal, Eric A. Fertuck, and Steven K. Huprich

Abstract Depressive disorders have a major impact on social functioning. In uncomplicated, episodic depression (i.e., major depressive disorder), transient symptoms of social withdrawal and loss of interest in activities are common functional impairments. However, in more complex forms of depression, social dysfunction can be chronic and pervasive, often leading to more severe and intractable functional impairments. This chapter presents a scoping review of the empirical literature that examines the impact of complex depression on five domains of social functioning: occupational functioning, romantic and sexual relationships, leisure activities, affiliation and attachment, and social support networks. Two case studies are presented that illustrate social dysfunction in two predominant forms of complex depression: chronic depressive disorders (CDD) and depression with personality disorder (DPD). These two forms of complicated depression encompass a range of complex depressive disorders as CDD focuses on persistent and non-remitting forms of depression (including dysthymia, pervasive depressive disorder, depressive personality disorder, and double depression), while DPD relates to episodic depression in the presence of co-occurring personality pathology. The limitations of included studies and the need for treatment development (e.g., lack of treatment studies, need for a focus on social dysfunction as a treatment target) for further investigation are discussed.

Keywords Complex depression · Social functioning · Chronic depression · Depressive personality disorder · Occupational functioning · Romantic functioning · Social support · Leisure activities · Affiliation and attachment

D. Duggal · E. A. Fertuck (✉)
City College and Graduate Center, City University of New York, New York, NY, USA
e-mail: efertuck@ccny.cuny.edu

S. K. Huprich
College of Human Medicine, Michigan State University, East Lansing, MI, USA

University of Detroit Mercy, Detroit, MI, USA

G. de la Parra et al. (eds.), *Depression and Personality Dysfunction*, Depression and Personality, https://doi.org/10.1007/978-3-030-70699-9_5

Depressive disorders, including major depressive disorder (MDD), pervasive depressive disorder (PDD), dysthymia, and other forms of "complex" depression, cause profound social dysfunction. Social functioning includes capacities for occupational engagement and commitment, cultivation and maintenance of romantic and sexual relations, nurturance of social support networks, affiliation and attachment, and appreciation and engagement with leisure activities (Chan et al., 2019; Weissman, 1975). Social dysfunction in uncomplicated major depressive disorder (uMDD) is well studied. uMDD is associated with often transient, episodic social withdrawal, social role dysfunction, increased dependency on others, and a lack of interest in interpersonal relations and sexuality (Kupferberg, Bicks, & Hasler, 2016). Prior studies have demonstrated the impact of depression on social functioning, most consistently noting impairments in interpersonal functioning and occupational abilities (Baune & Renger, 2014; Kamenov, Twomey, Cabello, Prina, & Ayuso-Mateos, 2017). Greater functional impairment results in feelings of demoralization, reinforcing depressive symptoms and creating a potentially vicious cycle (Kupferberg et al., 2016; Markowitz et al., 2007). Thus, individuals with ongoing social dysfunction are prone to recurrent depressive episodes (Knight & Baune, 2017).

A comprehensive empirical review of social dysfunction for chronic and complex forms of depression, to our knowledge, has not been conducted. This is significant from a public health perspective because the shorter- and longer-term social dysfunctions in complex depression may be more insidious and more chronically disabling than in uMDD. Specifically, complex depression may involve lower-grade depressive symptoms. However, the longer term and treatment refractory nature of complex depression may create more intractable social dysfunctions not seen in uMDD. This chapter, then, is a *scoping review* (a survey and evaluation of the findings, limitations, and future directions of an existing body of literature) (Munn et al., 2018) of the empirical literature along with representative case studies in two predominant forms of "complex" depression. The first form of complex depression, chronic depressive disorders (CDDs), will focus on social dysfunction studies of dysthymia, pervasive depressive disorder (PDD), depressive personality disorder, and chronic, non-remitting major depressive disorder (including double depression [i.e., dysthymia co-occurring with major depressive disorder]). These disorders share common features of less severe symptoms of depression than uMDD, coupled with a chronic and non-remitting course. The second form of complex depression, depression with personality disorder (DPD), includes personality disorders such as borderline personality disorder (BPD) that have a co-occurring lifetime depressive disorder. For BPD in particular, the rate of lifetime co-occurrence for depressive disorder ranges between 70% and 90% (see Fertuck, Chesin, & Johnston, 2018 for review). DPDs share the clinical features of personality pathology (emotional liability, self-disturbance, unstable or impaired interpersonal relations, and intense impulsive-aggression that impair social functioning) with pronounced depressive symptoms that can co-occur with this personality pathology. This scoping review will summarize and synthesize the CDD and DPD social dysfunction literature separately with an illustrative case for each. A synthesis and conclusion will follow.

5.1 Domains of Social Function in CDD and DPD

Investigators have operationalized the construct of social functioning, and, as a result, numerous psychometric instruments to assess the nature and extent of social deficits have been established (e.g., Birchwood, Smith, Cochrane, Wetton, & Copestake, 1990; Weissman, 1990). Despite this, there is a lack of consensus on how social functioning is optimally mesured, with some studies using self-report tools and others emphasizing clinician interview and observations. Additionally, studies that examine the relationship between complex depression and social functioning tend to utilize self-report measures that provide global functioning scores (e.g., Social Functioning Questionnaire [SFQ; Tyrer et al., 2011]), with only a few studies including measures that distinguish between the various domains of social functioning (e.g., Social Adjustment Scale – Self Report [SAS-SR]; (Weissman & Bothwell, 1976)). Thus, there is a need to differentiate how specific social functioning domains are impacted by complex forms of depressive disorders. In this chapter, we consider social dysfunction according to disruption in the following domains: occupational functioning, romantic and sexual relationships, leisure activities, affiliation and attachment, and social support networks. We define and summarize in the following section the significance of several domains of social functioning relevant to CDD and DPD.

Occupational Functioning Occupational functioning may be defined as the qualities required to effectively serve in an occupational position, including dealing with the physical, environmental, and psychological demands of a work setting (Combs & Heaton, 2016). Occupational functioning is reciprocally related to depression, as functional impairment is a major symptom of depressive disorders, and these deficits can, in turn, negatively impact the course of the pathology. Loss of a sense of self-efficacy, self-worth, and, in some cases, financial stability are typically noted deficits in work function that can be caused by and further reinforce symptoms of uMDD (Daremo, Kjellberg, & Haglund, 2015).

Romantic and Sexual Relations A meaningful and satisfying romantic relationship is important for both partners' psychological and physical sense of well-being, for instance, emotional intimacy in romantic relationships seems to buffer the impact of stressors and increase sexual satisfaction (van Lankveld et al., 2018). Romantic dysfunction can include experiences of partner dissatisfaction, conflicts, chronically stressful and unsupportive environments, and abuse (Daley, Burge, & Hammen, 2000) that can often result in depressive experiences (Davila, 2001). Conversely, depressive disorders seem to have a profoundly detrimental effect on the quality of romantic relationships (Sharabi, Delaney, & Knobloch, 2016). Individuals with uMDD can also demonstrate fixed patterns of communication that tend to burden or alienate their partners (Benazon & Coyne, 2000).

Leisure Activity Interest and engagement in leisure activities includes pleasurable or rewarding activities (e.g., hobbies, sports, creative pursuits, and intellectual pursuits) that individuals voluntarily engage with in the absence of other occupational or social responsibilities (Zhang & Zheng, 2017). Leisure activities are categorized into two broad domains: social activities that focus on interpersonal interactions (e.g., going out to dinner with friends) and self-focused activities where interpersonal interactions are not the primary focus (e.g., meditating, watching TV; Goodman, Geiger, & Wolf, 2016). While physical exercise can be considered as a form of leisure, most studies suggest that such activities display a different relationship with depressive symptoms (Goodman et al., 2016) and will not be included in our definition. Depressive disorders, particularly uMDD, are partly characterized by anhedonia, or the inability to derive pleasure from normally enjoyable activities during depressive episodes (i.e., activities commonly associated with leisure time) (Nydegger, 2008).

Affiliation and Attachment Affiliation refers to the individual's engagement in positive social interactions with others, whereas attachment is a selective affiliation that occurs in the context of a social bond. Additionally, Kupferberg et al. (2016) document the following social impairments in uMDD within this domain: social anhedonia, increased sensitivity to social rejection, increased altruistic punishment, and excessive use of social media at the cost of in-person activities. Individuals with depression tend to display diminished interest in social interactions that results in difficulties initiating, forming, and maintaining meaningful relationships with other people (Kupferberg et al., 2016). Additionally, uMDD seems to negatively impact the processing of social cues (Ehnvall et al., 2014), and individuals with uMDD are likely to behave in ways that elicit exclusionary events (Joiner & Katz, 1999). For instance, reduced eye contact, social withdrawal and isolation, or excessive reassurance-seeking can lead to greater potential of social rejection (De Rubeis et al., 2017) and consequently reinforce social withdrawal in individuals with uMDD.

Social Support Networks Social support networks can refer to emotional and physical resources provided by an individual's network (e.g., friends, family, community, religious groups, etc.) that can be either emotional or instrumental (Morelli, Lee, Arnn, & Zaki, 2015). The positive impact of strong social support and relationships on mental and physical health has been consistently documented (Leigh-Hunt et al., 2017). The literature on depression asserts the same. Perceived emotional support and large social networks (Santini, Koyanagi, Tyrovolas, & Haro, 2015), as well as the availability and extent of support, are associated with reductions in depressive symptoms (Moos, Cronkite, & Moos, 1998; Wang, Mann, Lloyd-Evans, Ma, & Johnson, 2018). Studies have also examined the bidirectional nature of this relationship, suggesting depressive symptoms can also cause reductions in access to and availability of social resources (Ren, Qin, Zhang, & Zhang, 2018). Social support networks have been assessed in a number of ways, ranging from the use of standardized social support network scales (e.g., Duke Social Support Index; Oddone, Hybels, McQuoid, & Steffens, 2011) to self-reported number of friends or close acquaintances (Oltmanns, Melley, & Turkheimer, 2002). Other assessments focus on the structure and function of networks. Network structures include the size, frequency of interactions, and availability of aid, while the function of the social network includes subjective experiences of feeling connected and useful to and satisfied by others (Santini et al., 2015).

5.2 Chronic Depressive Disorders (CDD) and Social Dysfunction

Several studies have investigated social dysfunction in chronic depressive disorders (CDD), which include dysthymia (DSM-IV), pervasive depressive disorder (PDD; DSM-5), depressive personality disorder, double depression (i.e., dysthymia or PDD co-occurring with MDD), and non-remitting major depressive disorder (without co-occurring *non*-depressive personality disorder). Though no longer in the DSM-5 or other diagnostic manuals, we include depressive personality disorder as a CDD based on its significant empirical validity (Huprich, 2012). Depressive personality disorder has been reformulated more dimensionally toward a construct of "malignant self-regard" (Huprich, 2014, 2020). The case study at the end of this CDD section of the chapter focuses on the social dysfunction in a case of malignant self-regard.

An early study compared individuals with depression (uMDD, dysthymia, and double depression) to those with chronic medical conditions (e.g., diabetes and arthritis) (Hays, Wells, Sherbourne, Rogers, & Spritzer, 1995). Those with any form of depression exhibited functional impairments in multiple domains that were comparable (and in some ways more severe) than chronic medical illnesses. At the 2-year follow-up, dysthymia was uniquely associated with increases in role limitations due to emotional problems relative to other forms of depression, which generally improved in this functional domain during follow-up. Hays et al. (1995) also document long-term impairments in functioning in dysthymia that are worse than other forms of depressive disorders. Further, the co-occurrence of dysthymia and MDD was associated with the most chronic functional impairments (i.e., double depression only improved on three of eight functional domains, the fewest domains of any group).

A subsequent study (Leader & Klein, 1996) directly compared social functioning in three groups: individuals with dysthymia, double depression, and episodic MDD (i.e., uMDD). While all three depressive groups exhibited significant social impairment, the double depression group was most impaired in both functioning and symptoms relative to the other two groups. Moreover, among individuals with dysthymia, those with more depressive symptoms had the most impaired social functioning, particularly in occupational functioning, extended family, and social role pursuits. While social role functioning was a prime focus in this study, it was noted that the diminished capacity to pursue and enjoy leisure activities was impaired in dysthymia relative to more acute depression. The authors concluded that CDD is comparable to acute depression in social dysfunction. A strength of the study was the use of semi-structured interviews of functioning rather than self-report.

A related study (Adler et al., 2004) investigated the impact of dysthymia on work functioning among employed primary care patients. Focusing on work functioning both on the job and assessed via absenteeism, these investigators compared individuals with dysthymia (without uMDD) to depression-free controls. Absenteeism was not different between groups, but on-the-job productivity was three times worse in the dysthymia group than the nondepressed group. The authors noted that a current episode of major depression had a more impairing impact on work performance than dysthymia in this cross-sectional design, indicating that severity of depression is the most debilitating factor to predict social dysfunction.

A prospective study that followed a community sample in Zurich for 20 years examined the characteristics of long-term depression versus uMDD (Angst, Gamma, Rössler, Ajdacic, & Klein, 2009). DSM-III-R criteria was used to diagnose a major depressive episode (MDE), while the long-term depression group was defined by the presence of depressive symptoms more days than not for over 2 years along with work or social impairments. Individuals with long-term depression were more often single, had fewer children, were more frequently unemployed, and less often in full-time employment than those diagnosed with uMDD as well as compared to individuals without a depression diagnosis.

Another naturalistic study examined the predictors of both course trajectories and outcomes in individuals with dysthymia over 10 years (Klein, Shankman, & Rose, 2008). Notably, functional impairment was an important outcome measure, in addition to depressive symptomatology. Their sample consisted of adult outpatients diagnosed with early-onset dysthymia with or without a co-occurring MDE. Social functioning was assessed using a modified version of the LIFE (Longitudinal Interval Follow-up Evaluation) semi-structured interview. This version specifically evaluates impairments in work, in school, as a homemaker, and as a parent. Neither pharmacotherapy nor psychotherapy significantly predicted the course of patients' social functioning. Six variables predicted both greater severity of depressive symptoms and more functional impairment at the 10-year follow-up: older age, lower education levels, concurrent anxiety disorder, higher familiar loading for chronic depression, poor maternal relationship, and a history of childhood sexual abuse. Finally, longer duration of dysthymia symptoms predicted greater functional impairment.

A cross-sectional study investigated the impact of CDD on multiple aspects of employee productivity and whether this impact varies depending on the specific work demands (Lerner et al., 2004). They compared individuals with depression (including dysthymia, uMDD, and double depression) to controls across employment sectors (e.g., managers, technical works, service industries, construction, transportation, etc.). Work functioning was evaluated by the Work Limitations Questionnaire (WLQ), a self-report questionnaire that assesses an employee's ability to perform specific job demands, including mental and interpersonal demands, physical demands, time management, and output demands. Depressed employees were two to three times more likely to report that health concerns interfered with their ability to meet job demands relative to controls. Employees with uMDD or double depression reported higher impairments than those with dysthymia across WLQ domains. The WLQ Productivity Loss Index, a summary score that estimates the amount of health-related productivity loss, provides additional support for the above finding. Dysthymic participants displayed the least on-the-job productivity loss, followed by double depression and then uMDD groups. Finally, employee absenteeism was also measured, with the control group missing a half-day average over a 2-week period compared to 1.4 days for the employees with dysthymia, 1.7 days for those with double depression, and 2.2 days for those with uMDD. The investigators also noted that more severe depressive symptoms and worse physical health related to higher WLQ scores as well as number of days missed at work. As the uMDD and double depression groups displayed greater symptom severity than the participants with dysthymia (determined by the Patient Health Questionnaire-9), this may explain the above pattern of results for the participants in the depressive groups.

Several studies have suggested the course and outcome of depressive disorders is impacted by concurrent social dysfunction. However, it appears that impaired social dysfunction can persist even after the remission of depressive symptoms (Rhebergen et al., 2010). In order to understand the trajectories of social functioning post-remission of a depressive disorder, the investigators followed a community population consisting of a control group and individuals with uMDD, dysthymia, or double depression for 3 years. Remission was defined by the absence of a clear depressive disorder (as determined by the Composite International Diagnostic Interview) after 1- and 3-year follow-ups. Social functioning was assessed using the Groningen Social Disability Score (GSDS) that includes three subscales: domains of social functioning, housekeeping, and leisure time functioning. At baseline, the level of social functioning was poorest in individuals with double depression, followed by those with uMDD and next those with dysthymic individuals. However, at the 3-year follow-up, the individuals with uMDD showed greatest improvement in all domains, followed by those with double depression and dysthymia. Thus, this study reinforces earlier findings that the long-term impact of CDDs on social functioning persists and is greater than uMDD, despite major symptom remission. The investigators speculate that this may be due to residual symptoms of depression and argued that depression recurrence may be partly a result of lingering social deficits. A limitation of the study noted by the investigators was the absence of premorbid assessment of social function, without which it is difficult to know the degree to which long-term social deficits can be accounted for by social functioning before illness onset.

Another cross-sectional study examined social functioning deficits in individuals with current uMDD as compared to those with dysthymia, other non-affective disorders, or no psychiatric diagnoses (Zlotnick, Kohn, Keitner, & Della Grotta, 2000). This study examined interpersonal functioning by assessing the quality of relationships with spouses, relatives, and other family members. Individuals with uMDD reported fewer positive interactions and more negative interactions with their spouse or live-in partner when compared to individuals with no diagnoses and those with non-affective disorder. However, no significant differences were noted in the quality of relationships across domains when the uMDD group was compared to the dysthymic group, suggesting that depression severity as well as the number of symptoms did not seem to have greater impact on interpersonal functioning. A major limitation of this study was the use of an unspecified quality of relationship measure that the authors noted has unreliable psychometric properties.

A prospective, longitudinal study of individuals with a dysthymia diagnosis over a 9-month period assessed the course of illness of a cohort of dysthymic patients, of which 18% showed symptom remission while the others did not (McCullough et al., 1988). It was noted that individuals with non-remitting dysthymia appeared shy or less sociable while being more compliant and submissive in relationships. These features may have related to feeling unsupported by interpersonal relationships, thereby maintaining dysthymic symptoms in participants.

A review of 19 studies examined the size and quality of social networks in individuals with chronic depression (Visentini, Cassidy, Bird, & Priebe, 2018). Included studies compared individuals with dysthymia to those with uMDD, other forms of psychopathology, and no psychiatric diagnoses across settings such as community, inpatient, and specialized tertiary settings. A variety of diagnostic terms were included (e.g., dysthymia, double depression, chronic depression, etc.) as long as chronic depression was characterized by a continuous 2-year (or longer) duration of depressed mood. Chronically depressed individuals display smaller social networks that are perceived as less satisfying when compared to the networks of healthy participants or those with other psychiatric diagnoses, particularly episodic depression. However, a major limitation of this review pertains to the variability in assessment measures for social functioning across the studies, making it difficult to compare results across studies.

Finally, there have been two studies investigating the impact of treatment and social dysfunction in CDD. The first was a psychopharmacological study (Friedman, Markowitz, Parides, Gniwesch, & Kocsis, 1999) that explored whether social functioning improvements persist after effective antidepressant (desipramine) treatment for dysthymia. To assess social dysfunction, the authors utilized a self-report version of the social adjustment scale (SAS; work, leisure time, family and children, and finances). They studied a cohort of patients with dysthymia who responded well to desipramine at 6 months of follow-up. While symptomatic reductions persisted, social functioning (including enjoyment of leisure time) only modestly improved during the follow-up period. In fact, only 24% of the patients had a "normative" level of social adjustment at 6-month follow-up. The authors note that social impairments are relatively neglected treatment foci relative to symptoms in dysthymia.

The second treatment study investigated the impact of antidepressant medication combined with psychotherapy on social dysfunction. This pioneering study (Hirschfeld et al., 2002) compared three treatments over 12 weeks: nefazodone alone, psychotherapy (Cognitive Behavioral Analysis System of Psychotherapy [CBASP]) alone, and the combination of these treatments for individuals with depressive episodes that were present for more than 2 years. Combined treatment was associated with greater functional improvement (in both work and social functioning) than either treatment alone. CBASP improved functioning independently of symptom change, and psychosocial gains were not explained simply by greater symptom reduction. Notably, the rate of improvement in functioning was slower than for symptom reduction, strongly suggesting that ongoing intervention is warranted to bolster functioning after symptoms have subsided.

An Illustrative Case of CDD and Social Dysfunction This case example (Huprich, 2019) is of a 27-year-old young professional, Mark, who sought treatment for chronic unhappiness and depression. He had been in brief mental health treatments while obtaining his undergraduate degree, though none of these seemed helpful. He initially denied wanting to consider medication but eventually tried, which yielded no therapeutic benefit. A more biologically oriented course of treatment was also tried, but this produced some deleterious side effects which led him to discontinue the treatment.

Mark often wondered if he could even be treated. He had transient suicidal ideation over the years and wondered if he would eventually kill himself, though he never acknowledged any imminent ideation or plans to do so. By contrast, he wondered if he was worth his therapist's time or effort, thinking that he did not deserve the time or attention given to him. His depressive symptoms intensified over the course of treatment, as he found his work situation more and more intolerable. While Mark was able to function adequately in a work setting, his work did not require a college degree and, thus, was below his potential relative to his level of education. At work, Mark complained he would make recommendations to his colleagues that were never implemented. He described these colleagues as apathetic about the work environment and as not wanting to invest the resources needed to improve their work situation. Mark's energy level decreased; he slept often, had little appetite, and struggled to awaken himself to go to work. While he eventually left his first job, a new position ultimately yielded the same results several months later: depression, apathy, and frustration at his ideas not being enacted and being questioned by a team of people charged with solving systemic problems and difficulties.

Mark's other dysfunction occurred in several ways. He had a limited support network. Though he enjoyed online games with friends out of state, his only immediate social support was his girlfriend and therapist. He pulled away from the gaming as his depressive symptoms increased. While his coworkers often shared the same concerns about the job environment as he did, Mark did not find them to be a source of support. Rather, he was reluctant to say anything to them, for fear of feeling worse. These ideas also highlight Mark's difficulties with affiliation and attachment. He often remained aloof and distant from others, even his therapist. Often approaching treatment with some formality and strong inhibition to directly express intense affects, he infrequently articulated emotions other than unhappiness or mild frustration. Even when discussing the therapeutic relationship, Mark seemed to recognize the genuine concern expressed by the therapist yet found a way to minimize its impact (e.g., "you are just doing your job").

With regard to his romantic attachments, Mark remained in a committed relationship with his girlfriend and seemed to be able to engage in somewhat regular sexual activity. However, he was reluctant to marry her, fearing that his depression would be so bad that she would ultimately reject him. While the relationship remained committed, he was not willing to have children, fearing that he would bring someone into the world to suffer as he did. Interestingly, he shared later in the course of treatment that his girlfriend was bisexual and was looking toward adding another person into their relationship. Such ideas did not concern him, nor did he feel typical jealousy or betrayal some may feel regarding a possible change in his romantic partner's sexual orientation.

Finally, Mark's leisure interests were very limited. Though he did participate in some online gaming, he reported no other hobbies or leisurely interests. In his depressive state, he would "surf the web" and watch YouTube© videos, which he never found other than mildly entertaining. Later in treatment, he seemed to take some interest in getting more physically active. However, outside of work and daily chores, he engaged very minimally with others.

Summary of CDD and Social Dysfunction Several highlights emerge in the literature on CDD and social dysfunction. First, in the long run, double depression may be the most profoundly impairing on social dysfunction compared to all other depressive disorders (Hays et al., 1995; Leader & Klein, 1996; Lerner et al., 2004; Zlotnick et al., 2000). Moreover, double depression is much more impairing to social dysfunction than common, chronic medical conditions such as diabetes and arthritis. The double "hit" of severe depressive episodes superimposed on chronic lower-grade depressive symptoms leads people to have entrenched and intensifying difficulties in work, interpersonal, and leisure domains. Moreover, the lack of consistently effective treatment options for double depression further compound the impact of the poor social functioning of this group. Secondly, for those with uMDD, while severity of depressive symptoms is the best predictor of short-term impairment in social dysfunction (Adler et al., 2004), over time such dysfunctions tend to *improve* significantly in uMDD. By contrast, for those with CDDs, while short-term social dysfunctions are less impaired (since symptom severity is less intense than uMDD), over time (2 years and beyond) social dysfunctions tend to *worsen* (Angst et al., 2009; Klein et al., 2008; Rhebergen et al., 2010). Thus, CDD may be more insidiously debilitating than uMDD. The incapacity to engage or enjoy any leisure activities emerged as a particularly pronounced area of social dysfunction in CDD (Friedman et al., 1999; Leader & Klein, 1996).

With regard to treatment, CDD appears to respond best to a combination of antidepressant medication and structured psychotherapy for both symptom reduction and social functioning (Hirschfeld et al., 2002). Further, in this study, psychotherapy had more of a positive impact on social functioning than antidepressant medication in CDD. Finally, CDD likely requires longer-term treatment to improve social dysfunction, which persists long after depressive symptoms improve (Friedman et al., 1999).

5.3 Depression with Personality Disorder (DPD) and Social Dysfunction

Impairments in social functioning are ubiquitous features of personality disorders (PDs) with some form of interpersonal dysfunction represented in each one's diagnostic criteria (APA, 2013). Different forms of personality pathology can exhibit specific patterns of interpersonal distress (e.g., unstable relationships due to a tendency to fluctuate between idealization and devaluation in borderline personality disorder; social inhibition or avoidance due to fear of criticism in avoidant personality disorder). However, the presence of any personality pathology impairs the individual's ability to function effectively in interpersonal settings. Additionally, PDs typically exhibit high rates of comorbidity with other psychopathology, most significantly depressive disorders, which exacerbates existing social impairments (Fertuck et al., 2018). In this section, we will consider studies that examine social dysfunction in individuals with personality pathology and episodic MDD.

A study investigating the impact of PDs on social functioning noted the compounding effects of depression (Newton-Howes, Psych, & Weaver, 2008). Using the Camberwell Assessment of Need and the SFQ, individuals across PD clusters reported greater social dysfunction and unmet social needs. uMDD was the only other disorder that similarly impacted social function in this sample, and the combined effect of PD and depression (i.e., DPD) was related to greater deterioration in social function.

A study examining interpersonal impairments among women compared three groups: those with current uMDD, formerly depressed (remitted uMDD), and those who were never depressed (Hammen & Brennan, 2002). An assessment of the severity of PD features was also conducted. The group of formerly depressed women had the most interpersonal impairment, in areas including marital stability, spousal injury and threatening control, and problems with children, friends, and extended family. This group also reported more stressful life events of an interpersonal nature and reported insecurity in their relations with others. The partners of the formerly depressed women similarly reported lower rates of marital satisfaction. Using the SCID-II interview, it was found that the formerly depressed group exhibited more borderline and dependent personality disorder features than the never-depressed group, suggesting that they exhibited a form of complex depression. It is possible that these personality features contributed to the maintenance of interpersonal dysfunction in the formerly depressed group.

A study investigating social and occupational disability in uMDD patients considered the contributing impact of co-occurring PDs (GÜleÇ & Hocaoğlu, 2011). Participants were divided into depressed and comparison groups using the Hamilton

Depression Rating Scale (HDRS). The Structured Clinical Interview for DSM-III-R; Axis II Disorders was then used to assess for PDs in both groups. The uMDD group displayed higher rates of co-occurring PDs (about 60%) compared to the non-uMDD group (10%). The Short Form-36 (SF-36) scale was used to measure quality of life based on eight dimensions: physical functioning, physical role limitations, emotional role limitations, social functioning, mental health, vitality, bodily pain, and general health perceptions. Depressed participants indicated greater deficits in the domains of physical role limitation, vitality, social functioning, emotional role limitation, and mental health than the non-uMDD group. Additionally, the investigators found that the participants with uMDD and co-occurring PDs showed greater impairments in these domains than those without a PD. Finally, the impact of PD clusters on specific social functioning subscales was examined: while Cluster A PDs showed no significant relationships with any domain, Cluster B PDs displayed a positive correlation with vitality and mental health domains, and Cluster C and Cluster NOS (including self-defeating and passive-aggressive PDs) were negatively correlated with emotional role limitation.

A naturalistic study investigated the compounding impact of co-occurring personality pathology on the social functioning and symptom severity of individuals with uMDD (Skodol et al., 2005). Individuals that met criteria for one of four PDs (schizotypal, borderline, avoidant, and obsessive-compulsive) were included in the uMDD with co-occurring PD group. Additionally, the study recruited from a variety of settings, including outpatient mental health, psychiatric inpatient, and other medical settings. The SF-36 was used to assess physical as well as social and emotional functioning. The latter was measured by four subscales: vitality, social functioning, emotional role limitations, and emotional well-being. These subscales address a wide range of concerns including impaired functioning of normal social activities with family, friends, and other social groups as well as concerns with work or other daily activities. Individuals with DPD displayed poorer functioning on all domains than individuals with uMDD only. In particular, domains of emotional role limitations, social functioning, and general health perceptions were poorest in DPD.

A related study examined the relationship between DPD and long-term social dysfunction (Markowitz et al., 2007). Using the DSM-IV-R diagnostic criteria, participants were divided into three study groups: individuals with uMDD alone, uMDD with persistent and co-occurring PD, and uMDD with remitted comorbid PD. Participants with schizotypal, borderline, avoidant, and obsessive-compulsive personality disorders were included. About 40% of the participants with PD remitted during the 2-year period as assessed by a modified, follow-along version of the Diagnostic Interview for DSM-IV Personality Disorders (remission was noted by the presence of two or fewer criteria over 12 consecutive months). Social functioning was assessed by the Longitudinal Interval Follow-up Evaluation (LIFE) psychosocial scales, which included items relating to employment; interactions with friends, partner, and parents; recreation; global social adjustment; and the DSM-IV Global Assessment of Functioning (GAF). At baseline, the uMDD-only group functioned at significantly higher levels compared to both the PD groups. However, at the 2-year follow-up, the uMDD with remitted PDs group improved significantly, almost catching up with the uMDD group, while the uMDD with non-remitting PD group showed least improvement across domains. The exception was parental relationships, wherein the remitted PDs group did not display significant improvement at follow-up. Finally, the individuals with non-remitting PDs displayed no significant changes in GAF scores over 2 years, remaining in the low 50s (reflective of moderate impairments in social, occupational, or school functioning).

A prospective study examining treatment outcome predictors of uMDD found that extant PDs and certain psychosocial variables were associated with non-complete remission of uMDD and, in some cases, persistence of moderate to severe depressive symptoms (Ezquiaga, García, Pallarés, & Bravo, 1999). Twenty-four percent of the sample displayed partial symptom remission and 17% showed no remission at the 12-month follow-up. The presence of a PD, smaller social network sizes, and less satisfaction with the quality of social support were all associated with the persistence of uMDD symptoms at follow-up. These relationships were reexamined in a subsequent study on a different sample of uMDD participants, wherein existing personality disorders predicted non-remission but not size of and satisfaction with social support networks (Ezquiaga et al., 2004). However, poor quality of life 6 months prior to the current MDE was also associated with lower rates of complete remission. The Quality of Life Scale was used to measure this variable on four dimensions: social support, general satisfaction, physical/psychological well-being, and absence of work overload/free time.

A study investigating the impact of co-occurring PDs on the treatment outcomes of uMDD followed participants in four treatment groups for 16 weeks: cognitive-behavioral therapy, interpersonal therapy, imipramine with case management, and placebo with case management (Shea, Widiger, & Klein, 1992). Social functioning was measured by the Social Adjustment Scale (SAS) that includes scales for social and leisure activities as well as occupational functioning. A majority of uMDD participants displayed co-occurring PD diagnoses (about 74% of the sample), and these individuals had worse outcomes in all social functioning domains except work function. Additionally, the presence of a PD was associated with residual uMDD symptoms posttreatment. The investigators noted that PD clusters or treatment type did not have a significant impact on these findings.

A treatment study similarly demonstrated the negative impact of co-occurring PDs on uMDD treatment and recovery (Patience, McGuire, Scott, & Freeman, 1995). Participants with uMDD were randomly assigned to four treatment groups: regular care with a general practitioner, psychopharmacological treatment with amitriptyline, cognitive-behavioral therapy, and counseling with a social worker. Follow-up assessments of depressive symptoms and social functioning were conducted at the end of treatment (16 weeks) and then at 18 months to determine long-term functioning. It was noted that, despite overall improvement posttreatment, depressed participants with PDs showed worse social functioning than depressed participants without a PD. However, at the 18-month follow-up, no differences were noted in self-reported social functioning between the groups. The investigators surmise that the presence of personality pathology likely delays recovery in individuals with uMDD, specifically with respect to functional impairments.

Most treatment studies examine the effect of a co-occurring PD on the trajectory of uMDD. However, this randomized controlled trial of three psychological treatments investigated the negative impact of comorbid uMDD on the recovery and psychosocial outcomes of individuals with PD (Renner, Bamelis, Huibers, Speckens, & Arntz, 2014). Remission from PDs was defined by no longer meeting the diagnostic criteria on the Structured Clinical Interview for DSM-IV Personality Disorders at 3-year follow-up. Participants mostly had Cluster C diagnoses (92%) and were assigned randomly to schema therapy, clarification-oriented psychotherapy, and treatment as usual groups. Baseline evaluations indicated that participants with co-occurring uMDD displayed lower Global Assessment of Functioning (GAF) scores as well as impaired social and occupational functioning. These participants also experienced lower rates of recovery from PDs posttreatment compared to participants without a comorbid uMDD diagnosis at baseline – an effect that did not differ between treatment conditions. Additionally, despite some improvement, the lower baseline social functioning levels noted in participants with uMDD do not catch up to the posttreatment functioning levels of participants without uMDD.

An Illustrative Case of DPD and Social Dysfunction Leah, as a 22-year-old college graduate of European descent, was diagnosed with BPD and recurrent MDD in her third year of undergraduate studies, having had two hospitalizations while completing her degree. She found herself regularly feeling hopeless and unmotivated. Leah had a boyfriend who appeared to offer regular support, though her mood state frequently remained dysphoric and uncertain about her future. Previous treatment in dialectical behavior therapy was not helpful, so she sought out treatment from a psychodynamically oriented clinician. In this treatment, Leah described sadness, helplessness, and pessimism, thinking that there was no meaning or purpose in her life, which thus led to her frequent suicidal ideation. Evenings were very problematic, as she would find her depressive feelings intensifying, even sometimes taking a belt and putting it around her neck, fantasizing about hanging herself. Leah believed that no one appreciated her misery but that after she died, she imagined others would finally understand how much she had suffered.

Leah had received high grades in a scientifically oriented degree. She moved home after graduation, which evoked strong ideas of being oppressed and disapproved of by her parents. She had very little identity of her own around her mother, complying with most everything she said. However, her resentment grew and was highest at night. Leah remained at her parents' home, believing that she could not leave without permission. She was evasive of the therapist's questions about her own ideas, only repeating what her mother's opinions were about her future and life outcome. Most notably, she considered that she should take a job out of state (which her mother strongly pressed for), even though she wanted to remain at home and stay in treatment with her therapist.

Like Mark (described earlier), Leah's only social support was her romantic partner (boyfriend), who happened to live hundreds of miles away. She had few other friends with whom she communicated, and most of her life was lived in isolation in her room at her parents' house. Though she had an older brother at home, their relationship was strained since Leah believed he did not care much about her suffering of distress. Leah seemed to appreciate the frequent weekly sessions with her therapist but did little to seek out other friendships. Likewise, her relationships toward others were detached and disinterested; however, once relationships moved into friendships, she believed she could share more intense ideas and feelings. Yet, she failed to incorporate the support of others, frequently questioning if they had her best interests in mind, including her therapist, who often found her to wait silently for him to offer ideas of support.

Leah had only one romantic partner, who was patient and committed to her. It was unclear to what extent they were sexually involved, and Leah never spoke about her sexuality or sexual interests. Leah's mood seemed dependent upon the support and availability of her boyfriend. In fact, one of her suicide attempts occurred after leaving a party early and feeling as if her boyfriend did not care. Hence, there was less interest in mutual romantic satisfaction but instead more of a need-gratifying orientation toward her boyfriend. By all accounts, the relationship was one of dependency and not mutual liking.

As one might imagine, Leah had no outside hobbies or activities. Like Mark, she would watch YouTube©, television, or movies, all from home. Even as a university student, it was unclear that Leah engaged in anything other than school and spending time with her boyfriend and a few people who lived in the same dormitory. Consequently, her life appeared empty, which corresponded to the lack of meaning she often described.

Summary of DPD and Social Dysfunction While the literature examining the relationship between DPD and social functioning is limited, a few major findings are noted in the above studies. First and most notably, DPD is associated with a far greater level of social dysfunction than other forms of psychopathology (Newton-Howes et al., 2008), and the combined effect of DPD is associated with significantly worse impairments than the independent effects of uMDD or PD across domains of social function (GÜleÇ & Hocaoğlu, 2011; Markowitz et al., 2007; Renner et al., 2014; Skodol et al., 2005). The synergistic impact of depression and personality pathology shows enduring and deleterious effects on social function even in the context of PD or uMDD remission (Hammen & Brennan, 2002; Markowitz et al., 2007). Given the early development and chronicity of interpersonal difficulties in PDs, it is unsurprising that functional impairment persists. Similar to CDD (described above), the lack of effective treatment options available for DPD further contributes to the maintenance of these impairments. Secondly, the relationship between DPD and social dysfunction was consistently observed across PD clusters and severity despite variations in their presentation (Hammen & Brennan, 2002; Markowitz et al., 2007; Skodol et al., 2005), which is indicative of the pervasive and intense nature of functional impairment in individuals with DPD. However, few studies examined the differential effects of PD clusters on social function domains, making it difficult to understand the specific pathological personality features that contribute to social impairments in these individuals.

Finally, extant personality disorders have a negative impact on the course and prognosis of social functioning in depressive disorders (Ezquiaga, García et al., 1999; Ezquiaga, García-López et al., 2004; Mulder, 2002; Shea et al., 1992). DPD individuals seem to benefit less from treatment and display persistent depressive symptoms as well as higher rates of recurrent episodes than individuals with depression and no PD (Ezquiaga, García et al., 1999; Ezquiaga, García-López et al., 2004; Hart, Craighead, & Craighead, 2001). The moderating effects of PDs on the maintenance of social impairments associated with uMDD and vice versa suggest that more long-term, targeted treatments may be needed to improve functional impairments in DPD.

5.4 Conclusions and Future Directions

While both CDD and DPD are associated with profound and chronic social dysfunction compared to uncomplicated MDD, this scoping review suggests two potentially contrasting trajectories of social dysfunction between CDD and DPD. The adult trajectory of social dysfunction in CDD – particularly double depression (Hays et al., 1995; Leader & Klein, 1996; Lerner et al., 2004; Zlotnick et al., 2000) – may be analogous to an incremental but pervasive decline over time. The analogy for CDD is to a long, gradual ramp ending in severe social dysfunction, touching nearly all domains (e.g., the case of Mark). By contrast, DPD has an adult trajectory that begins with significant impairment in multiple social functions (likely reflecting the impact of the PD, which typically has a late adolescent onset). However, rather than a gradual decline, DPD appears to exhibit plateaus and valleys, the valleys occurring when there is an intensification of depressive symptoms in the context of the PD, after which some improvement back to the relatively low baseline level of functioning can occur (e.g., the case of Leah). These potential trajectories of social dysfunction, a slow decline in CDD and a low plateau with even lower valleys in DPD, warrant further longitudinal investigation.

While there are no unambiguous comparisons between CDD and DPD in the literature, it appears that social dysfunction in DPD is associated with more turbulent relationship instability (Hammen & Brennan, 2002; Markowitz et al., 2007), whereas CDD is more associated with a lack of motivation or inhibition in pursuing social relations (Leader & Klein, 1996; Rhebergen et al., 2010). Both the case illustration (Leah) and the DPD literature suggest that disruption in close or romantic relationships precipitate worsening depressive symptoms and subsequent "valleys" in social functioning.

With regard to treatment implications, for both CDD and DPD, social dysfunctions are more treatment resistant than depressive symptoms themselves. Treatment development for CDD and DPD needs to target *both* symptom reduction and functional improvement. In terms of long-term improvement and stability of change, social functioning may be more important to nurture and sustain than symptomatic improvement. While data is limited to one study, it appears that structured psychotherapy confers the most benefit for social functioning, and combined psychotherapy and antidepressant medication for symptoms. Intervention for BPD (e.g., transference-focused psychotherapy [TFP]) (Radcliffe & Yeomans, 2019), for instance, requires that patients agree to explicit goals around occupational roles as a precondition for treatment, which may be worth incorporating in the treatment of CDD and DPD. Moreover, examining the impact of leisure activities (particularly aerobic exercise) on psychological well-being is a potential low-cost, alternative treatment for individuals with depression (Blumenthal et al., 2007) and anxiety (Martinsen, 2008) that is worth examining in CDD and DPD as adjunctive interventions. Engaging in recreational activities can distract individuals from the experience of depression and promote feelings of well-being by increasing perceptions of social support or self-improvement (Chang, Wray, & Lin, 2014).

The therapeutic alliance, which is generally regarded as one of the strongest predictors of treatment gain in psychotherapy (Horvath, Del Re, Flückiger, & Symonds, 2011; Wampold, 2015), is negatively impacted by depressive symptoms. However, the capacity to establish an early alliance in treatment of individuals with CDD predicted improvements in symptoms (Barber, Khalsa, & Sharpless, 2010; Klein et al., 2003). Additionally, strong early alliances that would be able to withstand and repair future alliance ruptures predicted significant improvements in symptoms of personality disorder and CDD (Strauss et al., 2006). Strains and ruptures in the alliance are frequently observed in the treatment of personality disorders and often lead to treatment noncompliance and premature termination (Jin, Sklar, Min Sen Oh, & Chuen Li, 2008). Thus, DPD seems to be associated with poorer working alliances and treatment compliance rates (Andreoli, Gressot, Aapro, Tricot, & Gognalons, 1989). One study found that more severe depression negatively impacts the therapeutic alliance in the treatment of BPD (Richardson-Vejlgaard, Broudy, Brodsky, Fertuck, & Stanley, 2013), suggesting that reducing depressive symptoms early on the treatment of PDs will enhance treatment outcomes as well.

Other high priority areas for future investigation include developing more refined measures of social dysfunction that are not confounded by symptom severity, since in CDD and DPD, social dysfunction can be difficult to disentangle from symptoms. Further, future investigations could better differentiate the domains of social dysfunction between uMDD, CDD, and DPD and over the course of these disorders. Relatedly, the impact of different expressions of DPD (i.e., BPD, narcissistic PD, or Cluster A PDs) on social dysfunctions has not been sufficiently investigated. Finally, potential gender, biological sex, social class, and cultural influences on social dysfunction in CDD and DPD are a ripe area of investigation.

References

Adler, D. A., Irish, J., McLaughlin, T. J., Perissinotto, C., Chang, H., Hood, M., … Lerner, D. (2004). The work impact of dysthymia in a primary care population. *General Hospital Psychiatry, 26*(4), 269–276. https://doi.org/10.1016/j.genhosppsych.2004.04.004

Andreoli, A., Gressot, G., Aapro, N., Tricot, L., & Gognalons, M. Y. (1989). Personality disorders as a predictor of outcome. *Journal of Personality Disorders, 3*(4), 307–320. https://doi.org/10.1521/pedi.1989.3.4.307

Angst, J., Gamma, A., Rössler, W., Ajdacic, V., & Klein, D. N. (2009). Long-term depression versus episodic major depression: Results from the prospective Zurich study of a community sample. *Journal of Affective Disorders, 115*(1–2), 112–121. https://doi.org/10.1016/j.jad.2008.09.023

Barber, J. P., Khalsa, S.-R., & Sharpless, B. A. (2010). The validity of the alliance as a predictor of psychotherapy outcome. In *The therapeutic alliance: An evidence-based guide to practice* (pp. 29–43). New York, NY: The Guilford Press.

Baune, B. T., & Renger, L. (2014). Pharmacological and non-pharmacological interventions to improve cognitive dysfunction and functional ability in clinical depression – A systematic review. *Psychiatry Research, 219*(1), 25–50. https://doi.org/10.1016/j.psychres.2014.05.013

Benazon, N. R., & Coyne, J. C. (2000). Living with a depressed spouse. *Journal of Family Psychology, 14*(1), 71–79. https://doi.org/10.1037/0893-3200.14.1.71

Birchwood, M., Smith, J., Cochrane, R., Wetton, S., & Copestake, S. (1990). The social functioning scale. The development and validation of a new scale of social adjustment for use in family intervention programmes with schizophrenic patients. *The British Journal of Psychiatry: the Journal of Mental Science, 157*, 853–859. https://doi.org/10.1192/bjp.157.6.853

Blumenthal, J. A., Babyak, M. A., Murali Doraiswamy, P., Watkins, L., Hoffman, B. M., Barbour, K. A., … Sherwood, A. (2007). Exercise and pharmacotherapy in the treatment of major depressive disorder. *Psychosomatic Medicine, 69*(7), 587–596. https://doi.org/10.1097/PSY.0b013e318148c19a

Chan, E. H. C., Kong, S. D. X., Park, S. H., Song, Y. J. C., Demetriou, E. A., Pepper, K. L., … Guastella, A. J. (2019). Validation of the social functioning scale: Comparison and evaluation in early psychosis, autism spectrum disorder and social anxiety disorder. *Psychiatry Research, 276*, 45–55. https://doi.org/10.1016/j.psychres.2019.03.037

Chang, P.-J., Wray, L., & Lin, Y. (2014). Social relationships, leisure activity, and health in older adults. *Health Psychology, 33*(6), 516–523. https://doi.org/10.1037/hea0000051

Combs, B., & Heaton, K. (2016). Occupational functionality: A concept analysis. *Workplace Health & Safety, 64*(8), 385–392. https://doi.org/10.1177/2165079916643099

Daley, S. E., Burge, D., & Hammen, C. (2000). Borderline personality disorder symptoms as predictors of 4-year romantic relationship dysfunction in young women: Addressing issues of specificity. *Journal of Abnormal Psychology, 109*(3), 451–460. https://doi.org/10.1037/0021-843X.109.3.451

Daremo, Å., Kjellberg, A., & Haglund, L. (2015, February 11). *Occupational performance and affective symptoms for patients with depression disorder* [Research Article]. Advances in Psychiatry; Hindawi. https://doi.org/10.1155/2015/438149.

Davila, J. (2001). Paths to unhappiness: The overlapping courses of depression and romantic dysfunction. In *Marital and family processes in depression: A scientific foundation for clinical practice* (pp. 71–87). Washington, DC: American Psychological Association. https://doi.org/10.1037/10350-004

De Rubeis, J., Lugo, R. G., Witthöft, M., Sütterlin, S., Pawelzik, M. R., & Vögele, C. (2017). Rejection sensitivity as a vulnerability marker for depressive symptom deterioration in men. *PLoS One, 12*(10). https://doi.org/10.1371/journal.pone.0185802

Ehnvall, A., Mitchell, P. B., Hadzi-Pavlovic, D., Parker, G., Frankland, A., Loo, C., … Perich, T. (2014). Rejection sensitivity and pain in bipolar versus unipolar depression. *Bipolar Disorders, 16*(2), 190–198. https://doi.org/10.1111/bdi.12147

Ezquiaga, E., García, A, Pallarés, T., & Bravo, M. F. (1999). Psychosocial predictors of outcome in major depression: A prospective 12-month study. *Journal of Affective Disorders, 52*(1–3), 209–216. https://doi.org/10.1016/s0165-0327(98)00057-3

Ezquiaga, E., García-López, A, de Dios, C., Leiva, A., Bravo, M., & Montejo, J. (2004). Clinical and psychosocial factors associated with the outcome of unipolar major depression: A one

year prospective study. *Journal of Affective Disorders, 79*(1), 63–70. https://doi.org/10.1016/S0165-0327(02)00346-4
Fertuck, E. A., Chesin, M. S., & Johnston, B. (2018). Borderline personality disorders and mood disorders. In B. Stanley & A. New (Eds.), *Borderline personality disorder*. New York, NY: Oxford University Press.
Friedman, R. A., Markowitz, J. C., Parides, M., Gniwesch, L., & Kocsis, J. H. (1999). Six months of desipramine for dysthymia: Can dysthymic patients achieve normal social functioning? *Journal of Affective Disorders, 54*(3), 283–286. https://doi.org/10.1016/S0165-0327(98)00129-3
Goodman, W. K., Geiger, A. M., & Wolf, J. M. (2016). Differential links between leisure activities and depressive symptoms in unemployed individuals. *Journal of Clinical Psychology, 72*(1), 70–78. https://doi.org/10.1002/jclp.22231
GÜleÇ, M. Y., & Hocaoğlu, Ç. (2011). Relationship between personality and disability in patients with major depressive disorder. *The Israel Journal of Psychiatry and Related Sciences, 48*(2), 123–128.
Hammen, C., & Brennan, P. A. (2002). Interpersonal dysfunction in depressed women: Impairments independent of depressive symptoms. *Journal of Affective Disorders, 72*(2), 145–156. https://doi.org/10.1016/S0165-0327(01)00455-4
Hart, A. B., Craighead, W. E., & Craighead, L. W. (2001). Predicting recurrence of major depressive disorder in young adults: A prospective study. *Journal of Abnormal Psychology, 110*(4), 633–643. https://doi.org/10.1037/0021-843X.110.4.633
Hays, R. D., Wells, K. B., Sherbourne, C. B., Rogers, W., & Spritzer, K. (1995). Functioning and well-being outcomes of patients with depression compared with chronic general medical illnesses. *Archives of General Psychiatry, 52*(1), 11. https://doi.org/10.1001/archpsyc.1995.03950130011002
Hirschfeld, R. M. A., Dunner, D. L., Keitner, G., Klein, D. N., Koran, L. M., Kornstein, S. G., … Keller, M. B. (2002). Does psychosocial functioning improve independent of depressive symptoms? A comparison of nefazodone, psychotherapy, and their combination. *Biological Psychiatry, 51*(2), 123–133. https://doi.org/10.1016/S0006-3223(01)01291-4
Horvath, A. O., Del Re, A. C., Flückiger, C., & Symonds, D. (2011). Alliance in individual psychotherapy. *Psychotherapy (Chicago, Ill.), 48*(1), 9–16. https://doi.org/10.1037/a0022186
Huprich, S. K. (2012). Considering the evidence and making the most empirically informed decision about depressive personality disorder in DSM-5. *Personality Disorders, Theory, Research, and Treatment, 3*(4), 470–482. https://doi.org/10.1037/a0027765
Huprich, S. K. (2014). Malignant self-regard: A self-structure enhancing the understanding of masochistic, depressive, and vulnerably narcissistic personalities. *Harvard Review of Psychiatry, 22*(5), 295–305. https://doi.org/10.1097/HRP.0000000000000019
Huprich, S. K. (2019). Personality-driven depression: The case for malignant self-regard (and depressive personalities). *Journal of Clinical Psychology, 75*(5), 834–845. https://doi.org/10.1002/jclp.22760
Huprich, S. K. (2020). Commentary on the special issue: Critical distinctions between vulnerable narcissism and depressive personalities. *Journal of Personality Disorders, 34*(Supplement), 207–209. https://doi.org/10.1521/pedi.2020.34.supp.207
Jin, J., Sklar, G. E., Min Sen Oh, V., & Chuen Li, S. (2008). Factors affecting therapeutic compliance: A review from the patient's perspective. *Therapeutics and Clinical Risk Management, 4*(1), 269–286.
Joiner, T. E., & Katz, J. (1999). Contagion of depressive symptoms and mood: Meta-analytic review and explanations from cognitive, behavioral, and interpersonal viewpoints. *Clinical Psychology: Science and Practice, 6*(2), 149–164. https://doi.org/10.1093/clipsy.6.2.149
Kamenov, K., Twomey, C., Cabello, M., Prina, A. M., & Ayuso-Mateos, J. L. (2017). The efficacy of psychotherapy, pharmacotherapy and their combination on functioning and quality of life in depression: A meta-analysis. *Psychological Medicine, 47*(3), 414–425. https://doi.org/10.1017/S0033291716002774

Klein, D. N., Schwartz, J. E., Santiago, N. J., Vivian, D., Vocisano, C., Castonguay, L. G., … Keller, M. B. (2003). Therapeutic alliance in depression treatment: Controlling for prior change and patient characteristics. *Journal of Consulting and Clinical Psychology, 71*(6), 997–1006. https://doi.org/10.1037/0022-006X.71.6.997

Klein, D. N., Shankman, S. A., & Rose, S. (2008). Dysthymic disorder and double depression: Prediction of 10-year course trajectories and outcomes. *Journal of Psychiatric Research, 42*(5), 408–415. https://doi.org/10.1016/j.jpsychires.2007.01.009

Knight, M. J., & Baune, B. T. (2017). Psychosocial dysfunction in major depressive disorder – Rationale, design, and characteristics of the cognitive and emotional recovery training program for depression (CERT-D). *Frontiers in Psychiatry, 8*. https://doi.org/10.3389/fpsyt.2017.00280

Kupferberg, A., Bicks, L., & Hasler, G. (2016). Social functioning in major depressive disorder. *Neuroscience & Biobehavioral Reviews, 69*, 313–332. https://doi.org/10.1016/j.neubiorev.2016.07.002

Leader, J. B., & Klein, D. N. (1996). Social adjustment in dysthymia, double depression and episodic major depression. *Journal of Affective Disorders, 37*(2–3), 91–101. FRANCIS.

Leigh-Hunt, N., Bagguley, D., Bash, K., Turner, V., Turnbull, S., Valtorta, N., & Caan, W. (2017). An overview of systematic reviews on the public health consequences of social isolation and loneliness. *Public Health, 152*, 157–171. https://doi.org/10.1016/j.puhe.2017.07.035

Lerner, D., Adler, D. A., Chang, H., Berndt, E. R., Irish, J. T., Lapitsky, L., … Rogers, W. H. (2004). The clinical and occupational correlates of work productivity loss among employed patients with depression. *Journal of Occupational and Environmental Medicine, 46*(Supplement), S46–S55. https://doi.org/10.1097/01.jom.0000126684.82825.0a

Markowitz, J. C., Skodol, A. E., Petkova, E., Cheng, J., Sanislow, C. A., Grilo, C. M., … McGlashan, T. H. (2007). Longitudinal effects of personality disorders on psychosocial functioning of patients with major depressive disorder. *The Journal of Clinical Psychiatry, 68*(02), 186–193. https://doi.org/10.4088/JCP.v68n0202

Martinsen, E. W. (2008). Physical activity in the prevention and treatment of anxiety and depression. *Nordic Journal of Psychiatry, 62*(Suppl 47), 25–29. https://doi.org/10.1080/08039480802315640

McCullough, J. P., Kasnetz, M. D., Braith, J. A., Carr, K. F., Cones, J. H., Fielo, J., & Martelli, M. F. (1988). A longitudinal study of an untreated sample of predominantly late onset characterological dysthymia. *The Journal of Nervous and Mental Disease, 176*(11), 658–667. https://doi.org/10.1097/00005053-198811000-00003

Moos, R. H., Cronkite, R. C., & Moos, B. S. (1998). The long-term interplay between family and extrafamily resources and depression. *Journal of Family Psychology, 12*(3), 326–343. https://doi.org/10.1037/0893-3200.12.3.326

Morelli, S. A., Lee, I. A., Arnn, M. E., & Zaki, J. (2015). Emotional and instrumental support provision interact to predict well-being. *Emotion (Washington, D.C.), 15*(4), 484–493. https://doi.org/10.1037/emo0000084

Mulder, R. T. (2002). Personality pathology and treatment outcome in major depression: A review. *The American Journal of Psychiatry, 159*(3), 359–371. https://doi.org/10.1176/appi.ajp.159.3.359

Munn, Z., Peters, M. D. J., Stern, C., Tufanaru, C., McArthur, A., & Aromataris, E. (2018). Systematic review or scoping review? Guidance for authors when choosing between a systematic or scoping review approach. *BMC Medical Research Methodology, 18*(1), 143. https://doi.org/10.1186/s12874-018-0611-x

Newton-Howes, G., Psych, M. R. C., Tyrer, P., & Weaver, T. (2008). Social functioning of patients with personality disorder in secondary care. *Psychiatric Services, 59*(9), 5.

Nydegger, R. (2008). Psychologists and hospice: Where we are and where we can be. *Professional Psychology: Research and Practice, 39*(4), 459–463. https://doi.org/10.1037/0735-7028.39.4.459

Oddone, C. G., Hybels, C. F., McQuoid, D. R., & Steffens, D. C. (2011). Social support modifies the relationship between personality and depressive symptoms in older adults. *The American*

Journal of Geriatric Psychiatry: Official Journal of the American Association for Geriatric Psychiatry, 19(2), 123–131.

Oltmanns, T. F., Melley, A. H., & Turkheimer, E. (2002). Impaired social functioning and symptoms of personality disorders assessed by peer and self-report in a nonclinical population. *Journal of Personality Disorders, 16*(5), 437–452.

Patience, D. A., McGuire, R. J., Scott, A. I. F., & Freeman, C. P. L. (1995). The Edinburgh primary care depression study: Personality disorder and outcome. *The British Journal of Psychiatry, 167*(3), 324–330. https://doi.org/10.1192/bjp.167.3.324

Radcliffe, J., & Yeomans, F. (2019). Transference-focused psychotherapy for patients with personality disorders: Overview and case example with a focus on the use of contracting: TFP for patients with personality disorders. *British Journal of Psychotherapy, 35*(1), 4–23. https://doi.org/10.1111/bjp.12421

Ren, P., Qin, X., Zhang, Y., & Zhang, R. (2018). Is social support a cause or consequence of depression? A longitudinal study of adolescents. *Frontiers in Psychology, 9*. https://doi.org/10.3389/fpsyg.2018.01634

Renner, F., Bamelis, L. L. M., Huibers, M. J. H., Speckens, A., & Arntz, A. (2014). The impact of comorbid depression on recovery from personality disorders and improvements in psychosocial functioning: Results from a randomized controlled trial. *Behaviour Research and Therapy, 63*, 55–62. https://doi.org/10.1016/j.brat.2014.09.006

Rhebergen, D., Beekman, A. T. F., de Graaf, R., Nolen, W. A., Spijker, J., Hoogendijk, W. J., & Penninx, B. W. J. H. (2010). Trajectories of recovery of social and physical functioning in major depression, dysthymic disorder and double depression: A 3-year follow-up. *Journal of Affective Disorders, 124*(1–2), 148–156. https://doi.org/10.1016/j.jad.2009.10.029

Richardson-Vejlgaard, R., Broudy, C., Brodsky, B., Fertuck, E., & Stanley, B. (2013). Predictors of psychotherapy alliance in Borderline Personality Disorder. *Psychotherapy Research, 23*(5), 539–546. https://doi.org/10.1080/10503307.2013.801001

Santini, Z. I., Koyanagi, A., Tyrovolas, S., & Haro, J. M. (2015). The association of relationship quality and social networks with depression, anxiety, and suicidal ideation among older married adults: Findings from a cross-sectional analysis of the Irish Longitudinal Study on Ageing (TILDA). *Journal of Affective Disorders, 179*, 134–141. https://doi.org/10.1016/j.jad.2015.03.015

Sharabi, L. L., Delaney, A. L., & Knobloch, L. K. (2016). In their own words: How clinical depression affects romantic relationships. *Journal of Social and Personal Relationships, 33*(4), 421–448. https://doi.org/10.1177/0265407515578820

Shea, M. T., Widiger, T. A., & Klein, M. H. (1992). Comorbidity of personality disorders and depression: Implications for treatment. *Journal of Consulting and Clinical Psychology, 60*(6), 857–868. https://doi.org/10.1037/0022-006X.60.6.857

Skodol, A. E., Grilo, C. M., Pagano, M. E., Bender, D. S., Gunderson, J. G., Shea, M. T., … Mcglashan, T. H. (2005). Effects of personality disorders on functioning and well-being in major depressive disorder. *Journal of Psychiatric Practice, 11*(6), 363–368.

Strauss, J. L., Hayes, A. M., Johnson, S. L., Newman, C. F., Brown, G. K., Barber, J. P., … Beck, A. T. (2006). Early alliance, alliance ruptures, and symptom change in a nonrandomized trial of cognitive therapy for avoidant and obsessive-compulsive personality disorders. *Journal of Consulting and Clinical Psychology, 74*(2), 337–345. https://doi.org/10.1037/0022-006X.74.2.337

Tyrer, P., Nur, U., Crawford, M., Karlsen, S., McLean, C., Rao, B., & Johnson, T. (2011). Social functioning questionnaire [data set]. *American Psychological Association*. https://doi.org/10.1037/t03074-000

van Lankveld, J., Jacobs, N., Thewissen, V., Dewitte, M., & Verboon, P. (2018). The associations of intimacy and sexuality in daily life: Temporal dynamics and gender effects within romantic relationships. *Journal of Social and Personal Relationships, 35*(4), 557–576.

Visentini, C., Cassidy, M., Bird, V. J., & Priebe, S. (2018). Social networks of patients with chronic depression: A systematic review. *Journal of Affective Disorders, 241*, 571–578. https://doi.org/10.1016/j.jad.2018.08.022

Wampold, B. E. (2015). How important are the common factors in psychotherapy? An update. *World Psychiatry, 14*(3), 270. https://doi.org/10.1002/wps.20238
Wang, J., Mann, F., Lloyd-Evans, B., Ma, R., & Johnson, S. (2018). Associations between loneliness and perceived social support and outcomes of mental health problems: A systematic review. *BMC Psychiatry, 18*. https://doi.org/10.1186/s12888-018-1736-5
Weissman, M. M. (1975). The assessment of social adjustment: a review of techniques. *Archives of General Psychiatry, 32*, 357–365.
Weissman, M. M., & Bothwell, S. (1976). Assessment of social adjustment by patient self-report. *Archives of General Psychiatry, 9*, 1111–1115.
Zhang, J., & Zheng, Y. (2017). How do academic stress and leisure activities influence college students' emotional well-being? A daily diary investigation. *Journal of Adolescence, 60*, 114–118. https://doi.org/10.1016/j.adolescence.2017.08.003
Zlotnick, C., Kohn, R., Keitner, G., & Della Grotta, S. A. (2000). The relationship between quality of interpersonal relationships and major depressive disorder: Findings from the National Comorbidity Survey. *Journal of Affective Disorders, 59*(3), 205–215. https://doi.org/10.1016/S0165-0327(99)00153-6

Chapter 6
Neurobiological Findings Underlying Personality Dysfunction in Depression: From Vulnerability to Differential Susceptibility

Alberto Botto and Caroline Leighton

Abstract The relationship between temperament as a manifestation of personality and mood disorders comes from Greek antiquity. Throughout history, the relationship between personality and depression has been conceptualized in at least four ways: (1) Personality is a predisposing or vulnerability factor for the development of depression. (2) Personality changes are a consequence of mood alteration resulting from depression. (3) Personality is a subclinical manifestation of depression (affective temperaments). And (4) personality characteristics influence the manner in which depression clinically manifests. Currently, there is a tendency to recover the concept of affective temperaments (depressive, hypertensive, cyclothymic, irritable, and anxious), considering them as subclinical manifestations of some disorder within the affective spectrum. These temperaments have been shown to be universal, with distinctive characteristics and without gender differences. Although in depressive illness there is important evidence regarding both functional and structural neurobiological alterations, much less is known about the biological findings of personality dysfunction in depression. One reason, in part, is that explanatory models are required that integrate various levels of analysis, including the different types of gene-environment relationships. In this chapter, we will review the relationship between personality and depression, then we will describe the main neurobiological findings underlying personality dysfunction in depression, and finally we will analyze the relationship between genes and environment in depression, taking into account the approach of differential sensitivity to environmental stimuli. We will conclude with some recommendations for future research.

Keywords Neurobiology · Personality · Affective temperaments · Depression · Gene-environment relationship

A. Botto (✉) · C. Leighton
Departamento de Psiquiatría y Salud Mental Campus Oriente, Facultad de Medicina, Universidad de Chile, Santiago, Chile

Millennium Institute for Research in Depression and Personality (MIDAP), Santiago, Chile

G. de la Parra et al. (eds.), *Depression and Personality Dysfunction*, Depression and Personality, https://doi.org/10.1007/978-3-030-70699-9_6

6.1 Introduction

Traditionally, it has been considered that personality (i.e., the habitual way of being and behaving of individuals) is composed of two fundamental aspects: the character and the temperament. Character is related to the way we see ourselves and behave based on learning and developing of our psychic life in interaction with others trough socialization. Temperament, on the other hand, is linked to biological based, innate attitudes, behaviors, and reactions to a series of environmental challenges and has genetic and neurobiological correlates that have been linked to critical processes, involving cognition, emotion, and behavior (Coccaro & Siever, 2005). However, for some authors, this distinction is questionable since personality traits would present all the characteristics of temperament, and they prefer to use the terms "personality" and "temperament" as if they were synonymous (Krueger & Johnson, 2008).

The relationship between temperament as a manifestation of personality and mood alterations comes from Greek antiquity (Berrios & Porter, 1995). At the beginning of the last century, Emil Kraepelin (2012) distinguished, within the forms of presentation of mood alterations, the affective episodes that broke into the continuity of life (and that generally came at the margin of external influences), from those manifestations – the so-called fundamental states – that persisted chronically independently of these episodes. These alterations consisted of certain singularities of the psychic life that were characterized by a permanent temperamental disposition before the experiences of life which he called "constitutions" and classified them into the following: depressive ("constitutional depression"), manic ("constitutional excitement"), and irritable and cyclothymic (successive alternation of depression and excitement). According to Kraepelin, the "depressive constitution" is characterized by a gloomy and insecure attitude, often accompanied by doubts and worries, with a tendency to sterile ruminations, especially of the hypochondriac type. Often the person feels overwhelmed and desperate, saying that "he has always felt this way." Everything seems serious to them, full of fears, feelings of guilt, and self-reproach. Each task is transformed into an unattainable enterprise, devoting themselves to their duties with abnegation but being unable to enjoy them. Many of these characteristics are manifested from youth in a more or less constant way, but it can also be the case in which they are imperceptibly transformed into affective episodes, which – Kraepelin says – reveals the intimate kinship that unites the manic-depressive illness with the depressive constitution, the latter corresponding to a preliminary state of the illness. The "manic constitution" or "constitutional excitement" is characterized by a higher-than-average intelligence, with a marked creativity, which can sometimes be altered by a tendency to distractibility and impulsivity, so that these subjects may appear as little reflective and rather superficial. In general, the mood is elevated, with greater self-confidence and high self-esteem, overvaluing their abilities and acting in an arrogant and provocative manner. They tend to be very sociable and communicative, easily adaptable to new situations, and therefore changeable and unpredictable, evidencing a scarce capacity for planning, which leads them to fleeting choices regarding their occupations and their interpersonal relationships. For the same reason, they usually maintain a conflictive relationship with their environment. There are often mood swings that can alternate with periods of distress and depression. However, in milder cases, they can be bright, vital, charming, and creative individuals close to genius. The "irritable constitution" is a combination of the first two. Individuals show a tendency to extreme oscillation in their moods, being very sensitive to life events. They are combative, unpredictable, and easily offended and can explode into insolence, anger, and aggression. Their mood is changing through periods of anxiety, moodiness, discouragement, and complaints of all kinds. Finally, the "cyclothymic constitution" is presented as a chronic and regular variation of mood in a manic or depressive sense. Unlike the irritable one, the cyclothymic alternates in its moods, appearing in one moment as full of joy and joviality and in another as completely dejected and depressed. These changes can last for weeks or months and can be the early manifestation of a manic-depressive psychosis.

Something similar was described by Kretschmer – with the picnic type in 1925 – and Sheldon – with the endomorphic constitution in 1940 – linking the affective psychosis with the cycloid temperament and a particular form of physical constitution characterized by an increase in volume in the visceral cavities, tendency to fat deposits in the lower part of the trunk, rather fine thorax, and thin limbs, with small hands and feet. However, at present, no clear evidence has been found regarding the association between bipolarity and body mass index (Ikeda et al., 2018).

Several decades later, in his text of 1946, Kurt Schneider referred to psychopathic personalities as "those personalities who suffer because of their abnormality or because of whose abnormality society suffers" and placed within them depressive psychopaths (Schneider, 1997). The fundamental state of mind of these subjects does not have such a direct relationship with temperament as in the case of hyperthymic psychopaths; however, they also suffer because of a constantly oppressed state of mind and a pessimistic and skeptical conception of life. They are insecure, anxious, lacking in self-confidence, flooded by multiple doubts and ponderings, and incapable of enjoying themselves, as if they were immersed in deep, grave, and heavy grief.

Later, Hubertus Tellenbach (1976) developed the concept of *typus melancholicus* to refer to a set of character traits that determine premorbid personality in melancholic depression. For Tellenbach, the essential constituent trait of the depressive is the fixation to a quest for order. These are characteristics of its meticulousness, scrupulosity, hypernomy (excessively rigid adaptation to social norms and established practices, leading to a stereotyped application of rules regardless of context), heteronomy (exaggerated influence of usual external practices, where each action of the subject is guided by impersonal motivations referred to socially established criteria), and intolerance to ambiguity, in addition to a permanent interest in the fulfillment of work tasks and an excessive concern for performance, especially in relations with others. The subject lives in a constant threat between the desire to fulfill and the high level of demands placed on himself, which easily triggers feelings of guilt and inadequacy. However, these temperamental dispositions only constitute the premorbid personality of depression. In order for the endogenous-melancholic transformation to occur – and thus become the depressive illness – it is necessary to have a special relationship with the lived world, what Tellenbach calls *situational constellations*.

Throughout life, people face two fundamental psychological challenges: (1) maintain close, reciprocal, and meaningful interpersonal relationships and (2) maintain a differentiated, coherent, realistic, and integrated sense of self. Based on these polarities (relationality and self-definition, respectively), Blatt (2008) has developed a theoretical model for understanding psychological development, personality organization, sources of psychopathology, and mechanisms of change in psychotherapy. This model is based on a conception of nonlinear, dialectical, and complex psychobiological development, in which the progress of certain domains allows the parallel advance of others, such as that occurs with the development of the sense of self and interpersonal relations. Its main assumption is that the quality of the depressive experience depends on the personality whose development occurs in a dialectical and synergic interaction between the tendency toward self-definition (identity) and interpersonal relatedness (Blatt & Luyten, 2009). These dimensions have been called, respectively, introyective (autonomy/perfectionism) and anaclitic (dependence/sociotropy). Both dimensions are associated with different personality structures, different relational and attachment styles, a vulnerability to specific environmental events (failure versus loss), a certain clinical presentation, and a characteristic response to pharmacological or psychotherapeutic treatments (Blatt, 2015). Each personality type is associated with a characteristic interpersonal style that enhances the risk of developing depression and influences the clinical presentation of its symptoms (Luyten, Blatt, & Corveleyn, 2005). Various pathological processes can arise from a disruption of this dialectical relationship at different levels of development and can manifest themselves in a variety of ways as with depression.

Currently, there is a tendency to recover the concept of *affective temperaments* (depressive, hypertimic, cyclothymic, irritable, and anxious), considering them as subclinical manifestations of some disorder within the affective spectrum (Akiskal & Akiskal, 2005). These temperaments have been shown to be universal, with distinctive characteristics and clear gender differences, where men scored significantly higher than women for hypertimic and irritable temperaments, while women scored significantly higher than men for cyclotimic, depressive, and anxious temperaments (Vazquez, Tondo, Mazzarini, & Gonda, 2012).

In brief, throughout history the relationship between personality and depression has been conceptualized in at least four ways (Hirschfeld, 2013): (1) Personality is a predisposing or vulnerability factor for the development of depression. (2) Personality changes are a consequence of mood swings resulting from depression. (3) Personality is a subclinical manifestation of depression (affective temperaments). And (4) personality characteristics influence the way depression clinically manifests itself (pathoplastic model). However, from a neurobiological point of view, the link between personality and depression depends on the approach we use. Thus, in the case of personality understood as a subclinical form of depression, it would be possible to raise the existence of etiological factors with a common neurobiological correlate, while in the case of the pathoplastic model, the presence of a shared neurobiological disorder would be less probably.

6.2 Neurobiology of Depression

Major depressive disorder has been linked to a series of neurobiological alterations ranging from dysfunction of the monoaminergic system and alteration of the hypothalamic-pituitary-adrenal (HPA) axis to alterations in the inflammatory pathways, mechanisms linked to neuroplasticity, neurogenesis, and even a series of epigenetic modifications (Malhi & Mann, 2018). Among the neurobiological systems investigated in relation to depression, most research has focused on the stress (Gold, 2015; Hammen, 2005) and reward system (Auerbach, Admon, & Pizzagalli, 2014). Genetics models of depression include a long series of genes involved in its etiopathogeny (Hong & Tsai, 2003). Frequently studied, the polymorphism (short or long variant) of the serotonin transporter encoder gene has been associated with depression. Individuals presenting one or two copies of the short allele of the gene have evidenced a higher tendency toward depressive symptoms and clinical depression and more frequent suicidal tendency in the face of adverse vital events than homozygous for the L-variant (Caspi et al., 2003). However, later investigations have failed to replicate the results (Gillespie, Whitfield, Williams, Heath, & Martin, 2005). As to the cognitive functions, depressed patients present a typical alteration of episodic memory (Ilsley, Moffoot, & O'Carroll, 1995), probably due to a hippocampal dysfunction (Bremner, 1999). In addition, the subtypes of depression (atypical versus melancholic) are related to specific alteration patterns (Austin, Mitchell, & Goodwin, 2001). Neuroanatomic and functional studies have shown decreased activity in the orbitofrontal cortex, alterations in the parahippocampal gyrus, and amygdala hyperactivity (Ebmeier, Donaghey, & Steele, 2006; Gillihan et al., 2010).

Traumatic childhood experiences may contribute to the appearance of adult depression, especially among individuals with genetic vulnerability (Risch et al., 2009). It has been suggested that the existence of different neurobiological subtypes of depression may depend on the presence or absence of early adverse events, which would also exert an influence on the response to treatment and the course of disease (Heim, Plotsky, & Nemeroff, 2004). Heim and Nemeroff (2001) have developed an etiopathogenic model of depression proposing that early adverse events, such as trauma or abandonment, trigger a long-term hyperactivation and sensibilization of the corticotropin-releasing factor (CRT) in the central nervous system (CNS), which leads to an increased endocrine, autonomic, and behavioral response to stress (vulnerable phenotype). In this regard, continuous exposure to stressful factors favors the appearance of a number of psychobiological changes, leading to an anxious or depressive clinical disorder. According to Hasler (2010), the clinically most relevant neurobiological hypotheses are as follows: (1) genetic vulnerability, (2) a dysfunction in the hypothalamus-pituitary-adrenal axis, (3) monoamine deficiency, (4) dysfunction in specific brain areas, (5) disequilibrium between neurotrophic and neurotoxic processes, (6) decreased GABA activity, (7) glutamate dysregulation, and (8) disruption of circadian rhythms. It has recently been suggested that a number of inflammatory processes have a role in the etiopathogeny of depression, both as precipitating and maintaining symptomatology factors. Some inflammatory markers could even prove useful in the diagnosis and prediction of treatment response (Krishnadas & Cavanagh, 2012).

Concerning to attachment theory, depression is thought to respond to a threat to affective bonds (and, in consequence, to our own *self*) in situations of separation, rejection, loss, or failure, leading to an altered awareness regarding the wishes and motivations of ourselves and others (Luyten, Fonagy, Lemma, & Target, 2012). Specifically, insecure attachment has been related to a higher vulnerability to develop depression and suicidal behavior (Grunebaum et al., 2010). Therefore, there is a close relationship between attachment, stress, and awareness in the etiopathogeny of depression (Heim, Newport, Mletzko, Miller, & Nemeroff, 2008).

Even though the first evolutionist hypotheses on the origin of depression were proposed years ago, they remain controversial to date (Nettle, 2004). Nesse (2000) developed a series of arguments in favor of the adaptive value of depression, where discouragement and its associated symptoms contribute to the management of inappropriate or potentially harmful situations, communicating the need for help, or acting as a signal of submission in social conflicts involving hierarchy when no chance exists of becoming victorious. On the other hand, a number of situations have been proposed to provoke different patterns of depressive symptoms aimed at solving the specific challenges posed by each situation (situation-symptom congruence hypothesis). Blame, rumination, fatigue, and pessimism tend to be associated to failure, while crying, sadness, and a need for social support are frequent after social losses (Keller & Nesse, 2006).

6.3 Neurobiology of Personality Traits in Depression

The neurobiology of temperament has been studied in several ways, including behavioral genetics, neuropsychopharmacology, molecular genetics, psychophysiology, and neuroimaging. Based on the affective neuroscience approach, Davis and Panksepp (2011) propose that the affective foundations of personality are found in the sub-neocortical "limbic" and "reptilian" areas of the central nervous system, where the most important evolutionary "roots" of personality would be based on six primary-process subcortical brain emotion systems (SEEKING, RAGE, FEAR, CARE, GRIEF, and PLAY). These systems would generate a type of affective valence within the brain in order to face the survival challenges that our ancestors faced for millennia. However, in humans, these "primary" systems are elaborated during development by "secondary" conditioning and "tertiary" thinking and self-reflection. More recently, it has been proposed to add to the study of personality neuroscience a perspective founded in the study of network maps of brain connectivity, which has been called the connectome paradigm (Markett, Montag, & Reuter, 2018).

In his seminal studies on the biological basis of personality, Eysenck (1963) postulated that personality is the result of an interplay between two dimensions: on the one hand introversion/extroversion and on the other hand stability/instability (also called emotionality or neuroticism). According to Eysenck, neuroticism was linked with intense emotional reactions to various stimuli which was associated with the activity of the autonomic nervous system, especially the sympathetic system. Furthermore, he proposed that extroversion would be linked to a rapid rise in cortical inhibition, its low dissipation, and its relatively high level (the opposite would be true of introversion). The brain structures related to these processes of excitation and inhibition would be the ascending reticular formation, an alternative pathway for ascending impulses from the periphery to the brain cortex. This proposal was reviewed by Gray (1970), who proposed that the physiological basis of introversion would consist not only in the activity of the ascending reticular system but also in the negative feedback loop, involving the orbitofrontal cortex, the medial septal area, and the hippocampus. Gray proposes that there are two major neurobehavioral systems that underlie behavior: the behavioral activation system (BAS), related to response of reward signals, and the behavioral inhibition system (BIS), which is particularly sensitive to punishment signals (for a complete review of neural correlates of these models, see (Kennis, Rademaker, & Geuze, 2013)). Some decades later, Siever and Davis (1991) proposed that the psychobiology of personality disorders could be formulated as a dimensional model based on the major psychiatric syndromes (from Axis I of DSM-III-R). Thus, they proposed the existence of four psychopathological dimensions: (1) *cognitive/perceptual organization*, (2) *impulsivity/aggression*, (3) *affective instability*, and (4) *anxiety/inhibition*. Alterations in each of these dimensions could occur on a *continuum* ranging from mild manifestations linked to personality to severe manifestations of a clinical syndrome, such schizophrenia or depression. Thus, each dimension was associated with the following: (1) Axis I disorder, (2) Axis II disorder, (3) biological indexes, (4) personality traits, and (5) defenses and coping strategies. For example, *affective instability* dimension was related with major mood disorders (Axis I); borderline and histrionic personality disorders (Axis II); neurobiological alterations related to REM latency, response to cholinergic and catecholaminergic challenges; personality traits, such environmental reactivity and transient affective changes; and finally, with defensive strategies such avoidance, compulsion, and dependent behaviors. Another prominent attempt to develop a psychobiological model of personality is that of Cloninger, Svrakic, and Przybeck (1993), who proposed a model of personality structure and development that accounts for the dimensions of both temperament and character. According Cloninger, the four temperamental dimensions (novelty seeking, harm avoidance, reward dependence, and persistence) are independently inherited, manifest early in life, and involve preconceptual biases in perceptual memory and habit formation. For its part, character dimensions mature in adulthood and influence personal and social life through learning about self-concept and correspond to self-directedness, cooperativeness, and self-transcendence.

Another model of personality classification that has been widely used is the so-called five-factor model (FFM), which states that personality is ordered hierarchically in a series of traits that can be summarized in five general characteristics: neuroticism, extraversion, conscientiousness, agreeableness, and openness to experience (Goldberg, 1990, 1993). Combining some of the previous models, more recently Whittle, Allen, Lubman, and Yucel (2006) have proposed that specific areas of the prefrontal cortex (dorsolateral prefrontal cortex, anterior cingulate, and orbitofrontal cortex) and limbic structures (amygdala, hippocampus, and nucleus *accumbens*) are related to three fundamental temperamental dimensions: negative affect, positive affect, and constraint. The authors propose that negative affect (manifested by inhibition, avoidance, and punishment sensitivity) is related to a circuit that links limbic-subcortical structures (like amygdala and ventral anterior cingulate cortex) involved in automatic processing of affective states with right hemisphere structures (hippocampus, dorsal anterior cingulate cortex, and dorsolateral prefrontal cortex) related to executive processes and involved with the integration of cognitive processes, affective input, and effortful regulation of affective states.

Based on Gray's psychobiological model, it has been hypothesized that depression would be associated with decreased BAS and/or heightened BIS sensitivity (Depue & Iacono, 1989). In addition, studies have linked high levels of harm avoidance and low levels of self-directedness in patients with depression compared with healthy controls (Celikel et al., 2009). Analyzing the patterns of neural activity in relation to various personality syndromes, using the functional magnetic resonance imaging paradigm in chronic depressive patients, Taubner, Wiswede, and Kessler (2013) found a positive correlation between a high score in "emotional-hostile-externalizing personality" and increased activity in the orbitofrontal cortex, ventral striatum, and temporal pole, areas that, as we saw, are directly linked to emotional processing. From the perspective of connectivity and network level correlates of personality (ranging from associations between single brain areas to whole-brain connectivity), the most studied traits have been neuroticism and avoidance (Markett et al., 2018), which have been associated with differential patterns of functional connectivity, originating in the amygdala and its subregions (neuroticism) and in the anterior insula (harm avoidance).

Unlike psychotic depression or melancholic depression (which has a recognizable genetic, neurobiological, and clinical profile), there are a number of so-called "atypical" or non-melancholic depressive conditions that have a marked reactivity to stressful life events and are related to personality styles and coping strategies (Parker, 2000). Moreover, personality styles can directly influence the level at which the individual is exposed to certain types of stressors, which could trigger the appearance of depressive states and be linked to the recurrence of the depressive disease (Liu, 2013). These personality styles can be determined by genetic variables and influence exposure to certain environments in what is known as gene-environment correlation (see below). Parker and Crawford (2007) have developed a model based on the notion of spectrum, where they propose that certain neurobiological processes shape personality styles, which are accentuated when the individual is stressed or depressed, and determine the clinical characteristics of non-melancholic (atypical) depression. The authors describe six dimensions of personality (anxious worrying, perfectionism, personal reserve, irritability/snappiness, social avoidance, and rejection sensitivity), each of which presents a specific pattern of symptoms and coping responses. An interesting aspect of this model is that it not only contributes to the understanding the role of personality in origin and clinical presentation of depression but also supports the importance of the differential indication of treatment, emphasizing the importance of psychotherapeutic interventions for the management of the personality in cases of non-melancholic depressions.

Despite the above, there is still much to know about the biological basis of personality in depression. For example, although the relationship between stress, alterations in HPA axis, and the hippocampus is relevant in the pathogenesis of depression, there is no strong evidence regarding the link between these alterations and personality that can be categorically linked to depression (Foster & MacQueen, 2008). In relation to monoaminergic systems, the evidence is also contradictory. Both for dopamine (a neurotransmitter linked to the reward system, which in turn has been linked to extroversion) and serotonin (linked to neuroticism), the results have not been sufficiently consistent, and this is probably because the study of the relationship between monoamines, personality traits, and depression requires a more complex approach that includes the analysis of neural circuits linked to complex behaviors (Shao & Zhu, 2020). Discrepancies in studies of the biological basis of personality in depression are likely to be due, at least in part, to the fact that depression is a multidetermined clinical phenomenon that requires study from diverse perspectives. In that sense, one particularly interesting area is the research of the relationship between genes and the environment.

6.4 Gene-Environment Relationship in Depression

Recent decades have witnessed a clear shift in the study of psychopathology from models emphasizing either genetic (Hong & Tsai, 2003) or environmental (Brown & Harris, 1978) factors to models incorporating various relationships between the genome and the environment (Dick, 2011; Rutter, 2007; Uher, 2008), including cultural variables and gene-culture coevolution (Chiao & Blizinsky, 2010; Way & Lieberman, 2010).

Every human being is unique, despite sharing over 99% of genetic material with the rest of the human species. The answer of what makes us distinctively different from other human beings lies in the continuous reciprocal interaction between the environment and our biology. Such gene-environment relations are thought to result from both gene-environment correlations (rGE) and gene-environment interactions (GxE). Recent theoretical models stress the fact that a person's relationship with his environment from the moment of conception can be assumed to play a crucial role in this uniqueness (Heim & Nemeroff, 2001, 2002; Nemeroff, 1998). The inheritance of our personality traits is polygenic and needs environmental factors to express itself. In order to illustrate how this relationship between the environment and genes can operate, we will proceed to briefly explain how genes function. Genes contain the information for protein synthesis (coding genes) or a noncoding RNA (RNA genes). They consist of a promoter region (sequence that regulates gene expression) and then the sequence that is transcribed. One way to induce variation in genetic structure is through polymorphisms. Polymorphisms are variations in the DNA sequence by substitution, deletion, or insertion. Not all genetic polymorphisms lead to an alteration in the sequence of a protein or its expression levels, i.e., many are silent and have no phenotypic expression. Genetic polymorphism is the presence in the same population of two or more alleles at a locus, with a significant frequency, where the minimum frequency is usually 1%. Polymorphisms that affect the coding or regulatory sequences, and therefore significantly change the structure of the protein or the mechanism of regulation of its expression, can give rise to different phenotypes. It is the differences in sequence that, together with environmental differences, contribute to phenotypic divergence. They are part of the biological foundations of plasticity and differential response to environmental stimuli and serve as an example to explain the relationship between genes and environment in the etiopathogenesis of mental disorders. Therefore, we are not all affected equally by the environment. The phenotype can be defined as a set of morphological, functional, biochemical, behavioral, and other characteristics of a living being, i.e., expression of the genotype according to a certain environment.

The genome regulates gene expression basically through three mechanisms, all of which are closely intertwined: (1) based on the regulation of transcription factors that bind to the promoter sequences, (2) epigenetic modification mechanisms, and (3) control of accessibility to promoters determined by the degree of chromatin condensation.

An example of polymorphism, which induces a different response in the carrier according to the environment it is related to, is the polymorphism of the promoter region of the serotonin transporter gene (5HTTLPR), and being one of the most studied, many of the examples and investigations that we will describe refer to it. The polymorphism is an insertion/deletion of 44 bp that determines two allelic variants, a short allele (S) with 14 repetitions and a long one (L) with 16 repetitions. The short form has been associated with less than 40% of gene expression compared to the long allele, resulting in decreased expression of the transport protein in the neuronal membrane. This results in a slower performance of the serotonin transporter and an increase in the availability of serotonin in the synaptic space. This has been associated with certain personality traits, such as neuroticism and with greater vulnerability to anxious depressive conditions.

6.4.1 Gene-Environment Correlation (rGE)

Research on gene-environment correlation (rGE) explores the role of genes in the exposure to environmental factors (Kendler & Eaves, 1986; Kendler et al., 1995). rGE refers to the tendency of individuals to select and generate their environment based on genetic features that influence behavior, thoughts, and feelings. It explains why some people attract certain situations into their lives that actively create stress, while others create satisfying lives, depending on their personalities, which, in turn, depend in part on their genes (Plomin, DeFries, McClearn, & Rutter, 1997). Three types of rGE have been described in the literature: (a) passive, (b) reactive, provocative or evocative, and (c) active or selective (Jaffee & Price, 2008).

(a) Passive rGE refers to the situation in which children inherit from their parents not only a genetic constitution but also the environment in which they are raised (i.e., they inherit intellectual curiosity and the means to satisfy it). The association between genetically related individuals is a requirement for passive rGE.
(b) Evocative, provocative, or reactive rGE refers to the tendency of certain genetically influenced behaviors or temperamental features to elicit certain types of responses from people within their environment, (e.g., a child with a difficult temperament is more likely to elicit negative parenting behaviors). Fighting with your partner may cause someone to become depressed, but it's equally possible that people who are prone to depression tend to trigger arguments with significant others, questioning the direction of the effect.
(c) Active or selective rGE refers to the active generation of certain environments based on genetic tendencies. This refers to the association between genetic features of the individual and the environmental niches that the individual selects or generates (e.g., a child with intellectual curiosity will tend to find intellectually rich environments, while a child with behavioral disorder will seek peers with similar behaviors; that is, people who are more extroverted may seek very different social environments from those who are shy and withdrawn) (Plomin et al., 1997).

6.4.2 Gene-Environment Interaction (GxE)

Gene-environment interaction (GxE) refers to an individual's genetic sensitivity to environmental factors. Explains why people respond differently to environmental factors, some becoming depressed and others becoming stronger, after being exposed to similar life events (Plomin et al., 1997). Until relatively recently, GxE were thought to be rare in psychiatry, but research over the past decades has proven its existence both for medical diseases, (Morales & Duffy, 2019; Raby, 2019) as for mental disorders, shifting research toward a focus on GxE (Moffitt, Caspi, & Rutter, 2005; Rutter, 2010). One of the earliest studies of GxE was reported by Kendler and colleagues (Kendler et al., 1995), who found that stressful life events increased the risk of developing depression more in people with a high genetic risk for depression (i.e., with a twin with depression) than in people with a low genetic risk for depression (i.e., with a twin without depression). This study overthrew the concept of reactive or endogenous depression, because those individuals with a greater genetic risk for depression were shown to be also more reactive to negative environmental events. In 2003, Caspi and colleagues (2003) published a groundbreaking study, which reported that carrying the short allele of the 5HTTLPR gene interacted with both early and recent negative events to predict depression and suicidal thoughts. Yet, findings have not always been consistent. Two meta-analyses (Munafo, 2012; Risch et al., 2009), for instance, failed to corroborate an interaction between the 5HTTLPR gene and stressful life events in predicting depression. By contrast, a meta-analysis by Uher and McGuffin (Uher, 2014) did find evidence for an interaction between the 5HTTLPR gene and adversity in predicting depression. Differences between these studies' conclusions may be due to differences in their methodology and inclusion criteria. But it is clear that there still is controversy regarding the role of GxE and rGE in psychiatric disorders.

There is now increasing consensus that most common psychiatric disorders, such as depression and anxiety, are best explained as complex disorders, involving dysfunctions in several biological systems in interaction with environmental factors. Gene-environment correlations and interactions are not mutually exclusive. A polymorphism may correlate with some traits that generate changes in the environment (mediation model) and at the same time interact with the environment to generate a new result (moderation model). An example of such a mediational model is the finding that the short allele of the 5HTTLPR gene has been shown to correlate with neuroticism (Greenberg et al., 2000; Sen, Burmeister, & Ghosh, 2004), which in turn has been shown to be related to a tendency to have a negative interpretation bias related to life events (John & Gross, 2004) and therefore a more pessimistic and depressive interpretation of life events (correlational explanation with a mediation model of the relationship between the HTTLPR gene and depression). But this same polymorphism can be associated with the environment in an interaction model, that is, through the moderation of environmental effects. Studies suggest that carriers of the short 5HTTLPR gene allele may interact with negative life events to predict higher levels of depression (Caspi et al., 2003), but they may also interact with social support to lower levels of depression more than noncarriers of the short 5HTTLPR gene (Kaufman et al., 2004; Kim et al., 2014).

6.5 Psychopathology Models on Gene-Environment Relationship

The potential interactions between genetic, neurochemical, and cognitive factors have only recently been demonstrated. The combination of findings from behavioral genetics and cognitive neuroscience opens new opportunities to integrate research results. It is suggested that a comprehensive study of the psychological and biological correlates of mental disorders may grant a new way to understand how we get mentally ill (Beck, 2008). Since the last decade, investigators propose that the future of clinical research and therapeutic efforts should focus on the study of processes of vulnerability (Corveleyn & Blatt, 2005). It becomes especially urgent to accommodate these new proposals and integrate biological, psychological, and environmental findings if we look at the results of meta-analytic review about the effectiveness of treatments with empirical support (Gaynes et al., 2008; Kirsch, 2019; van der Lem, van der Wee, van Veen, & Zitman, 2012; Westen, Novotny, & Thompson-Brenner, 2004). Because the low rates of response to treatment, researchers agree on the need to change research strategies to target from the beginning the question of which patients require what type of treatment (e.g., pharmacotherapy or psychotherapy, brief or long term) being necessary to then identify dimensions related to patient treatment.

In the 1990s, empirical studies on the interaction between genes and environment began in psychiatry. These investigations were designed to determine vulnerable to stress phenotypes. They conclude that some people carrying particular polymorphisms are more vulnerable to the effects of stressful environment.

6.5.1 Diathesis-Stress Model/Vulnerable Phenotype Model

The diathesis-stress model of mental diseases proposes that stress activates a latent predisposition or diathesis, which then manifests itself as some form of psychopathology. This model assumes that a predisposition is necessary but not an enough condition for the development of a mental disorder and that the interaction with stress activates the diathesis to increase the risk of developing a mental disorder (Zuckerman, 1999). Originally, the predisposition was presumed to be a genetic condition that was observable in certain biological traits; since then, the concept of diathesis has been expanded to include factors such as cognitive or social predispositions (Abela, 2001; Monroe & Simons, 1991). Under this broader concept, biological and psychological traits can be considered diathesis, i.e., the necessary precursors to develop the disorder. As such, in this theory, stress vulnerability is a predisposition or diathesis. This extension of the concept of vulnerability to stress has some conceptual problems, for example, a negative cognitive scheme that makes an individual more vulnerable to stress and anxiety can itself be influenced by genetic, social, or both (Zuckerman, 1999).

Stress not only can be defined as “a specific response of the body to a demand” (Lanfumey, Mongeau, Cohen-Salmon, & Hamon, 2008) but also can be described as “any environmental internal external change, or altering maintenance homeostasis” (Leonard, 2005). Its role as a risk factor for presenting psychopathology has been extensively studied. For this purpose, stress can be subdivided into three categories: acute stress, chronic stress, and stress in early life.

In the diathesis-stress model, events that occur within the previous year of onset of the disorder are considered stressors or acute stress. Generally, life events that involve loss or humiliation have proved depressogenic (OR: 5.64) (Kendler, Karkowski, & Prescott, 1999). Mild chronic stress studies have shown in animals and humans that stress is related with neurobiological changes, like those seen in depressed individuals (Grippo, Beltz, & Johnson, 2003; Tennant, 2002). Finally, stress in early life, such as childhood trauma (physical, sexual, or emotional abuse) and alterations in attachment, has shown to produce permanent biological changes that confer increased vulnerability to psychopathology (Gutman & Nemeroff, 2003; Heim & Binder, 2012; Heim et al., 2008) and even different response to treatment, responding better to psychotherapy than drugs on chronic depressed women with a history of trauma (Nemeroff et al., 2003).

The distinction between early or remote and recent events is important for this model. This distinction is equally important for the psychoanalytic theory, where it is considered that childhood events are predisposing factors for mental disorders in adults. Prior to the 1990s, stress was considered as a nonspecific and continuous concept, measured as high or low levels. The predisposition to stress was assumed as a threshold, below which the disorder is not expressed, no matter how severe was the stressor, and above which the disorder is expressed if you have sufficient levels of stress to activate the latent predisposition (Monroe & Simons, 1991). The vulnerable phenotype model, instead, incorporates the concept that early adverse experience can have lifelong effects on physical and psychological functioning and become a vulnerability or diathesis for mental disorders. The vulnerable phenotype model illustrates independent and interactive effects of genes and early environment in the development of the phenotype of the individual (Rutter et al., 1997). The GxE interaction is implicit in the stress diathesis model and the vulnerable phenotype model. Adverse childhood experiences can exacerbate genetic vulnerability to stress. This can result in a phenotype that is hypersensitive to future exposures to stress and has an increased risk of developing psychopathology. Early social support and coping styles interact with the genetically determined temperament (Scarr & McCartney, 1983) and can act as buffers against the effect of early adversity in the development of the phenotype. Evidence from animal and human studies supports the model of vulnerable phenotype, suggesting that early adversity induces neurobiological changes and that these changes inhibit the ability of the central nervous system to regulate stress and emotions. This deregulation is accompanied by an increase in the rate of psychiatric disorders (Claes, 2004; Heim & Nemeroff, 2002; Shea, Walsh, Macmillan, & Steiner, 2005). Individuals carrying the vulnerable genotype are more sensitive to adverse environments presenting a worse outcome than noncarriers of the vulnerable genotype. The latter are considered resistant to negative environments (resilient).

The problem of the diathesis-stress model is that it is limited by its focus on stress, which excludes other aspects of the environment that may interact with biological factors. As it was conceptualized to explain psychopathology, the focus is on environmental stressors that can contribute to the development of mental disorders, leaving out environmental factors that can prevent, delay, or treat mental disorders and promote resilience and health. This is the case of the polymorphism of the promoter region of the serotonin transporter (5HTTLPR) gene, which the short allele variant would be more vulnerable to stressful environments. This model of psychopathology, in recent years, has shifted, including positive aspects of the environment and considering these "vulnerable" alleles as "prosocial or plastic" alleles, that is, more sensitive to both negative and positive environment. The model changes from vulnerability to stress to different sensitivity to the environment. That is, if the relationship between genotype and environment shows that carriers of the short allele of the serotonin transporter are more sensitive to environment. That is, the influence of the environment to predict symptoms is stronger on plastic allele carriers.

6.5.2 Differential Susceptibility to Environment

Over recent years, investigators have reported about the relationship of certain genes, especially the serotonin transporter gene and increased sensitivity to environmental events. Taylor, Way, and Lieberman (Way & Lieberman, 2010; Way & Taylor, 2010) have proposed the hypothesis that these polymorphisms predispose to greater social sensitivity, i.e., they would be prosocial genes, while Pluess and Belsky (Belsky et al., 2009; Belsky & Pluess, 2009) proposed that these kinds of genes confer differential susceptibility to the environment and would be plastic genes, malleable by the environment (Fox, Zougkou, Ridgewell, & Garner, 2011). Previously, Ellis and Boyce (Ellis & Boyce, 2008), from an evolutionary perspective, proposed the model of biological sensitivity to context. Bringing together their theories, they proposed that these genes confer differential sensitivity to environment. Therefore, health and illness depend on the interaction between environmental and biological factors. That is, the genes (as biological factors) would give us more or less sensitivity to environmental factors, and the environment, as if it's positive or negative, would shape the individual, for worse or for better.

Unlike the vulnerable phenotype model, in which the presence of the short allele HTTLPR gene confers susceptibility to adverse environmental factors, in this model, the presence of this allele may provide greater sensitivity to the environment. This means that the short allele actually increases the sensitivity to the environment more generally, so exposition to adverse environments leads to worse outcomes, while supporters and positive environments lead to advantages (Bakermans-Kranenburg & van, 2015; Homberg & Lesch, 2011; Perez-Perez et al., 2018; Stocker et al., 2017). This model includes the previous models of stress diathesis and vulnerable phenotype but takes a more integrated vision of the environment (not only the negative aspects). "It seems that these models (diathesis stress and vulnerable phenotype) are only half the story" (Way & Taylor, 2010). The serotonin transporter gene has been the most studied gene as plastic, known by its interaction with stress (environment) to develop psychopathology. Taylor's study (2006) on prediction of depressive symptoms, according to early family environment and recent life events, showed that homozygotes short allele carriers, when they described a family atmosphere of low-risk and low number of recent stressors, presented the lower depressive symptoms rates of the sample, whereas if they described a high-risk family environment and many recent stressful events, they had the highest depressive symptoms rates of the sample. This indicates that individuals homozygous for the short allele are more sensitive to life events, both positive and negative ones, than the other genotypes. Way & Taylor (2010) studied whether the nature of recent life events influences this interaction. He distinguished recent events between social events (i.e., end of romantic relationship, conflict with family or friends, death of a loved one) and nonsocial events (receiving a low grade, job loss, car accident). He noted that the relationship between genotype SS, life events, and depression remains significant for recent social events, but it was lost for recent nonsocial events, supporting the subtle difference between prosocial alleles instead of plastic alleles that he proposed. For individuals carrying the short allele, social support appears to be an important factor in maintaining their well-being. Kilpatrick et al. (2007) observed that subjects homozygous for the short allele that were exposed to a hurricane had no greater risk for depression than those homozygous for the long allele, when they had a good perceived social support. However, if they perceived a bad social support, they had 4.5 times greater risk of depression. Kaufman (Kaufman et al., 2004) found that social support moderated the risk for depression associated with the short allele and child abuse. Children with a history of abuse and SS genotype reported higher levels of depression. Maltreated children with the SS genotype and an absence of positive support had depression scores that were approximately twice as high as those of maltreated children with the SS genotype and positive social support. The authors conclude that the availability and frequency of social support may promote resilience even in children with high genetic vulnerability to depression and who have experienced adversity in childhood.

Individuals carrying more plastic alleles may be more sensitive to the detection of biological and socially relevant information from the environment, which is a critical function for social interaction and emotional functioning. The association of increased amygdala reactivity and short allele 5HTTLPR genotype has been demonstrated both with scary faces and with other negative emotions, like anger and grief (Dannlowski et al., 2008), and with positive emotions, such as joy (Domschke et al., 2006), both in healthy population and patients with depression and panic disorder. This indicates, again, sensitivity to socially relevant information rather than only specific threat keys (Canli & Lesch, 2007). Several studies on cognitive function, especially on voluntary attention and working memory in healthy individuals, have shown that carriers of the short allele perform better (Anderson, Bell, & Awh, 2012; Enge, Fleischhauer, Lesch, Reif, & Strobel, 2011). Studies on emotional biases have shown that carriers of the S allele have a strong tendency toward negative material, especially related to threat (Beevers, Wells, Ellis, & McGeary, 2009), and greater difficulty disengaging from emotional, positive, and negative stimuli (Beevers, Gibb, McGeary, & Miller, 2007; Beevers et al., 2011; Fox, Ridgewell, & Ashwin, 2009), and this was even observed in a meta-analysis (Pergamin-Hight, Bakermans-Kranenburg, van Ijzendoorn, & Bar-Haim, 2012). While plasticity can operate toward negative and positive information, attention would respond more to negative bias, maybe related to neuroticism trait related to this polymorphism. Studies in healthy volunteers submitted to learning paradigms show greater and faster learning in short allele carriers (Fox et al., 2011).

Cultural factors may also come into play here. For instance, some GxE seem quite robust in Western cultures but have not been replicated in Eastern cultures (Leighton, Botto, Silva, Jiménez, & Luyten, 2017). Further, GxE may also differ along the course of development, with some interactions observed at some points during development but not during other developmental stages, and some may be gender dependent.

Unlike the vulnerability model, the differentiated sensitivity to the environment is a model that includes an evolutionary perspective, which considers the potential disadvantages and advantages of individual differences. This evolutionary perspective may be better able to explain the observation that many of the genetic variants included in studies of GxE candidate genes in psychiatry are "common" variants (i.e., have a high frequency in the general population). If there were genetic variants associated exclusively with an increased risk for the development of psychopathology in the presence of adversity, it could be expected that the frequency of these genes would decrease over time (and that the genetic variants associated with resilience would increase). However, this has not been observed; many of these variations are very frequent. It is thought that this type of genetic variation could allow faster adaptation to environmental changes and favor the reproduction of the species.

6.6 Conclusions

Regardless of whether we call it "personality," "temperament," or "character," clinically it is evident that there are certain typologies regarding the way of being and behaving of individuals that are determined by a mood tone and that do not constitute (either by their intensity or their quality) a characteristic mood disorder (manifested by lack of reactivity, an episodic and recurrent course, and with complete interepisodic restitution). Despite the abundant research on the various personality types and their associated traits (both normal and pathological), little is known about the biological basis of these traits. In the case of the relationship between personality and mood disorders, this is especially evident. This may have several explanations. Firstly, it should be noted that, unlike phenomena such as delirium or hallucinations, sadness and depressed mood are part of a set of emotional experiences that are present in everyone's daily life and, therefore, can be difficult to classify immediately as pathological. Another important aspect relates to the diagnosis of depression. We know that there are different clinical subtypes of depression that, under the perspective of a spectrum, can be considered from more chronic, more reactive, and less recurrent manifestations (and, therefore, more linked to personality) to less reactive, more episodic, and recurrent depressions, which would have a more evident genetic and biological component and, therefore, less related to personality (Ghaemi, Vohringer, & Vergne, 2012). It is important to note that many of the personality traits involved in depression have also been associated with other disorders, such as anxiety disorders (Kotov, Watson, Robles, & Schmidt, 2007), so it is difficult to attribute a specificity to them; rather, they would be a general risk factor for various forms of psychopathology. In addition, it's known that personality is not a stable construct but varies throughout life, which can influence how you approach your study scientifically if not considering a life cycle perspective.

As summarized by Klein, Kotov, and Bufferd (2011), the study of the relationship between personality and depression may have a number of implications for research and clinical practice: (1) personality traits associated with the expression and regulation of emotional experiences could be considered as intermediate phenotypes and therefore contribute to a more focalized study of the genetic and biological basis of depression; (2) the study of personality may be useful to distinguish subgroups of depressive disorders that differ in their etiopathogenesis and developmental trajectories; (3) the analysis of the relationship between personality and depressive disorders may facilitate the understanding of the proximal processes involved in the emergence of mood disorders; (4) the study of personality traits may guide in the indication of treatments and predict the therapeutic response; (5) the identification of personality traits that could be considered at risk would allow the development of prevention strategies in the most vulnerable population.

Finally, we now know that the psychosocial environment (including psychotherapeutic interventions) produces modifications in the central nervous system and many of these can be mediated by epigenetic mechanisms (Jimenez et al., 2018). These processes influence the entire life cycle and can act as a molecular bridge between nature and nurture. Therefore, it is necessary to have studies that analyze the relationship between personality and depression from multiple perspectives, having a comprehensive view that integrates the various types of relationships between genes and the environment, including models that, beyond vulnerability, consider the perspective of differentiated sensitivity to environmental stimuli (Leighton et al., 2017). Moreover, as McNaughton (2020) recently suggests, research on explanatory models of personality constructs and the relationship between personality traits, basic emotions, and their disorders should take an evolutionary approach, starting with the study of conserved neutral-level modulators and only then invoke emergent, higher order (i.e., cognitive or behavioral disfunctions) explanations.

References

Abela, J. R. (2001). The hopelessness theory of depression: A test of the diathesis-stress and causal mediation components in third and seventh grade children. *Journal of Abnormal Child Psychology, 29*(3), 241–254. Retrieved from http://www.ncbi.nlm.nih.gov/pubmed/11411786

Akiskal, K. K., & Akiskal, H. S. (2005). The theoretical underpinnings of affective temperaments: Implications for evolutionary foundations of bipolar disorder and human nature. *Journal of Affective Disorders, 85*(1–2), 231–239. https://doi.org/10.1016/j.jad.2004.08.002

Anderson, D. E., Bell, T. A., & Awh, E. (2012). Polymorphisms in the 5-HTTLPR gene mediate storage capacity of visual working memory. *Journal of Cognitive Neuroscience, 24*(5), 1069–1076. https://doi.org/10.1162/jocn_a_00207

Auerbach, R. P., Admon, R., & Pizzagalli, D. A. (2014). Adolescent depression: Stress and reward dysfunction. *Harvard Review of Psychiatry, 22*(3), 139–148. https://doi.org/10.1097/HRP.0000000000000034

Austin, M. P., Mitchell, P., & Goodwin, G. M. (2001). Cognitive deficits in depression: Possible implications for functional neuropathology. *The British Journal of Psychiatry: The Journal of Mental Science, 178*, 200–206. Retrieved from http://bjp.rcpsych.org/content/178/3/200.full.pdf

Bakermans-Kranenburg, M. J., & van, I. M. H. (2015). The hidden efficacy of interventions: Genexenvironment experiments from a differential susceptibility perspective. *Annual Review of Psychology, 66*, 381–409. https://doi.org/10.1146/annurev-psych-010814-015407

Beck, A. T. (2008). The evolution of the cognitive model of depression and its neurobiological correlates. *The American Journal of Psychiatry, 165*(8), 969–977. https://doi.org/10.1176/appi.ajp.2008.08050721

Beevers, C. G., Gibb, B. E., McGeary, J. E., & Miller, I. W. (2007). Serotonin transporter genetic variation and biased attention for emotional word stimuli among psychiatric inpatients. *Journal of Abnormal Psychology, 116*(1), 208–212. https://doi.org/10.1037/0021-843x.116.1.208

Beevers, C. G., Marti, C. N., Lee, H. J., Stote, D. L., Ferrell, R. E., Hariri, A. R., & Telch, M. J. (2011). Associations between serotonin transporter gene promoter region (5-HTTLPR) polymorphism and gaze bias for emotional information. *Journal of Abnormal Psychology, 120*(1), 187–197. https://doi.org/10.1037/a0022125

Beevers, C. G., Wells, T. T., Ellis, A. J., & McGeary, J. E. (2009). Association of the serotonin transporter gene promoter region (5-HTTLPR) polymorphism with biased attention for emotional stimuli. *Journal of Abnormal Psychology, 118*(3), 670–681. https://doi.org/10.1037/a0016198

Belsky, J., Jonassaint, C., Pluess, M., Stanton, M., Brummett, B., & Williams, R. (2009). Vulnerability genes or plasticity genes? *Molecular Psychiatry, 14*(8), 746–754. https://doi.org/10.1038/mp.2009.44

Belsky, J., & Pluess, M. (2009). Beyond diathesis stress: Differential susceptibility to environmental influences. *Psychological Bulletin, 135*(6), 885–908. https://doi.org/10.1037/a0017376

Berrios, G., & Porter, R. (1995). *A history of clinical psychiatry*. London, UK: The Athlone Press.

Blatt, S. (2005). Therapeutic implications. In *Experiences of depression. Theoretical, clinical and research perspectives* (pp. 255–295). Washington, DC: American Psychological Association.

Blatt, S. (2008). *Polarities of experience. Relatedness and self-definition in personality development, psychopathology, and the therapeutic process*. Washington, DC: American Psychological Association.

Blatt, S. (2015). Depression. In P. Luyten, L. Mayes, P. Fonagy, M. Target, & S. Blatt (Eds.), *Handbook of psychodynamic approaches to psychopathology* (pp. 131–151). New York, NY: The Guilford Press.

Blatt, S. J., & Luyten, P. (2009). A structural-developmental psychodynamic approach to psychopathology: Two polarities of experience across the life span. *Development and Psychopathology, 21*(3), 793–814. https://doi.org/10.1017/S0954579409000431

Bremner, J. D. (1999). Does stress damage the brain? *Biological Psychiatry, 45*(7), 797–805. Retrieved from http://www.biologicalpsychiatryjournal.com/article/S0006-3223(99)00009-8/abstract

Brown, G., & Harris, T. (1978). *Social origins of depression. A study of psychiatric disorder in women*. New York, NY: Free Press.

Canli, T., & Lesch, K. P. (2007). Long story short: The serotonin transporter in emotion regulation and social cognition. *Nature Neuroscience, 10*(9), 1103–1109. https://doi.org/10.1038/nn1964

Caspi, A., Sugden, K., Moffitt, T. E., Taylor, A., Craig, I. W., Harrington, H., ... Poulton, R. (2003). Influence of life stress on depression: Moderation by a polymorphism in the 5-HTT gene. *Science, 301*(5631), 386. Retrieved from http://search.ebscohost.com/login.aspx?direct=true&db=a9h&AN=10422967&lang=es&site=ehost-live

Celikel, F. C., Kose, S., Cumurcu, B. E., Erkorkmaz, U., Sayar, K., Borckardt, J. J., & Cloninger, C. R. (2009). Cloninger's temperament and character dimensions of personality in patients with major depressive disorder. *Comprehensive Psychiatry, 50*(6), 556–561. https://doi.org/10.1016/j.comppsych.2008.11.012

Chiao, J. Y., & Blizinsky, K. D. (2010). Culture-gene coevolution of individualism-collectivism and the serotonin transporter gene. *Proceedings of the Royal Society B: Biological Sciences, 277*(1681), 529–537. https://doi.org/10.1098/rspb.2009.1650

Claes, S. J. (2004). Corticotropin-releasing hormone (CRH) in psychiatry: From stress to psychopathology. *Annals of Medicine, 36*(1), 50–61.

Cloninger, C. R., Svrakic, D. M., & Przybeck, T. R. (1993). A psychobiological model of temperament and character. *Archives of General Psychiatry, 50*(12), 975–990. https://doi.org/10.1001/archpsyc.1993.01820240059008

Coccaro, E., & Siever, L. (2005). Neurobiology. In J. Oldham, A. Skodol, & D. Bender (Eds.), *Textbook of personality disorders* (pp. 155–169). Arlington, TX: American Psychiatric Publishing, Inc.

Corveleyn, J. L. P., & Blatt, S. J. (2005). *The theory and treatment of depression: Towards a dynamic interactionism model*. Leuven, Belgium: Leuven University Press.

Dannlowski, U., Ohrmann, P., Bauer, J., Deckert, J., Hohoff, C., Kugel, H., … Suslow, T. (2008). 5-HTTLPR biases amygdala activity in response to masked facial expressions in major depression. *Neuropsychopharmacology: Official Publication of the American College of Neuropsychopharmacology, 33*(2), 418–424. https://doi.org/10.1038/sj.npp.1301411

Davis, K. L., & Panksepp, J. (2011). The brain's emotional foundations of human personality and the affective neuroscience personality scales. *Neuroscience and Biobehavioral Reviews, 35*(9), 1946–1958. https://doi.org/10.1016/j.neubiorev.2011.04.004

Depue, R. A., & Iacono, W. G. (1989). Neurobehavioral aspects of affective disorders. *Annual Review of Psychology, 40*, 457–492. https://doi.org/10.1146/annurev.ps.40.020189.002325

Dick, D. M. (2011). Gene-environment interaction in psychological traits and disorders. *Annual Review of Clinical Psychology, 7*, 383–409. https://doi.org/10.1146/annurev-clinpsy-032210-104518

Domschke, K., Braun, M., Ohrmann, P., Suslow, T., Kugel, H., Bauer, J., … Deckert, J. (2006). Association of the functional -1019C/G 5-HT1A polymorphism with prefrontal cortex and amygdala activation measured with 3 T fMRI in panic disorder. *The International Journal of Neuropsychopharmacology/Official Scientific Journal of the Collegium Internationale Neuropsychopharmacologicum (CINP), 9*(3), 349–355. https://doi.org/10.1017/s1461145705005869

Ebmeier, K. P., Donaghey, C., & Steele, J. D. (2006). Recent developments and current controversies in depression. *Lancet, 367*(9505), 153–167. https://doi.org/10.1016/S0140-6736(06)67964-6

Ellis, B. J., & Boyce, W. T. (2008). Biological sensitivity to context. *Current Directions in Psychological Science, 17*(3), 183–187.

Enge, S., Fleischhauer, M., Lesch, K. P., Reif, A., & Strobel, A. (2011). Serotonergic modulation in executive functioning: Linking genetic variations to working memory performance. *Neuropsychologia, 49*(13), 3776–3785. https://doi.org/10.1016/j.neuropsychologia.2011.09.038

Eysenck, H. J. (1963). Biological basis of personality. *Nature, 199*, 1031–1034. https://doi.org/10.1038/1991031a0

Foster, J. A., & MacQueen, G. (2008). Neurobiological factors linking personality traits and major depression. *Canadian Journal of Psychiatry, 53*(1), 6–13. https://doi.org/10.1177/070674370805300103

Fox, E., Ridgewell, A., & Ashwin, C. (2009). Looking on the bright side: Biased attention and the human serotonin transporter gene. *Proceedings of the Royal Society B: Biological Sciences, 276*(1663), 1747–1751. https://doi.org/10.1098/rspb.2008.1788

Fox, E., Zougkou, K., Ridgewell, A., & Garner, K. (2011). The serotonin transporter gene alters sensitivity to attention bias modification: Evidence for a plasticity gene. *Biological Psychiatry, 70*(11), 1049–1054. https://doi.org/10.1016/j.biopsych.2011.07.004

Gaynes, B. N., Rush, A. J., Trivedi, M. H., Wisniewski, S. R., Spencer, D., & Fava, M. (2008). The STAR*D study: Treating depression in the real world. *Cleveland Clinic Journal of Medicine, 75*(1), 57–66.

Ghaemi, S. N., Vohringer, P. A., & Vergne, D. E. (2012). The varieties of depressive experience: Diagnosing mood disorders. *The Psychiatric Clinics of North America, 35*(1), 73–86. https://doi.org/10.1016/j.psc.2011.11.008

Gillespie, N. A., Whitfield, J. B., Williams, B., Heath, A. C., & Martin, N. G. (2005). The relationship between stressful life events, the serotonin transporter (5-HTTLPR) genotype and major depression. *Psychological Medicine, 35*(1), 101–111.

Gillihan, S. J., Rao, H., Wang, J., Detre, J. A., Breland, J., Sankoorikal, G. M., ... Farah, M. J. (2010). Serotonin transporter genotype modulates amygdala activity during mood regulation. *Social Cognitive and Affective Neuroscience, 5*(1), 1–10. https://doi.org/10.1093/scan/nsp035

Gold, P. W. (2015). The organization of the stress system and its dysregulation in depressive illness. *Molecular Psychiatry, 20*(1), 32–47. https://doi.org/10.1038/mp.2014.163

Goldberg, L. R. (1990). An alternative "description of personality": The big-five factor structure. *Journal of Personality and Social Psychology, 59*(6), 1216–1229. https://doi.org/10.1037//0022-3514.59.6.1216

Goldberg, L. R. (1993). The structure of phenotypic personality traits. *The American Psychologist, 48*(1), 26–34. https://doi.org/10.1037//0003-066x.48.1.26

Gray, J. A. (1970). The psychophysiological basis of introversion-extraversion. *Behaviour Research and Therapy, 8*(3), 249–266. https://doi.org/10.1016/0005-7967(70)90069-0

Greenberg, B. D., Li, Q., Lucas, F. R., Hu, S., Sirota, L. A., Benjamin, J., ... Murphy, D. L. (2000). Association between the serotonin transporter promoter polymorphism and personality traits in a primarily female population sample. *American Journal of Medical Genetics, 96*(2), 202–216.

Grippo, A. J., Beltz, T. G., & Johnson, A. K. (2003). Behavioral and cardiovascular changes in the chronic mild stress model of depression. *Physiology & Behavior, 78*(4–5), 703–710.

Grunebaum, M. F., Galfalvy, H. C., Mortenson, L. Y., Burke, A. K., Oquendo, M. A., & Mann, J. J. (2010). Attachment and social adjustment: Relationships to suicide attempt and major depressive episode in a prospective study. *Journal of Affective Disorders, 123*(1–3), 123–130. https://doi.org/10.1016/j.jad.2009.09.010

Gutman, D. A., & Nemeroff, C. B. (2003). Persistent central nervous system effects of an adverse early environment: Clinical and preclinical studies. *Physiology & Behavior, 79*(3), 471–478. https://doi.org/10.1016/s0031-9384(03)00166-5. PMID: 12954441.

Hammen, C. (2005). Stress and depression. *Annual Review of Clinical Psychology, 1*, 293–319. https://doi.org/10.1146/annurev.clinpsy.1.102803.143938

Hasler, G. (2010). Pathophysiology of depression: Do we have any solid evidence of interest to clinicians? *World Psychiatry: Official Journal of the World Psychiatric Association (WPA), 9*(3), 155–161. Retrieved from http://www.ncbi.nlm.nih.gov/pmc/articles/PMC2950973/pdf/wpa030155.pdf

Heim, C., & Binder, E. B. (2012). Current research trends in early life stress and depression: Review of human studies on sensitive periods, gene-environment interactions, and epigenetics. *Experimental Neurology, 233*(1), 102–111. https://doi.org/10.1016/j.expneurol.2011.10.032

Heim, C., & Nemeroff, C. B. (2001). The role of childhood trauma in the neurobiology of mood and anxiety disorders: Preclinical and clinical studies. *Biological Psychiatry, 49*(12), 1023–1039. https://doi.org/10.1016/s0006-3223(01)01157-x

Heim, C., & Nemeroff, C. B. (2002). Neurobiology of early life stress: Clinical studies. *Seminars in Clinical Neuropsychiatry, 7*(2), 147–159.

Heim, C., Newport, D. J., Mletzko, T., Miller, A. H., & Nemeroff, C. B. (2008). The link between childhood trauma and depression: Insights from HPA axis studies in humans. *Psychoneuroendocrinology, 33*(6), 693–710. https://doi.org/10.1016/j.psyneuen.2008.03.008

Heim, C., Plotsky, P. M., & Nemeroff, C. B. (2004). Importance of studying the contributions of early adverse experience to neurobiological findings in depression. *Neuropsychopharmacology: Official Publication of the American College of Neuropsychopharmacology, 29*(4), 641–648. https://doi.org/10.1038/sj.npp.1300397

Hirschfeld, R. M. (2013). Personality and mood disorders. In M. Keller (Ed.), *Clinical guide to depression and bipolar disorder. Findings from the collaborative depression study* (Vol. First, pp. 135–140). Washington, DC: American Psychiatric Publishing.
Homberg, J. R., & Lesch, K. P. (2011). Looking on the bright side of serotonin transporter gene variation. *Biological Psychiatry, 69*(6), 513–519. https://doi.org/10.1016/j.biopsych.2010.09.024
Hong, C., & Tsai, T. (2003). The genomic approaches to major depression. *Current Pharmacogenomics, 1*, 67–74.
Ikeda, M., Tanaka, S., Saito, T., Ozaki, N., Kamatani, Y., & Iwata, N. (2018). Re-evaluating classical body type theories: Genetic correlation between psychiatric disorders and body mass index. *Psychological Medicine, 48*(10), 1745–1748. https://doi.org/10.1017/S0033291718000685
Ilsley, J. E., Moffoot, A. P., & O'Carroll, R. E. (1995). An analysis of memory dysfunction in major depression. *Journal of Affective Disorders, 35*(1–2), 1–9. Retrieved from http://www.jad-journal.com/article/0165-0327(95)00032-I/abstract
Jaffee, S. R., & Price, T. S. (2008). Genotype-environment correlations: Implications for determining the relationship between environmental exposures and psychiatric illness. *Psychiatry, 7*(12), 496–499. https://doi.org/10.1016/j.mppsy.2008.10.002
Jimenez, J. P., Botto, A., Herrera, L., Leighton, C., Rossi, J. L., Quevedo, Y., … Luyten, P. (2018). Psychotherapy and genetic neuroscience: An emerging dialog. *Frontiers in Genetics, 9*, 257. https://doi.org/10.3389/fgene.2018.00257
John, O. P., & Gross, J. J. (2004). Healthy and unhealthy emotion regulation: Personality processes, individual differences, and life span development. *Journal of Personality, 72*(6), 1301–1333. https://doi.org/10.1111/j.1467-6494.2004.00298.x
Kaufman, J., Yang, B. Z., Douglas-Palumberi, H., Houshyar, S., Lipschitz, D., Krystal, J. H., & Gelernter, J. (2004). Social supports and serotonin transporter gene moderate depression in maltreated children. *Proceedings of the National Academy of Sciences of the United States of America, 101*(49), 17316–17321. https://doi.org/10.1073/pnas.0404376101
Keller, M. C., & Nesse, R. M. (2006). The evolutionary significance of depressive symptoms: Different adverse situations lead to different depressive symptom patterns. *Journal of Personality and Social Psychology, 91*(2), 316–330. https://doi.org/10.1037/0022-3514.91.2.316
Kendler, K. S., & Eaves, L. J. (1986). Models for the joint effect of genotype and environment on liability to psychiatric illness. *The American Journal of Psychiatry, 143*(3), 279–289. Retrieved from http://search.proquest.com.ezproxy.puc.cl/docview/220469699?accountid=16788
Kendler, K. S., Karkowski, L. M., & Prescott, C. A. (1999). Causal relationship between stressful life events and the onset of major depression. *The American Journal of Psychiatry, 156*(6), 837–841.
Kendler, K. S., Kessler, R. C., Walters, E. E., MacLean, C., Neale, M. C., Heath, A. C., & Eaves, L. J. (1995). Stressful life events, genetic liability, and onset of an episode of major depression in women. *The American Journal of Psychiatry, 152*(6), 833–842.
Kennis, M., Rademaker, A. R., & Geuze, E. (2013). Neural correlates of personality: An integrative review. *Neuroscience and Biobehavioral Reviews, 37*(1), 73–95. https://doi.org/10.1016/j.neubiorev.2012.10.012
Kilpatrick, D. G., Koenen, K. C., Ruggiero, K. J., Acierno, R., Galea, S., Resnick, H. S., … Gelernter, J. (2007). The serotonin transporter genotype and social support and moderation of posttraumatic stress disorder and depression in hurricane-exposed adults. *The American Journal of Psychiatry, 164*(11), 1693–1699. https://doi.org/10.1176/appi.ajp.2007.06122007
Kim, J. M., Stewart, R., Kim, S. W., Kang, H. J., Kim, S. Y., Lee, J. Y., … Yoon, J. S. (2014). Interactions between a serotonin transporter gene, life events and social support on suicidal ideation in Korean elders. *Journal of Affective Disorders, 160*, 14–20. https://doi.org/10.1016/j.jad.2014.02.030
Kirsch, I. (2019). Placebo effect in the treatment of depression and anxiety. *Frontiers in Psychiatry, 10*, 407. https://doi.org/10.3389/fpsyt.2019.00407

Klein, D. N., Kotov, R., & Bufferd, S. J. (2011). Personality and depression: Explanatory models and review of the evidence. *Annual Review of Clinical Psychology, 7*, 269–295. https://doi.org/10.1146/annurev-clinpsy-032210-104540

Kotov, R., Watson, D., Robles, J. P., & Schmidt, N. B. (2007). Personality traits and anxiety symptoms: The multilevel trait predictor model. *Behaviour Research and Therapy, 45*(7), 1485–1503. https://doi.org/10.1016/j.brat.2006.11.011

Kraepelin, E. (2012). *La locura maníaco-depresiva*. Madrid, Spain: Ergon.

Krishnadas, R., & Cavanagh, J. (2012). Depression: An inflammatory illness? *Journal of Neurology, Neurosurgery, and Psychiatry, 83*(5), 495–502. https://doi.org/10.1136/jnnp-2011-301779

Krueger, R. F., & Johnson, W. (2008). Behavioral genetics and personality: A new look at the integration of nature and nurture. In O. P. John, R. W. Robins, & L. A. Pervin (Eds.), *Handbook of personality: Theory and research* (3rd ed., pp. 287–310). New York, NY: Guilford.

Lanfumey, L., Mongeau, R., Cohen-Salmon, C., & Hamon, M. (2008). Corticosteroid-serotonin interactions in the neurobiological mechanisms of stress-related disorders. *Neuroscience and Biobehavioral Reviews, 32*(6), 1174–1184. https://doi.org/10.1016/j.neubiorev.2008.04.006

Leighton, C., Botto, A., Silva, J. R., Jiménez, J. P., & Luyten, P. (2017). Vulnerability or sensitivity to the environment? Methodological issues, trends, and recommendations in gene–environment interactions research in human behavior. *Frontiers in Psychiatry, 8*, 106. https://doi.org/10.3389/fpsyt.2017.00106

Leonard, B. E. (2005). The HPA and immune axes in stress: The involvement of the serotonergic system. *European Psychiatry: The Journal of the Association of European Psychiatrists, 20*(Suppl 3) (Journal Article), S302–S306.

Liu, R. T. (2013). Stress generation: Future directions and clinical implications. *Clinical Psychology Review, 33*(3), 406–416. https://doi.org/10.1016/j.cpr.2013.01.005

Luyten, P., Blatt, S., & Corveleyn, J. (2005). Towards integration in the theory and treatment of depression? The time is now. In J. Corveleyn, P. Luyten, & S. Blatt (Eds.), *The theory and treatment of depression. Towards a dynamic interactionism model* (Vol. First, pp. 253–284). Leuven, Belgium: Leuven University Press.

Luyten, P., Fonagy, P., Lemma, A., & Target, M. (2012). Depression. In A. Bateman & P. Fonagy (Eds.), *Handbook of mentalizing in mental health practice* (Vol. First, pp. 385–417). Washington, DC: American Psychiatric Association.

Malhi, G. S., & Mann, J. J. (2018). Depression. *Lancet, 392*(10161), 2299–2312. https://doi.org/10.1016/S0140-6736(18)31948-2

Markett, S., Montag, C., & Reuter, M. (2018). Network neuroscience and personality. *Personal Neuroscience, 1*, e14. https://doi.org/10.1017/pen.2018.12

McNaughton, N. (2020). Personality neuroscience and psychopathology: Should we start with biology and look for neural-level factors? *Personal Neuroscience, 3*, e4. https://doi.org/10.1017/pen.2020.5

Moffitt, T. E., Caspi, A., & Rutter, M. (2005). Strategy for investigating interactions between measured genes and measured environments. *Archives of General Psychiatry, 62*(5), 473–481. https://doi.org/10.1001/archpsyc.62.5.473

Monroe, S. M., & Simons, A. D. (1991). Diathesis-stress theories in the context of life stress research: Implications for the depressive disorders. *Psychological Bulletin, 110*(3), 406–425. Retrieved from http://psycnet.apa.org/journals/bul/110/3/406/

Morales, E., & Duffy, D. (2019). Genetics and gene-environment interactions in childhood and adult onset asthma. *Frontiers in Pediatrics, 7*, 499. https://doi.org/10.3389/fped.2019.00499

Munafo, M. R. (2012). The serotonin transporter gene and depression. *Depression and Anxiety, 29*(11), 915–917. https://doi.org/10.1002/da.22009

Nemeroff, C. B. (1998). The neurobiology of depression. *Scientific American, 278*(6), 42–49.

Nemeroff, C. B., Heim, C. M., Thase, M. E., Klein, D. N., Rush, A. J., Schatzberg, A. F., ... Keller, M. B. (2003). Differential responses to psychotherapy versus pharmacotherapy in patients with chronic forms of major depression and childhood trauma. *Proceedings of the National*

Academy of Sciences of the United States of America, 100(24), 14293–14296. https://doi.org/10.1073/pnas.2336126100

Nesse, R. M. (2000). Is depression an adaptation? *Archives of General Psychiatry, 57*(1), 14–20.

Nettle, D. (2004). Evolutionary origins of depression: A review and reformulation. *Journal of Affective Disorders, 81*(2), 91–102. https://doi.org/10.1016/j.jad.2003.08.009

Parker, G. (2000). Classifying depression: Should paradigms lost be regained? *The American Journal of Psychiatry, 157*(8), 1195–1203. https://doi.org/10.1176/appi.ajp.157.8.1195

Parker, G. B., & Crawford, J. (2007). A spectrum model for depressive conditions: Extrapolation of the atypical depression prototype. *Journal of Affective Disorders, 103*(1–3), 155–163. https://doi.org/10.1016/j.jad.2007.01.022

Perez-Perez, B., Cristobal-Narvaez, P., Sheinbaum, T., Kwapil, T. R., Ballespi, S., Pena, E., … Barrantes-Vidal, N. (2018). Interaction between FKBP5 variability and recent life events in the anxiety spectrum: Evidence for the differential susceptibility model. *PLoS One, 13*(2), e0193044. https://doi.org/10.1371/journal.pone.0193044

Pergamin-Hight, L., Bakermans-Kranenburg, M. J., van Ijzendoorn, M. H., & Bar-Haim, Y. (2012). Variations in the promoter region of the serotonin transporter gene and biased attention for emotional information: A meta-analysis. *Biological Psychiatry, 71*(4), 373–379. https://doi.org/10.1016/j.biopsych.2011.10.030

Plomin, R., DeFries, J., McClearn, G., & Rutter, M. (1997). *Behavioral genetics*. New York, NY: W. H. Freeman.

Raby, B. A. (2019). Asthma severity, nature or nurture: Genetic determinants. *Current Opinion in Pediatrics, 31*(3), 340–348. https://doi.org/10.1097/mop.0000000000000758

Risch, N., Herrell, R., Lehner, T., Liang, K. Y., Eaves, L., Hoh, J., … Merikangas, K. R. (2009). Interaction between the serotonin transporter gene (5-HTTLPR), stressful life events, and risk of depression: A meta-analysis. JAMA: The Journal of the American Medical Association, 301(23), 2462–2471. https://doi.org/10.1001/jama.2009.878

Rutter, M. (2007). Gene-environment interdependence. *Developmental Science, 10*(1), 12–18. https://doi.org/10.1111/j.1467-7687.2007.00557.x

Rutter, M. (2010). Gene-environment interplay. *Depression and Anxiety, 27*(1), 1–4. https://doi.org/10.1002/da.20641

Rutter, M., Dunn, J., Plomin, R., Simonoff, E., Pickles, A., Maughan, B., … Eaves, L. (1997). Integrating nature and nurture: Implications of person–environment correlations and interactions for developmental psychopathology. *Development and Psychopathology, 9*(02), 335–364. Retrieved from https://doi.org/10.1017/S0954579497002083

Scarr, S., & McCartney, K. (1983). How people make their own environments: A theory of genotype greater than environment effects. *Child Development, 54*(2), 424–435.

Schneider, K. (1997). *Psicopatología clínica*. Madrid, Spain: Fundación Archivos de Neurobiología.

Sen, S., Burmeister, M., & Ghosh, D. (2004). Meta-analysis of the association between a serotonin transporter promoter polymorphism (5-HTTLPR) and anxiety-related personality traits. *American Journal of Medical Genetics. Part B, Neuropsychiatric Genetics, 127B*(1), 85–89. https://doi.org/10.1002/ajmg.b.20158

Shao, X., & Zhu, G. (2020). Associations among monoamine neurotransmitter pathways, personality traits, and major depressive disorder. *Frontiers in Psychiatry, 11*, 381. https://doi.org/10.3389/fpsyt.2020.00381

Shea, A., Walsh, C., Macmillan, H., & Steiner, M. (2005). Child maltreatment and HPA axis dysregulation: Relationship to major depressive disorder and post traumatic stress disorder in females. *Psychoneuroendocrinology, 30*(2), 162–178. https://doi.org/10.1016/j.psyneuen.2004.07.001

Siever, L. J., & Davis, K. L. (1991). A psychobiological perspective on the personality disorders. *The American Journal of Psychiatry, 148*(12), 1647–1658. https://doi.org/10.1176/ajp.148.12.1647

Stocker, C. M., Masarik, A. S., Widaman, K. F., Reeb, B. T., Boardman, J. D., Smolen, A., … Conger, K. J. (2017). Parenting and adolescents' psychological adjustment: Longitudinal moderation by adolescents' genetic sensitivity. *Development and Psychopathology, 29*(4), 1289–1304. https://doi.org/10.1017/s0954579416001310

Taubner, S., Wiswede, D., & Kessler, H. (2013). Neural activity in relation to empirically derived personality syndromes in depression using a psychodynamic fMRI paradigm. *Frontiers in Human Neuroscience, 7*, 812. https://doi.org/10.3389/fnhum.2013.00812

Taylor, S. E., Way, B. M., Welch, W. T., Hilmert, C. J., Lehman, B. J., & Eisenberger, N. I. (2006). Early family environment, current adversity, the serotonin transporter promoter polymorphism, and depressive symptomatology. *Biological Psychiatry, 60*(7), 671–676. https://doi.org/10.1016/j.biopsych.2006.04.019

Tellenbach, H. (1976). *La Melancolía. Visión histórica del problema: endogeneidad, tipología, patogenia y clínica*. Madrid, Spain: Morata.

Tennant, C. (2002). Life events, stress and depression: A review of recent findings. *Australian and New Zealand Journal of Psychiatry, 36*(2), 173–182. https://doi.org/10.1046/j.1440-1614.2002.01007.x

Uher, R. (2008). The implications of gene-environment interactions in depression: Will cause inform cure? *Molecular Psychiatry, 13*(12), 1070–1078. https://doi.org/10.1038/mp.2008.92

Uher, R. (2014). Gene-environment interactions in severe mental illness. *Frontiers in Psychiatry, 5*, 48.

van der Lem, R., van der Wee, N. J., van Veen, T., & Zitman, F. G. (2012). Efficacy versus effectiveness: A direct comparison of the outcome of treatment for mild to moderate depression in randomized controlled trials and daily practice. *Psychotherapy and Psychosomatics, 81*(4), 226–234. https://doi.org/10.1159/000330890

Vazquez, G. H., Tondo, L., Mazzarini, L., & Gonda, X. (2012). Affective temperaments in general population: A review and combined analysis from national studies. *Journal of Affective Disorders, 139*(1), 18–22. https://doi.org/10.1016/j.jad.2011.06.032

Way, B. M., & Lieberman, M. D. (2010). Is there a genetic contribution to cultural differences? Collectivism, individualism and genetic markers of social sensitivity. *Social Cognitive and Affective Neuroscience, 5*(2–3), 203–211. https://doi.org/10.1093/scan/nsq059

Way, B. M., & Taylor, S. E. (2010). Social influences on health: Is serotonin a critical mediator? *Psychosomatic Medicine, 72*(2), 107–112. https://doi.org/10.1097/PSY.0b013e3181ce6a7d

Westen, D., Novotny, C. M., & Thompson-Brenner, H. (2004). The empirical status of empirically supported psychotherapies: Assumptions, findings, and reporting in controlled clinical trials. *Psychological Bulletin, 130*(4), 631–663. https://doi.org/10.1037/0033-2909.130.4.631

Whittle, S., Allen, N. B., Lubman, D. I., & Yucel, M. (2006). The neurobiological basis of temperament: Towards a better understanding of psychopathology. *Neuroscience and Biobehavioral Reviews, 30*(4), 511–525. https://doi.org/10.1016/j.neubiorev.2005.09.003

Zuckerman, M. (1999). *Vulnerability to psychopathology: A biosocial model*. Washington, DC: American Psychological Association.

Chapter 7
The Functional Domain of Self-Criticism

Ulrike Dinger, Christina A. Löw, and Johannes C. Ehrenthal

Abstract Self-criticism has been identified as a core dimension of depressive experience. At the same time, the ability to regulate self-esteem and maintain a realistic and positive view of the self is an important aspect of personality functioning. Thus, the functional domain of self-criticism overlaps with both depression and personality dysfunction. The chapter will first provide an overview of commonalities and differences between self-criticism, depression, and personality dysfunction. Empirical studies are reviewed to shed light on the overlap as well as the unique aspects of the three constructs. A particular focus will be placed on the impact of personality dysfunction from a perspective of the Structural Integration Axis of the Operationalized Psychodynamic Diagnosis System (OPD-2), which highly overlaps with the levels of functioning from the DSM-5 Alternative Model of Personality Disorders. Secondly, we review clinical theory and empirical research on self-criticism as a predictor of psychotherapy outcome. The findings demonstrate that pronounced self-criticism has a meaningful impact on the treatment process and needs to be addressed specifically and adaptively for successful outcomes.

Keywords Self-criticism · Personality dysfunction · Depression · Outcome predictors

U. Dinger (✉)
Department for General Internal Medicine and Psychosomatics, University Hospital Heidelberg, Heidelberg, Germany
e-mail: Ulrike.Dinger-Ehrenthal@med.uni-heidelberg.de

C. A. Löw
Department for General Internal Medicine and Psychosomatics, University Hospital Heidelberg, Heidelberg, Germany

Psychologisches Institut, Universität Heidelberg, Heidelberg, Germany

J. C. Ehrenthal
Department of Psychology, University of Cologne, Cologne, Germany

G. de la Parra et al. (eds.), *Depression and Personality Dysfunction*, Depression and Personality, https://doi.org/10.1007/978-3-030-70699-9_7

7.1 The Construct of Self-Criticism

A critical view of the self is highly prevalent in depression. As early as Freud's seminal writing *Mourning and Melancholia*, he described the phenomenon of self-criticism as moralistic superego attacks on the ego (Freud, 1917). Freud further described the characteristics of the depressive experience, already alluding to a self-critical stance therein:

> The distinguishing mental features of melancholia are a profoundly painful dejection, cessation of interest in the outside world, loss of the capacity to love, inhibition of all activity, *and a lowering of the self-regarding feelings to a degree that finds utterance in self-reproaches and self-revilings, and culminates in delusional expectation of punishment* (emphasis added, p. 244).

A more detailed examination of the construct of self-criticism later occurred in Sid J. Blatt's two-polarities model of personality development (Blatt, 1974, 2006; Blatt & Zuroff, 1992). In his cognitive-developmental theory, he adopted the idea of two very fundamental psychological dimensions – *interpersonal relatedness* and *self-definition* – and linked them to variations in normal personality development and to differences in psychopathology. According to Blatt, normal personality development evolves through a complex dialectic interaction between relatedness (the development of increasingly mature, intimate, mutually satisfying, reciprocal, interpersonal relationships), and self-definition (the development of an increasingly differentiated, integrated, realistic, essentially positive sense of self or identity) across the lifespan. Developmental disruptions are assumed to cause a defensive, markedly exaggerated preoccupation with one of these basic configurations at the expense of the other. These imbalances might be mild as in normal personality variations or more distinct, resulting in severe personality pathology.

Blatt (2008) coined the term self-criticism to refer to an exaggerated emphasis on the developmental line of self-definition. Thus, self-critical individuals are particularly concerned with issues of self-definition such as self-worth, autonomy, and self-control, while they neglect interpersonal relationships. They can be very competitive, driven by high ambitions, perfectionism, and an effort to avoid failures. At the same time, they cannot feel lasting satisfaction in reaction to successes and thus permanently raise the bar for achievements (Blatt, 1995, 1998; Blatt, Shahar, & Zuroff, 2001). Furthermore, self-critical individuals fear to be criticized by others and to lose others' appreciation. As a consequence, they frequently experience feelings of unworthiness, failure, guilt, inferiority, and shame (Blatt & Luyten, 2009; Whelton & Greenberg, 2005).

In a similar vein, the cognitive school of psychotherapy postulated two basic dimensions of vulnerability to depression that can be related to Blatt's conceptualizations of relatedness and self-definition (Beck, 1983). While *sociotropy* refers to a person's tendency to focus on interpersonal relationships, the fear of being disappointed or abandoned, and includes wishes for intimacy, acceptance, and support, *autonomy* refers to an individual's need for independence and control, the fear of personal failure or defeat, and associated self-reproaches. Although measures of sociotropy correlate with interpersonal relatedness, autonomy does not converge with Blatt's understanding of self-criticism (Blaney & Kutcher, 1991; Rude & Burnham, 1993). As opposed to self-criticism, autonomy implies rather positive than negative premorbid self-evaluations and can be understood as a construct emphasizing aspects of counterdependency rather than unrelenting self-scrutiny (Blaney & Kutcher, 1991; Zuroff, Mongrain, & Santor, 2004). Thus, even though both two-polarities models overlap significantly, Blatt, Quinlan, Pilkonis, and Shea (1995) defined the construct of self-criticism more narrowly in terms of negative self-evaluations associated with active self-bashing. While not explicitly using the term self-criticism, the cognitive approach still implies the concept of self-critical thoughts and beliefs within Beck's conceptualization of the depressive triad (Beck, Rush, Shaw, & Emery, 1979), which was formulated even before the idea of the sociotropy-autonomy dichotomy emerged. The depressive triad postulates three types of negative automatic thoughts present in depression: negative views about (1) the self, (2) the world, and (3) the future. The negative views about the self imply self-critical thoughts such as "I am worthless and inadequate," which are assumed to be activated in specific situations that trigger the underlying (self-critical) core belief (Beck & Alford, 2009).

7.1.1 Development of Self-Criticism

Within psychodynamic as well as in cognitive approaches, self-criticism is thought to develop as a result of repetitive, early life experiences with significant others, which lead to the development of mental representations or cognitive schemas (Beck, 1996; Blatt, 1974). In line with psychoanalytic object relations theories, Blatt and colleagues (Blatt, 1974; Blatt & Lerner, 1983) assume that early parent-child interactions lead to the formation of mental representations of self and others, which gain complexity throughout the life span and which are composed of affective, cognitive, and motivational features. Specifically, self-critical traits are assumed to originate in the experience of children with parental criticism in a harsh and punitive family environment (Flett, Hewitt, Oliver, & Macdonald, 2002). Similarly, Beck (1967) attributes the development of negative core beliefs and cognitions about the self to critical and disapproving caregivers. Later on, he also spoke of modes or schemas with cognitive, affective, behavioral, and motivational elements that have their origin in early childhood experience and become more elaborate and abstract over time (Beck, 1996). Empirical associations between self-criticism and childhood experiences linked a self-critical stance with parental rejection, overprotection, and unfairness (Campos, Besser, & Blatt, 2013; Irons, Gilbert, Baldwin, Baccus, & Palmer, 2006; Katz & Nelson, 2007).

The assumptions that the predisposition for self-criticism is formed in early infancy and that the cognitive-affective mental structures underlying self-criticism differentiate over the course of development raise the question of whether self-criticism should be rather understood as a trait-like construct or as a more variable state. While Blatt originally spoke of self-criticism as a relatively stable trait, which is however amenable to change within psychotherapy (Blatt & Behrends, 1987), together with colleagues, he later elaborated on a state-trait model of self-criticism (Zuroff, Blatt, Sanislow III, Bondi, & Pilkonis, 1999). This model posits that the availability (i.e., content and structure) of self-critical representations might be rather stable, while the accessibility of these representations can fluctuate due to current mood, social context, and biological factors. Empirical support for this model was recently provided by Zuroff, Sadikaj, Kelly, and Leybman (2016), who showed that self-criticism displayed both trait-like variance between persons and daily fluctuations around individuals' mean scores. Within cognitive theory at first sight, self-criticism is conceptualized as a rather transient set of thoughts, beliefs, and attitudes toward the self as part of the depressive triad (Beck et al., 1979). However, from the very beginning, Beck defined core beliefs as relatively stable cognitive patterns, and with the adaption of his theory and the introduction of modes that entail cognitive, affective, behavioral, and motivational elements, he moved even closer to a theory of personality development (Beck, 1996). Hence, within both the psychodynamic and cognitive tradition, self-criticism can refer to a relatively stable trait as well as to state-like components such as self-critical automatic thoughts or attitudes.

7.1.2 Measurement of Self-Criticism

The different approaches toward self-criticism described above are also visible in the multiplicity of available assessment instruments. To date, self-criticism is typically measured by self-report questionnaires. One of the most extensively used scales assessing self-criticism, the Depressive Experiences Questionnaire (DEQ), was developed in the research group around Blatt in the mid-1970s (Blatt, D'Afflitti, & Quinlan, 1976). The DEQ self-criticism subscale includes items that reflect a discrepancy between a person's self-image and his or her ideals as well as an associated active self-bashing. Item examples are as follows: "I often find that I don't live up to my own standards or ideals," "There is a considerable gap between how I am now and how I would like to be," and "I tend to be very self-critical." Another widely used scale for self-criticism, the Dysfunctional Attitude Scale (DAS; Weissman & Beck, 1978), is based on Beck's conception of cognitive dysfunctions and was developed to assess pervasive negative attitudes of depressed people toward the self. Item examples are as follows: "If I fail at my work, then I am a failure as a person" and "If I do not do as well as other people, it means I am an inferior human being." More recent instruments try to distinguish between different subtypes of self-criticism (Gilbert, Clarke, Hempel, Miles, & Irons, 2004; Thompson & Zuroff, 2004). For example, the Forms of Self-Criticizing/Attacking and Self-Reassuring Scale (FSCRS; Gilbert et al., 2004) differs between a component of self-criticism that relates to dwelling on mistakes and a sense of inadequacy (*inadequate self*; e.g., "I remember and dwell on my failings" or "There is a part of me that feels I am not good enough") and a second, more aggressive component that relates to the urge to hurt the self and feel disgust or hate toward the self (*hated self*; e.g., "I have become so angry with myself that I want to hurt or injure myself" or "I have a sense of disgust with myself").

7.1.3 Perfectionism and Self-Esteem

Self-criticism overlaps with other constructs related to self-evaluation such as perfectionism and self-esteem. In the past, *perfectionism* and self-criticism were even used interchangeably or merged into the term *self-critical perfectionism* (Blatt, Zuroff, Hawley, & Auerbach, 2010; Blatt et al., 1995; Shahar, Blatt, & Zuroff, 2007). The work of Dunkley and colleagues was helpful with regard to disentangling the confusion of terms (Dunkley & Blankstein, 2000; Dunkley, Blankstein, Masheb, & Grilo, 2006; Dunkley, Zuroff, & Blankstein, 2006). They found that different measures of perfectionism and self-criticism load on two higher-order dimensions they called *personal standards perfectionism* and *self-critical* or *evaluative concerns perfectionism*. While personal standards perfectionism refers to the setting of and striving for high standards for oneself, self-critical perfectionism refers to overly critical evaluations of one's own behavior, an inability to derive satisfaction from successful performance, and chronic concerns about others' criticism and expectations. Based on findings that associated self-critical perfectionism consistently with psychopathology, while personal standards showed weak or nonexistent associations with psychopathology (Dunkley, Blankstein, et al., 2006; Dunkley, Zuroff, & Blankstein, 2006; Stoeber & Otto, 2006), it was concluded that the setting of and striving for high standards is not in itself pathological but that the tendency to critically evaluate the self is pathological and maladaptive. The researchers further found the DEQ self-criticism subscale to be the primary indicator of the self-critical perfectionism dimension (Dunkley, Zuroff, & Blankstein, 2003). Thus, most researchers in the field view self-critical perfectionism and self-criticism as identical, whereas the construct of perfectionism involves further facets such as personal standards (Dunkley, Zuroff, & Blankstein, 2006; Shahar, 2015).

The content overlap between self-criticism and self-esteem is also worth a consideration. Self-esteem is one of the most widely investigated personality and self-concept constructs in psychology (Baumeister, 1993; Hewitt, 2002; Kernis, 2006; Rosenberg, 1965; Swann & Bosson, 2010). The first influential definition of self-esteem was formulated by William James (1890), who viewed self-esteem in terms of the ratio of successes to pretentions in important areas of life. He argued that self-esteem becomes visible in the gap between the real self and the ideal self. This definition comes very close to the items of the DEQ self-criticism subscale that reflect a discrepancy between a person's self-image and his or her ideals. Later approaches to self-esteem stressed the aspect of personal worth and the judgment of the value of the self (Donnellan, Trzesniewski, & Robins, 2011; Kernis & Waschull, 1995; Rosenberg, 1965; Sedikides & Gress, 2003). For example, Rosenberg (1965), one of the most prominent theoreticians in the field of self-esteem, stated that self-esteem refers to an individual's overall evaluation of his or her worth as a person. This cognitive self-appraisal in self-esteem is accompanied by an emotional experience toward the self (Crocker & Park, 2012; Leary & Baumeister, 2000). MacDonald and Leary (2012) even put this affective component at the heart of their definition of self-esteem, speaking of an affectively laden self-evaluation, which basically reflects how a person feels about him- or herself. While such an affective self-evaluation is clearly present in self-esteem as well as in self-criticism, it becomes clear from the definitions above that self-esteem refers to how a person generally or most typically feels about him- or herself, while self-criticism specifically refers to critically evaluating and attacking the self. In fact, associations between self-criticism and self-esteem range between −.44 and −.68 (Abela, Webb, Wagner, Ho, & Adams, 2006; Dunkley & Grilo, 2007), suggesting an overlap between both constructs but no perfect congruency. Possibly, self-criticism and self-esteem might even interact in predicting clinical outcomes. Abela et al. (2006) found that individuals with high levels of self-criticism and low levels of self-esteem reported greater elevations in depressive symptoms following elevations in hassles than did individuals with only one or neither of these vulnerability factors. They concluded that self-criticism is a vulnerability factor for depression but only for individuals with low self-esteem.

Altogether, the lack of a clear-cut definition of the term self-criticism poses a challenge to the study of the construct. However, the most comprehensive one might be a combination of definitions from the two research groups around Sidney J. Blatt and David M. Dunkley, who state that self-criticism involves constant and harsh self-scrutiny, overly critical evaluations of one's own behavior, an inability to derive satisfaction from successful performance, ongoing concerns over mistakes, and negative reactions to perceived failures in terms of active self-bashing and hostility toward the self (Blatt & Luyten, 2009; Dunkley & Kyparissis, 2008; Dunkley et al., 2003).

7.2 Self-Criticism as Part of the Depressive Experience

The original clinical description of self-critical phenomena in depressive patients by Freud was intertwined with the description of melancholia and depression. In Freud's view, the main difference between mourning and melancholia is the loss of self-respect, which manifests in self-accusations and self-hate (Freud, 1917). As a consequence, later clinical theories of depression evolved around the view of the self and further described how the clinical experience of self-criticism contributes to the development and shapes the clinical expression of depression (e.g., Abraham, Jacobson, and others). Building on this previous work, Sid Blatt's further development of two pathways leading to depression has been labeled as the "double helix theory of depression" (Auerbach, 2015). Thus, although the relevance of the two dimensions relatedness and self-definition was later extended to other disorders as well, the theory originated from the description of depressed patients. Blatt proposed that one of the two forms of depression is primarily shaped by the experience of self-criticism, which further indicates the high importance of this domain for depressive disorders. As outlined above, this conceptualization is in agreement with cognitive theory and therapy, which puts negative views of the self as part of the depressive triad at the core target of the treatment (Beck, 1967). Notably, different theoretical traditions view self-criticism as integral part of depressive psychopathology.

A closer look at the criteria for depressive disorders in the main classification systems further underscores the special importance of self-criticism for depression. The DSM-5 (American Psychiatric Association, 2013) as well as the ICD-10 (World Health Organization, 1993) both include feelings of worthlessness (DSM-5) and reduced self-esteem and ideas of unworthiness (both ICD-10) as part of the symptoms of a depressive episode. In comparison, feelings of dependency (which are of similar theoretical importance for the development of depression according to the theories outlined above) are not included in any of the major classification systems.

Additional support for the clinical relevance of impairments in the functional domain of self-criticism for the clinical description of depression comes from the repeated finding that self-critical subtypes of depression are especially severe and may require special care during treatment. For example, clinical literature associates self-criticism with an increased risk for serious, lethal suicide attempts. According to this line of thought, self-critical and perfectionistic patients primarily experience diminished self-worth during a depressive episode, which is accompanied by intense feelings of guilt, shame, and worthlessness (e.g., Campos et al., 2013). These intense negative inner experiences may lead to more severe overall symptoms and have a negative impact on treatment outcome (Blatt, 1995).

7.2.1 Regulation of Self-Esteem as an Aspect of Personality Functioning

While self-criticism in itself received considerable attention, recent developments in the dimensional assessment of personality disorders suggest that personality functioning may be closely related to the phenomenon as well. Personality functioning as an approach to assess personality disorders was reintroduced into mainstream psychiatry with the Alternative Model for the Assessment of Personality Disorders of the DSM-5 (Bender, Morey, & Skodol, 2011) as well as the personality disorders section of the ICD-11 (Tyrer et al., 2011). It provides a number of empirically derived and clinically relevant core psychological abilities with regard to the self and others that help a given individual to cope with internal as well as external demands. The DSM-5 AMPD focuses on self-worth from a general positive self-evaluation and the ability to correctly assess the self and to regulate self-esteem via reduced self-esteem with critical and biased self-view to a more pronounced vulnerability and idealization and devaluation of either the self and to fragile self-esteem with a distorted self-view, strong self-contempt, and/or self-glorification. The ICD-11 also focuses on the ability to maintain an overall positive and stable sense of self-worth and its impairment, where the self-view may be characterized by self-contempt or by grandiosity or eccentricity up to a generally poor self-worth and predominant self-defeating behaviors. DSM-5 and ICD-11 are currently in the process of being evaluated also with regard to self-worth and personality functioning (Tyrer et al., 2019; Zimmermann et al., 2019).

In addition to DSM-5 and ICD-11, there are other models that have already been related to clinical decision-making and intervention strategies for about 25 years, such as the Operationalized Psychodynamic Diagnosis System (OPD-2; Task Force OPD, 2008). Axis IV of the OPD-2 describes personality functioning as 24 facets organized in four areas of abilities related to perception, regulation, communication, and attachment, again toward to the self and others. It is conceptually and empirically related to the DSM-5 AMPD and other similar approaches (Ehrenthal & Benecke, 2019; Jauk & Ehrenthal, in press). In the OPD system, self-esteem and self-worth are present on three axes:

1. It appears as a phenomenon of interpersonal patterns (Axis II) with an experience to belittle, devalue, and embarrass either with regard toward the self or another person. The OPD would take this as a rather descriptive information and try to determine the factors that drive this behavior, which can be motivational insecurities, personality function, a mixture of both, or a secondary regulatory defensive pattern in the service of other factors.
2. It appears as part of a mostly nonconscious motivational conflict (Axis III). Here insecurities about the value of one's own person are compensated either by a more "passive" habitual self-presentation as a person of less worth compared to others, often related to shame, or by an "active," enforced, yet fragile self-confidence toward others, often related to "narcissistic rage." Importantly, the conflictual topic usually becomes relevant in specific situations related to self-esteem such as evaluations, promotions, criticism, review, and the like.
3. It is related to basic psychological capacities (Axis IV). In the OPD-2, in addition to self-reflection and identity, regulation of self-esteem is seen as a key feature of personality functioning. It describes the ability to restore an adequate level of self-esteem after related challenges and is at least conceptually seen as independent from impulse control, which is partly backed by research findings that show that instabilities in self-worth and affective instability are probably not the same phenomenon (Santangelo et al. 2020). Importantly, from the perspective of the OPD, regulation of self-worth can be relatively independent from self-worth conflicts but also occurs with other motivational insecurities and is seen as a separate target for psychotherapeutic interventions. The impact of impairment of these regulatory capacities is therefore not necessarily bound to certain topics but rather shows themselves whenever the psychological system of the individual is challenged by internal or external demands (Ehrenthal & Benecke, 2019; Ehrenthal & Grande, 2014).

Relevant for the understanding of self-criticism are therefore at least three perspectives. Firstly, all of the abovementioned models of personality functioning incorporate psychological capabilities related to self-esteem and regulation of self-worth. In other words, the phenomenon of self-criticism can be observed in interpersonal patterns toward the self and others, which are either driven by motives and motivational conflicts or formed by specific deficits of personality functioning. Secondly, the specific form and impact of self-criticism on other variables may be shaped by levels of personality functioning. If especially capacities of the self, such as self-perception and self-regulation, but also self-soothing abilities are not available, the handling of self-criticism is much more difficult than with relatively intact psychological tools. In other words, self-criticism in an individual with high levels of personality functioning looks differently from and has usually less detrimental consequences than self-criticism in individuals with generally low levels of personality functioning.

7.2.2 Empirical Research on the Overlap Between Self-Criticism, Depression, and Personality Functioning

Empirical research shows that self-criticism overlaps both with depression severity (i.e., depression symptoms) and with personality functioning. Typical empirical studies on the overlap report on the covariance of questionnaires, which are answered at the same time by patients and/or participants. Regarding the correlation between self-criticism and depression severity, numerous studies have been published that demonstrate a positive correlation between the two constructs. Two studies may serve as illustrative examples: Luyten et al. (2007) investigated four samples (patients with major depressive disorder, mixed psychiatry inpatients, university students, and a sample of nonclinical participants from the community) and found a consistent, positive, moderate to high association between depressive symptoms (measured with three different depression scales) and self-criticism (measured with the DEQ) in all four samples. Dinger et al. (2015) reported a similar pattern of correlations for two depressed samples (inpatients from Germany and psychotherapy outpatients in the United States) and further showed that the moderate correlation between the BDI-II and the DEQ was mainly driven by the high correlation with the BDI cognitive subscale. This finding drew attention to the significant overlap of item content in cognitively oriented depression scales with the DEQ, which aims to assess more stable dimension of experience. Thus, it is not entirely clear if the observed associations originate from particularly severe depression symptoms of self-critical individuals or if self-critical attitudes receive particularly high attention in cognitively oriented measures such as the BDI, which might inflate the observed association. Of note, Dinger et al. (2015) reported significantly lower associations between self-reported self-criticism and observer ratings of depression severity (Hamilton Scale).

Studies on the overlap between personality functioning and depression severity also report positive associations between the two constructs. For example, de la Parra, Dagnino, Valdés, and Krause (2017) found a high correlation of self-criticism (DEQ) and personality functioning (OPD-SQ total score) in a combined sample of Chilean outpatient's and university students. Similarly, Dagnino et al. (2018) report a moderate to high correlation between OPD-SQ and the self-criticism scale of the DEQ in a sample of Chilean psychotherapy outpatients. In addition to the conceptual overlap between self-criticism and the capacity for self-regulation of the OPD structure axis, the empirical studies showed specific impairments in self-critical individuals. More specifically, self-criticism is associated with pronounced difficulties in the capacities to *regulate object relationships* and to *attach to internal objects* (Dagnino et al., 2018; de la Parra et al., 2017; Schauenburg & Dinger, 2018).

The empirical findings support the theoretical and clinical perspective that self-criticism is a relevant aspect of the depressive experience as well as an integral aspect of personality dysfunction. As further complication, measures of symptoms (e.g., depression) typically correlate in a low to moderate range with measures of personality dysfunction (Ehrenthal et al., 2012). Thus, a comprehensive analysis of all three constructs is in order to analyze their respective degree of overlap and distinct characteristics. To do so, the study by Schauenburg and Dinger recruited 80 inpatients with a major depressive disorder in a German psychosomatic university hospital. Of these, 44 patients were diagnosed with a comorbid borderline personality disorder (see Dinger et al. in press for further details). At the beginning of their inpatient treatment, patients responded to the BDI-II for depression severity, the OPD-SQ for personality functioning, and the DEQ for self-criticism. The findings showed that each variable overlaps uniquely with the other two, and there is additional shared variance between the three scales. However, more than half of the variance of each instrument is not shared with the other two constructs, which indicates that the separate assessment of the three variables is justified and provides unique information (see Fig. 7.1).

7.3 Self-Criticism as Predictor of Therapy Outcome

As a consequence of the strong link between self-criticism and depression (Blatt, Quinlan, Chevron, McDonald, & Zuroff, 1982; Carver & Ganellan, 1983; Cox, McWilliams, Enns, & Clara, 2004; Mongrain & Leather, 2006; Zuroff, Santor, & Mongrain, 2005), the construct and its role with regard to psychotherapy outcome gained increasing attention since the mid-1990s. One of the first studies investigating the predictive value of self-criticism for therapy outcome was the National Institute of Mental Health (NIMH) Treatment of Depression Collaborative Research Program (TDCRP, Blatt et al., 1995). The TDCRP was a multisite coordinated study that compared the effectiveness of three forms of treatment for outpatients with major depression – interpersonal therapy, cognitive-behavioral therapy, and pharmacotherapy plus clinical management – and a placebo control plus clinical management. Results indicated that self-critical individuals experienced poorer

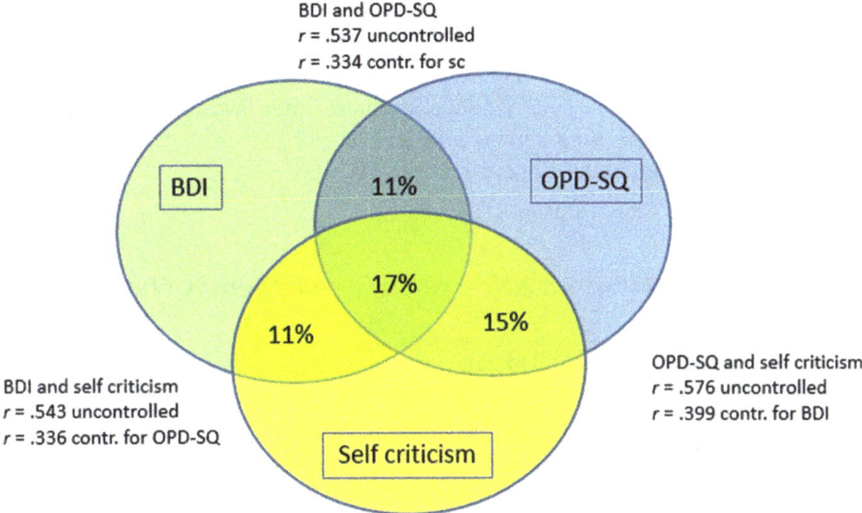

Fig. 7.1 Overlap between depression (BDI), personality functioning (OPD-SQ), and self-criticism (DEQ)

outcomes across all four treatment conditions. Specifically, increased pretreatment levels of self-criticism, as measured by the Dysfunctional Attitude Scale (Weissman & Beck, 1978), significantly interfered with treatment outcome at termination, as measured by posttreatment depression severity scores.

In another frequently cited study, depressed outpatients were randomly assigned to receive either interpersonal therapy, cognitive-behavioral therapy, or pharmacotherapy with clinical management (Marshall, Zuroff, McBride, & Bagby, 2008). Higher pretreatment levels of self-criticism, as measured with the Depressive Experiences Questionnaire (Blatt et al., 1976), predicted higher posttreatment depression levels among individuals treated with interpersonal therapy. In other words, self-criticism was also associated with poorer response to treatment but only for individuals in interpersonal therapy. The authors further found a trend toward self-criticism, predicting better response to pharmacotherapy. In a similar vein, Rector, Bagby, Segal, Joffe, and Levitt (2000) found that highly self-critical patients were more likely to have poor response to treatment. However, this was only the case for individuals treated with cognitive therapy and not for those treated with pharmacotherapy.

Overall, this selection of studies suggests a detrimental effect of self-criticism on treatment outcome, albeit differential effects for different treatment modalities seem to be present. Marshall et al. (2008) attributed these diverging findings to differences in study settings and instruments for self-criticism used. Another explanation might be that treatment methods in fact differently affect the relationship between self-criticism and therapy outcome. In line with this, Blatt and colleagues argue that self-critical patients are more responsive to long-term, intensive, insight-oriented treatments (Blatt & Zuroff, 2005). This assumption is based on the results from the TDCRP that showed self-critical individuals doing less well in brief outpatient treatment as well as the finding that the therapeutic progress among patients with high levels of self-criticism was disrupted in the latter half of the treatment process, possibly due to their anticipation of the forced termination after the 16th treatment session (Blatt et al., 2010). Further support comes from investigations that found self-critical patients showing significantly greater positive changes in open-ended psychoanalysis (Blatt, 1992; Blatt & Ford, 1994).

7.3.1 Meta-Analysis on Self-Criticism and Therapy Outcome

In order to permit a well-founded conclusion about self-criticism as a predictor of therapy outcome, we conducted a comprehensive meta-analysis on the relationship between pretreatment self-criticism and various forms of psychotherapy outcome (Löw, Schauenburg, & Dinger, 2020). The main advantage of this approach is that we do not further have to rely on findings from single studies but that conclusions can be drawn from a quantitative synthesis of relevant findings across a variety of different studies. Thus, the main goal of our meta-analysis was to estimate the magnitude and direction of the overall correlation between self-criticism and therapy outcome, summarizing what researchers have found out about this association up until today. Our definition of self-criticism corresponds with the conceptualizations of the construct by Blatt and Dunkley (see Blatt & Luyten, 2009; Dunkley & Kyparissis, 2008; Dunkley et al., 2003). Since we view self-criticism in terms of a cognitive-affective mental structure, which forms in early child-caregiver dyads and which further differentiates and changes within relationship experiences later in life (see e.g., Blatt, 1974; Blatt & Behrends, 1987), also including the therapeutic relationship, we were particularly interested in treatment outcomes following psychotherapeutic interventions. However, we considered a broad range of therapy outcomes, including primary symptom-related outcomes as well as secondary outcomes such as quality of life, interpersonal and psychological functioning, and psychological stress reactivity. We further included only studies with a longitudinal design, where self-criticism was assessed previous to or in the beginning of treatment and outcome was assessed after treatment.

Based on a systematic literature search and a set of strict inclusion criteria, we could identify 52 longitudinal studies (59 independent effect sizes), which involved 3610 patients. The overall association between pretreatment self-criticism and psychotherapy outcome across all studies was $r = -.21$, suggesting that the higher the level of self-criticism in the beginning of treatment, the poorer the psychotherapeutic outcome. The magnitude of this relationship can be evaluated as small to moderate (Cohen, 1992). A low degree of variability in study outcomes further suggested high comparability of single studies. Thus, on a meta-analytic level, it could be confirmed that self-criticism predicts poor therapy outcome across different treatment modalities, study designs, mental health issues, and outcome measures. However, the association between self-criticism and outcomes varied by type of mental health problem, indicating stronger associations for certain disorders (e.g., eating disorders). The type of treatment also moderated the association, showing the largest negative association between self-criticism and treatment outcome for interpersonal therapies, closely followed by other therapies, which mostly consisted of psychodynamic and emotion-focused therapies, and the lowest negative association for cognitive-behavioral therapies. At first sight, the latter finding challenges the assumption that self-critical patients respond better to psychoanalytic long-term treatment (Blatt & Zuroff, 2005). However, just a very small proportion of primary studies actually included intensive long-term treatments, so the question of which treatment duration fits self-critical patients best cannot be answered yet.

Although the meta-analysis established self-criticism as a small to moderately strong, robust predictor of therapy outcome, based on the correlational nature of primary data, we cannot assume that pretreatment self-criticism *causes* poor treatment response. The exclusive inclusion of longitudinal studies at least added a temporal order, but as described above third variables could still affect the association. Moreover, a handful of studies suggest that we should not only rely on pretreatment self-criticism but also on how self-criticism changes over the course of treatment and how this affects outcome. For example, Rector et al. (2000) found that, while high pretreatment self-criticism was associated with less well response to cognitive psychotherapy, the degree to which self-criticism was successfully reduced in treatment was shown to be the best predictor of outcome. Similarly, the reduction of self-criticism within a psychodynamic therapy was linked with the rate of decrease in symptomatic distress over time (Lowyck, Luyten, Vermote, Verhaest, & Vansteelandt, 2016). However, there are also studies that did not find an association between change in self-criticism over time and therapy outcome (Chui, Zilcha-Mano, Dinger, Barrett, & Barber, 2016; O'Connor, Lavoie, Desaulniers, & Audet, 2018; see systematic review of relevant studies in Löw et al., 2020). In order to better understand the potentially causal impact of self-criticism on treatment outcome and the reciprocal relationships between self-criticism and outcomes over the course of therapy, future research should use prospective designs with multiple measurement points, also taking into account further process and confounding variables. However, the meta-analysis presented here provides a significant contribution to the role of self-criticism in predicting the outcome of psychotherapy.

7.3.2 *Self-Criticism and the Therapeutic Process*

One possible explanation for the relationship between self-criticism and poor psychotherapy outcome can be withdrawn from Blatt's two-polarities model of personality and his conceptualization of self-criticism, which state that an exaggerated preoccupation with issues of self-definition, self-worth, and self-criticism goes at the expense of learning how to build intimate and mutually satisfying interpersonal relationships (Blatt, 1974, 2006). Such deficits in interpersonal relatedness are reflected in too distant, cold, cynical, and even overtly hostile interpersonal behaviors of self-critical individuals as well as in a lack of self-disclosure in intimate relationships (Dinger et al., 2015; Dunkley & Kyparissis, 2008; Mongrain, Lubbers, & Struthers, 2004; Zuroff & Duncan, 1999; Zuroff & Fitzpatrick, 1995). Translating these findings into the therapeutic situation, analyses based on the TDCRP data showed that pretreatment self-criticism interfered with patients' participation in the therapeutic alliance (Zuroff et al., 2000). Furthermore, the disruptions in the therapeutic alliance as a consequence of higher levels of self-criticism significantly interfered with therapeutic outcome (Shahar, Blatt, Zuroff, Krupnick, & Sotsky, 2004). The authors did not only identify self-critical patient's difficulties in relating constructively to their therapist but also their problems with establishing and maintaining satisfying social relationships outside of treatment. Specifically, Shahar et al. (2004) found that pretreatment self-criticism predicted a less positive social network over the course of therapy, which in turn predicted less reduction of symptoms at termination. On the whole, these results suggest that relationship difficulties may mediate the association between self-criticism and psychotherapy outcomes.

In addition to the relationship difficulties that generally go along with high levels of self-criticism, the problem might aggravate for those individuals with additional low personality dysfunction. As specified above, personality functioning overlaps with self-criticism, which appears to be specifically related to the capacities to *regulate relationships* and to *attach to internal objects* (Dagnino et al., 2018; de la Parra et al., 2017; Schauenburg & Dinger, 2018). This pattern of personality dysfunctions again reflects self-critical individuals' deficits in the interpersonal realm and even further highlights the profound scars within personality structure as a consequence of an emphasis on the developmental line of self-definition. It might help to clarify why it is so challenging to build and maintain positive alliances with self-critical patients. The difficulties in the domain of attachment (e.g., the capacity to enter a relationship with trust) and for relationship regulation (e.g., the capacity to hold back on devaluating, cynical comments) can explain why self-critical patients generally tend to behave in a cold or even cynical manner toward others (e.g., Dinger et al., 2015). This is likely to apply to the therapeutic relationship as well, where self-critical patients may be challenged by the necessity to open up toward the therapist and allow a certain degree of closeness.

We argue that in addition to the common variance between self-criticism and personality functioning, the unique variance of personality functioning appears to be important. More specifically, personality dysfunction in general may be a moderator of the association between self-criticism and alliance, with more problems arising for patients with severe personality dysfunction. Clinical and empirical evidence show that patients with severe personality dysfunction, e.g., those with borderline personality disorder, have profound difficulties to engage in a positive and helpful working alliance (e.g., Kivity et al. 2020; Levy et al., 2010; Levy et al. 2017). Thus, we argue that while self-criticism may always be a challenge for the establishment of a positive therapeutic relationship (i.e., regardless of the degree of personality dysfunction), the lack of capacities to deal with interpersonal challenge (e.g., to be able to self-reflect on these difficulties or to be able to communicate the associated emotions) will lead to even greater problems for self-critical individuals with lower levels of personality dysfunction in psychotherapy.

7.4 Clinical Implications

As outlined above, patient self-criticism is an influential and challenging variable in the psychotherapeutic treatment of depression, especially for the development of a secure and trusting relationship. One can further assume that patient agency, i.e., the experience of oneself as positively influential in the therapeutic process, may be hindered in self-critical individuals (Huber, Born, et al., 2019; Huber, Nikendei, et al., 2019). The first consequence that arises from this assumption is a focus on assessment. Clinicians need to know about their patients' harsh and ungracious view of the self in order to tailor their relationship offer and therapeutic strategy toward this issue. As specified above, there are several self-report instruments that can be used either as screening tools (e.g., DEQ short forms with only 12 items, Krieger et al., 2014) or as more detailed measures to differentiate between adaptive and maladaptive forms of self-criticism (e.g., the FSCRS, Gilbert et al., 2004). Ideally, standardized self-reports are complemented by therapists' individual assessment of the self-image, which should be part of regular intake interviews. Particularly informative are patients' responses to therapists' request to describe themselves. In addition, typical relationship difficulties (detached, cold, or critical interpersonal behavior) are likely to occur in the therapeutic relationship with highly self-critical patients, so a monitoring of the interpersonal "messages" toward the therapist as well as patients' tendency to belittle or bash him- or herself during therapy needs to be noticed, taken seriously, and examined in more detail.

If self-criticism has been established as a relevant aspect of the current or chronic clinical problem of the patient, the next step should be directed toward a deepened understanding of possible sources of or risk factors for this issue (see 7.2.1 Regulation of Self-Esteem as an Aspect of Personality Functioning). In line with the OPD-2, the distinction between directly related motivational conflicts or secondary coping strategies for other motivational conflicts, on the one hand, and self-criticism as an epiphenomenon of low personality functioning, on the other hand, is crucial for tailoring the therapeutic approach (Task Force OPD, 2008). In the first case of more "neurotic levels" of good to moderately impaired personality functioning, a self-critical patient may benefit from an attentive and curious therapist, who remains alert to relationship difficulties and connects those with the phenomenon of profound self-criticism. In psychodynamic therapies, these patients are typically treated with longer-term therapy, which aims to change the negative inner representation of the self. Importantly, patients with higher levels of personality functioning can be expected to take responsibility for the therapeutic process. This means that, although the therapist nevertheless needs to display a high degree of sensitivity to the patient's experience of their relationship and the therapy in general, patients can be expected to regulate the view of her- or himself as well as associated emotions in a tolerable corridor. However, it is important to monitor own impulses and motives toward progress, as one of the challenges is to avoid reinforcing self-critical tendencies by identifying with the patient's wish to be a "perfect client." In other words, therapists usually should try to slow down, be mindful about subtle interpersonal signals of insecurity as well as trust, and even consider evaluating tendencies of "imperfection" such as temporarily coming unprepared into sessions, as possible markers of progress.

On the contrary, self-critical patients with lower levels of personality functioning are likely to need more active co-regulation of their inner states, as their capacities to tolerate negative affects, to self-reflect, and to self-soothe will be impaired. Thus, therapists need to collaboratively anticipate with their clients at which points harsh self-scrutiny is likely to appear and explicitly address and try to improve the impaired related structural abilities. Generally, a parental therapeutic stance is helpful, which implies more activity and presence of the therapist to limit regressive phenomena and associated anxiety and to foster interpersonal learning (Dahl et al., 2014; Ehrenthal & Dinger, 2018; Rudolf, 2020).

The meta-analysis and review by Löw et al. (2020) did not indicate that a specific form of treatment was more effective than another for self-critical patients. However, several third-wave CBT treatments specifically aim to increase self-compassion and mindfulness as a buffer against maladaptive, self-critical perfectionism (e.g., acceptance and commitment therapy, mindfulness-based cognitive therapy, compassion-focused therapy). These treatments are effective in increasing self-compassion but not generally more effective than other bona fide therapies (Wilson et al., 2019). Future research will show if these specific treatments are differentially more effective for self-critical patients. On the other hand, approaches with less RCT-based evidence that draw on general strategies for dealing with self-criticism or build intervention strategies that target related areas of personality functioning, for example, psychodynamic treatments, should be put to empirical tests to establish a more competitive evidence based that allows for a better comparison. However, given the variety of phenomena usually associated with the topic, most research is needed on the integration of core principles for reducing self-criticism into established therapy programs. This would also fit in with current ideas of individualized treatment planning along the lines of cross-diagnostic, specific functional impairments. Thus, we would like to end this chapter with a call for further research on helpful therapeutic stances, specific interventions, treatment modules, or other psychotherapy components that prove to be helpful for the severe distress and the challenging relationship difficulties of self-critical individuals.

References

Abela, J. R. Z., Webb, C. A., Wagner, C., Ho, M.-H. R., & Adams, P. (2006). The role of self-criticism, dependency, and hassles in the course of depressive illness: A multiwave longitudinal study. *Personality and Social Psychology Bulletin, 32*(3), 328–338. https://doi.org/10.1177/0146167205280911

American Psychiatric Association. (2013). *Diagnostic and statistical manual of mental disorders* (5th ed.). Washington, DC: Publisher.

Auerbach, J. (2015). Sidney Blatt's contributions to personality assessment. *Journal of Personality Assessment, 98*, 1–4. https://doi.org/10.1080/00223891.2015.1107728

Baumeister, R. F. (1993). *Self-esteem: The puzzle of low self-regard*. New York, NY: Plenum Press.
Beck, A. T. (1967). *Depression: Clinical, experimental and theoretical aspects*. New York, NY: Hoeber.
Beck, A. T. (1983). Cognitive therapy of depression: New perspectives. In P. J. Clayton & J. E. Barrett (Eds.), *Treatment of depression: Old controversies and new approaches* (pp. 265–290). New York, NY: Raven.
Beck, A. T. (1996). Beyond belief: A theory of modes, personality, and psychopathology. In P. Salkovskis (Ed.), *Frontiers of cognitive therapy* (pp. 1–25). New York, NY: Guilford.
Beck, A. T., & Alford, B. A. (2009). *Depression: Causes and treatment* (2nd ed.). Baltimore, MD: University of Pennsylvania Press.
Beck, A. T., Rush, A. J., Shaw, B. F., & Emery, G. (1979). *Cognitive therapy of depression*. New York, NY: Guilford.
Bender, D. S., Morey, L. C., & Skodol, A. E. (2011). Toward a model for assessing level of personality functioning in DSM-5, part I: A review of theory and methods. *Journal of Personality Assessment, 93*(4), 332–346. https://doi.org/10.1080/00223891.2011.583808
Blaney, P. H., & Kutcher, G. S. (1991). Measures of depressive dimensions: Are they interchangeable? *Journal of Personality Assessment, 56*, 502–512.
Blatt, S. J. (1974). Levels of object representation in anaclitic and introjective depression. *Psychoanalytic Study of the Child, 29*, 107–157.
Blatt, S. J. (1992). The differential effect of psychotherapy and psychoanalysis with anaclitic and introjective patients: The Menninger psychotherapy research project revisited. *Journal of the American Psychoanalytic Association, 40*(3), 691–724. https://doi.org/10.1177/000306519204000303
Blatt, S. J. (1995). The destructiveness of perfectionism: Implications for the treatment of depression. *American Psychologist, 50*(12), 1003–1020. https://doi.org/10.1037/0003-066X.50.12.1003
Blatt, S. J. (1998). Contributions of psychoanalysis to the understanding and treatment of depression. *Journal of the American Psychoanalytic Association, 46*, 723–752.
Blatt, S. J. (2006). A fundamental polarity in psychoanalysis: Implications for personality development, psychopathology, and the therapeutic process. *Psychoanalytic Inquiry, 26*(4), 494–520. https://doi.org/10.1080/07351690701310581
Blatt, S. J. (2008). *Polarities of experiences: Relatedness and self-definition in personality development, psychopathology, and the therapeutic process*. Washington, DC: American Psychological Association.
Blatt, S. J., & Behrends, R. S. (1987). Internalization, separation-individuation, and the nature of therapeutic action. *The International Journal of Psychoanalysis, 68*(2), 279–297.
Blatt, S. J., D'Afflitti, J. P., & Quinlan, D. M. (1976). Experiences of depression in normal young adults. *Journal of Abnormal Psychology, 85*(4), 383–389. https://doi.org/10.1037/0021-843X.85.4.383
Blatt, S. J., & Ford, R. Q. (1994). *Therapeutic change: An object relations perspective*. New York, NY: Plenum.
Blatt, S. J., & Lerner, H. D. (1983). The psychological assessment of object representation. *Journal of Personality Assessment, 47*(1), 7–28. https://doi.org/10.1207/s15327752jpa4701_2
Blatt, S. J., & Luyten, P. (2009). A structural-developmental psychodynamic approach to psychopathology: Two polarities of experience across the life span. *Development and Psychopathology, 21*(3), 793–814. https://doi.org/10.1017/S0954579409000431
Blatt, S. J., Quinlan, D. M., Chevron, E. S., McDonald, C., & Zuroff, D. (1982). Dependency and self-criticism: Psychological dimensions of depression. *Journal of Consulting and Clinical Psychology, 50*, 113–124. https://doi.org/10.1037/0022-006X.50
Blatt, S. J., Quinlan, D. M., Pilkonis, P. A., & Shea, M. T. (1995). Impact of perfectionism and need for approval on the brief treatment of depression: The National Institute of Mental Health Treatment of Depression Collaborative Research Program revisited. *Journal of Consulting and Clinical Psychology, 63*(1), 125–132. https://doi.org/10.1037/0022-006X.63.1.125

Blatt, S. J., Shahar, G., & Zuroff, D. C. (2001). Anaclitic (sociotropic) and introjective (autonomous) dimensions. *Psychotherapy: Theory, Research, Practice, Training, 38*(4), 449–454. https://doi.org/10.1037/0033-3204.38.4.449

Blatt, S. J., & Zuroff, D. C. (1992). Interpersonal relatedness and self-definition: Two prototypes for depression. *Clinical Psychology Review, 12*(5), 527–562. https://doi.org/10.1016/0272-7358(92)90070-O

Blatt, S. J., & Zuroff, D. C. (2005). Empirical evaluation of the assumptions in identifying evidence based treatments in mental health. *Clinical Psychology Review, 25*(4), 459–486. https://doi.org/10.1016/j.cpr.2005.03.001

Blatt, S. J., Zuroff, D. C., Hawley, L. L., & Auerbach, J. S. (2010). Predictors of sustained therapeutic change. *Psychotherapy Research, 20*(1), 37–54. https://doi.org/10.1080/10503300903121080

Campos, R. C., Besser, A., & Blatt, S. J. (2013). Recollections of parental rejection, self-criticism and depression in suicidality. *Archives of Suicide Research, 17*(1), 58–74. https://doi.org/10.1080/13811118.2013.748416

Carver, C. S., & Ganellan, R. (1983). Depression and components of self-punitiveness: High standards, self-criticism, and overgeneralization. *Journal of Abnormal Psychology, 92*, 330–337. https://doi.org/10.1037/0021-843X.92.3.330

Chui, H., Zilcha-Mano, S., Dinger, U., Barrett, M. S., & Barber, J. P. (2016). Dependency and self-criticism in treatments for depression. *Journal of Counseling Psychology, 63*(4), 452–459. https://doi.org/10.1037/cou0000142

Cohen, J. (1992). A power primer. *Psychological Bulletin, 112*(1), 155–159.

Cox, B. J., McWilliams, L. A., Enns, M. W., & Clara, I. P. (2004). Broad and specific personality dimensions associated with major depression in a nationally representative sample. *Comprehensive Psychiatry, 45*, 246–253. https://doi.org/10.1016/j.comppsych.2004.03.002

Crocker, J., & Park, L. E. (2012). Contingencies of self-worth. In M. R. Leary & J. P. Tangney (Eds.), *Handbook of self and identity* (pp. 309–326). New York, NY: The Guilford Press.

Dagnino, P., Valdés, C., de-la-Fuente, I., Harismendy, M. d. l. Á., Gallardo, A. M., Gómez-Barris, E., & de-la-Parra, G. (2018). Impacto de la Personalidad y el Estilo Depresivo en los Resultados Psicoterapéuticos de Pacientes con Depresión [The impact of personality and depressive style on the psychotherapeutic outcomes of depressed patients]. *Psykhe: Revista de la Escuela de Psicología, 27*(2), 1–15.

Dahl, H.-S. J., Røssberg, J. I., Crits-Christoph, P., Gabbard, G. O., Hersoug, A. G., Perry, J. C., … Høglend, P. A. (2014). Long-term effects of analysis of the patient–therapist relationship in the context of patients' personality pathology and therapists' parental feelings. *Journal of Consulting and Clinical Psychology, 82*(3), 460–471. https://doi.org/10.1037/a0036410

de la Parra, G., Dagnino, P., Valdés, C., & Krause, M. (2017). Beyond self-criticism and dependency: Structural functioning of depressive patients and its treatment. *Research in Psychotherapy, 20*, 236. https://doi.org/10.4081/ripppo.2017.236

Dinger, U., Barrett, M. S., Zimmermann, J., Schauenburg, H., Wright, A. G., Renner, F., … Barber, J. P. (2015). Interpersonal problems, dependency, and self-criticism in major depressive disorder. *Journal of Clinical Psychology, 71*(1), 93–104. https://doi.org/10.1002/jclp.22120

Donnellan, M. B., Trzesniewski, K. H., & Robins, R. W. (2011). Self- esteem: Enduring issues and controversies. In T. Chamorro-Premuzic, S. von Stumm, & A. Furnham (Eds.), *The Wiley-Blackwell handbook of individual differences* (pp. 718–746). Chichester, UK: Wiley-Blackwell.

Dunkley, D. M., & Blankstein, K. R. (2000). Self-critical perfectionism, coping, hassles, and current distress: A structural equation modeling approach. *Cognitive Therapy and Research, 24*, 713.

Dunkley, D. M., Blankstein, K. R., Masheb, R. M., & Grilo, C. M. (2006). Personal standards and evaluative concerns dimensions of "clinical" perfectionism: A reply to Shafran et al. (2002, 2003) and Hewitt et al. (2003). *Behaviour Research and Therapy, 44*(1), 63–84. https://doi.org/10.1016/j.brat.2004.12.004

Dunkley, D. M., & Grilo, C. M. (2007). Self-criticism, low self-esteem, depressive symptoms, and over-evaluation of shape and weight in binge eating disorder patients. *Behaviour Research and Therapy, 45*(1), 139–149. https://doi.org/10.1016/j.brat.2006.01.017

Dunkley, D. M., & Kyparissis, A. (2008). What is DAS self-critical perfectionism really measuring? Relations with the five-factor model of personality and depressive symptoms. *Personality and Individual Differences, 44*, 1295–1305. https://doi.org/10.1016/j.paid.2007.11.022

Dunkley, D. M., Zuroff, D. C., & Blankstein, K. R. (2003). Self-critical perfectionism and daily affect: Dispositional and situational influences on stress and coping. *Journal of Personality and Social Psychology, 84*(1), 234–252. https://doi.org/10.1037/0022-3514.84.1.234

Dunkley, D. M., Zuroff, D. C., & Blankstein, K. R. (2006). Specific perfectionism components versus self-criticism in predicting maladjustment. *Personality and Individual Differences, 40*(4), 665–676. https://doi.org/10.1016/j.paid.2005.08.008

Ehrenthal, J. C., Dinger, U., Horsch, L., Komo-Lang, M., Klinkerfuß, M., Grande, T., et al. (2012). Der OPD-strukturfragebogen (OPD-SF): erste ergebnisse zu reliabilität und validität. Psychother. Psychosom. Med. Psychol. 62, 25–32. https://doi.org/10.1055/s-0031-1295481.

Ehrenthal, J. C. & Grande, T. (2014). Fokusorientierte Beziehungsgestaltung in der Psychotherapie von Persönlichkeitsstörungen – ein integratives Modell. PiD - Psychotherapie im Dialog, 3, 80–85.

Ehrenthal, J. C., & Dinger, U. (2018). Strukturdiagnostik in der Praxis – von der Indikation zur Therapieplanung. *Ärztliche Psychotherapie, 14*, 32–40.

Ehrenthal, J. C. & Benecke, C. (2019). Tailored treatment planning for individuals with personality disorders: The OPD approach. In: U. Kramer (Ed.). Case Formulation for Personality Disorders: Tailoring Psychotherapy to the Individual Client. Cambridge, MA: Elsevier, pp. 291–314.

Flett, G. L., Hewitt, P. L., Oliver, J. M., & Macdonald, S. (2002). Perfectionism in children and their parents: A developmental analysis. In G. L. Flett & P. L. Hewitt (Eds.), *Perfectionism: Theory, research, and treatment* (pp. 89–132). Washington, DC: American Psychological Association.

Freud, S. (1917). *Mourning and melancholia* (Standard edition 14) (pp. 243–248). New York, NY: Vintage.

Gilbert, P., Clarke, M., Hempel, S., Miles, J. N. V., & Irons, C. (2004). Criticizing and reassuring oneself: An exploration of forms, styles and reasons in female students. *British Journal of Clinical Psychology, 43*(1), 31–50. https://doi.org/10.1348/014466504772812959

Hewitt, J. P. (2002). The social construction of self-esteem. In C. R. Snyder & S. Lopez (Eds.), *Handbook of positive psychology* (pp. 135–147). New York, NY: Oxford University Press.

Huber, J., Born, A.-K., Claaß, C., Ehrenthal, J. C., Nikendei, C., Schauenburg, H., & Dinger, U. (2019). Therapeutic Agency, In-Session Behavior and Patient-Therapist Interaction. *Journal of Clincial Psychology, 75*, 66–78.

Huber, J., Nikendei, C., Ehrenthal, J. C., Schauenburg, H., Dinger, U. (2019). Therapeutic Agency Inventory. *Psychotherapy Research, 29*(7), 919–934.

Irons, C., Gilbert, P., Baldwin, M. W., Baccus, J., & Palmer, M. (2006). Parental recall, attachment relating and self-attacking/self-reassurance: Their relationship with depression. *The British Journal of Clinical Psychology, 12*, 297–308. https://doi.org/10.1348/014466505X68230

James, W. (1890). *The principles of psychology*. New York, NY: Holt.

Jauk, I., & Ehrenthal, J. C. (in press). Self-reported levels of personality functioning from the Operationalized Psychodynamic Diagnosis (OPD) system and emotional intelligence likely assess the same latent construct. *Journal of Personality Assessment*. https://doi.org/10.1080/00223891.2020.17750891

Katz, J., & Nelson, R. A. (2007). Family experiences and self-criticism in college students: Testing a model of family stress, past unfairness, and self-esteem. *The American Journal of Family Therapy, 35*(5), 447–457. https://doi.org/10.1080/01926180601057630

Kernis, M. H. (2006). *Self-esteem issues and answers: A sourcebook of current perspectives*. New York, NY: Psychology Press.

Kernis, M. H., & Waschull, S. B. (1995). The interactive roles of stability and level of self-esteem: Research and theory. In M. P. Zanna (Ed.), *Advances in experimental social psychology* (Vol. 27, pp. 93–141). San Diego, CA: Academic Press.

Kivity, Y., Levy, K. N., Kolly, S., Kramer, U. (2020). The therapeutic alliance over 10 sessions of therapy for Borderline Personality Disorder: Agreement and congruence analysis and relation to outcome. *Journal of Personality Disorders, 34*(1), 1–21, 2020.

Krieger, T., Zimmermann, J., Beutel, M. B., Wiltink, J., Schauenburg, H., & grosse Holtforth, M. (2014). Ein Vergleich verschiedener Kurzversionen des Depressive Experiences Questionnaire (DEQ) zur Erhebung von Selbstkritik und Abhängigkeit. *Diagnostica, 60*(3), 126–139.

Leary, M. R., & Baumeister, R. F. (2000). The nature and function of self-esteem: Sociometer theory. In M. P. Zanna (Ed.), *Advances in experimental social psychology* (Vol. 32, pp. 1–62). New York, NY: Academic Press.

Levy, K. N., Beeney, J. E., Wasserman, R. H., & Clarkin, J. F. (2010). Conflict begets conflict: Executive control, mental state vacillations, and the therapeutic alliance in treatment of borderline personality disorder. Psychotherapy Research, 20, 413–422.

Levy, K. N., Scala, J. W., & Ellison, W. D. (2017). The therapeutic alliance in the treatment of borderline personality disorder: A metaanalysis. Manuscript in preparation.

Löw, C. A., Schauenburg, H., & Dinger, U. (2020). Self-criticism and psychotherapy outcome: A systematic review and meta-analysis. *Clinical Psychology Review, 75*, 101808.

Lowyck, B., Luyten, P., Vermote, R., Verhaest, Y., & Vansteelandt, K. (2016). Self-critical perfectionism, dependency, and symptomatic distress in patients with personality disorder during hospitalization-based psychodynamic treatment: A parallel process growth modeling approach. *Personality Disorders, Theory, Research, and Treatment, 8*(3), 268–274. https://doi.org/10.1037/per0000189

Luyten, P., Sabbe, B., Blatt, S. J., Meganck, S., Jansen, B., De Grave, C., … Corveleyn, J. (2007). Dependency and self-criticism: Relationship with major depressive disorder, severity of depression, and clinical presentation. *Depression and Anxiety, 24*(8), 586–596. https://doi.org/10.1002/da.20272

MacDonald, G., & Leary, M. R. (2012). Individual differences in self-esteem. In M. R. Leary & J. P. Tangney (Eds.), *Handbook of self and identity* (pp. 354–377). New York, NY: The Guilford Press.

Marshall, M. B., Zuroff, D. C., McBride, C., & Bagby, R. M. (2008). Self-criticism predicts differential response to treatment for major depression. *Journal of Clinical Psychology, 64*(3), 231–244. https://doi.org/10.1002/jclp.20438

Mongrain, M., & Leather, F. (2006). Immature dependence and self-criticism predict the recurrence of major depression. *Journal of Clinical Psychology, 62*(6), 705–713. https://doi.org/10.1002/jclp.20263

Mongrain, M., Lubbers, R., & Struthers, W. (2004). The power of love: Mediation of rejection in roommate relationships of dependents and self-critics. *Personality and Social Psychology Bulletin, 30*(1), 94–105. https://doi.org/10.1177/0146167203258861

O'Connor, K., Lavoie, M., Desaulniers, B., & Audet, J. S. (2018). Cognitive psychophysiological treatment of bodily-focused repetitive behaviors in adults: An open trial. *Journal of Clinical Psychology, 74*(3), 273–285. https://doi.org/10.1002/jclp.22501

Rector, N. A., Bagby, R. M., Segal, Z. V., Joffe, R. T., & Levitt, A. (2000). Self-criticism and dependency in depressed patients treated with cognitive therapy or pharmacotherapy. *Cognitive Therapy and Research, 24*(5), 571–584. https://doi.org/10.1023/A:1005566112869

Rosenberg, M. (1965). *Society and the adolescent self-image*. Princeton, NJ: Princeton University Press.

Rude, S. S., & Burnham, B. L. (1993). Do interpersonal and achievement vulnerabilities interact with congruent events to predict depression? Comparison of the DEQ, SAS, DAS, and combined scales. *Cognitive Therapy and Research, 17*, 531–548.

Rudolf, G. (2020). *Structure-oriented psychotherapy [Strukturbezogene Psychotherapie].* Stuttgart, Germany: Schattauer.

Santangelo, P. S., Kockler, T. D., Zeitler, M. L.., Knies, R., Kleindienst, N., Bohus, M., & Ebner-Priemer, U. (2020). Self-esteem instability and affective instability in everyday life after remission from borderline personality disorder. *Borderline Personality Disorder amd Emotion Dysregulation 7*, 25(2020). https://doi.org/10.1186/s40479-020-00140-8

Schauenburg, H., & Dinger, U. (2018). *How does self-criticism overlap with personality functioning and depression severity?* Paper presented at the Society for Psychotherapy Research (SPR), 49th International Annual Meeting, Amsterdam.

Sedikides, C., & Gress, A. P. (2003). Portraits of the self. In M. A. Hogg & J. Cooper (Eds.), *Sage handbook of social psychology* (pp. 110–138). London, UK: Sage.

Shahar, G. (2015). *Erosion: The psychopathology of self-criticism.* New York, NY: Oxford University Press.

Shahar, G., Blatt, S. J., & Zuroff, D. C. (2007). Satisfaction with social relations buffers the adverse effect of (mid-level) self-critical perfectionism in brief treatment for depression. *Journal of Social and Clinical Psychology, 26*(5), 540–555. https://doi.org/10.1521/jscp.2007.26.5.540

Shahar, G., Blatt, S. J., Zuroff, D. C., Krupnick, J. L., & Sotsky, S. M. (2004). Perfectionism impedes social relations and response to brief treatment for depression. *Journal of Social and Clinical Psychology, 23*(2), 140–154. https://doi.org/10.1521/jscp.23.2.140.31017

Stoeber, J., & Otto, K. (2006). Positive conceptions of perfectionism: Approaches, evidence, challenges. *Personality and Social Psychology Review, 10*, 295–319. https://doi.org/10.1207/s15327957pspr1004_2

Swann, W. B., & Bosson, J. K. (2010). Self and identity. In S. T. Fiske, D. T. Gilbert, & G. Lindzey (Eds.), *Handbook of social psychology* (Vol. 1, 5th ed., pp. 589–628). Hoboken, NJ: Wiley.

Task Force OPD. (2008). *Operationalized psychodynamic diagnosis OPD-2.* Göttingen, Germany/Toronto, ON: Hogrefe.

Thompson, R., & Zuroff, D. C. (2004). The levels of self-criticism scale: Comparative self-criticism and internalized self-criticism. *Personality and Individual Differences, 36*(2), 419–430. https://doi.org/10.1016/S0191-8869(03)00106-5

Tyrer, P., Crawford, M., Mulder, R., Blashfield, R., Farnam, A., Fossati, A., Kim, Y., Koldobsky, N., Lecic-Tosevski, D., Ndetei, D., Swales, M., Clark, L. A., & Reed, G. M. (2011). The rationale for the reclassification of personality disorder in the 11th revision of the International Classification of Diseases (ICD-11). *Personality and Mental Health, 5*(4), 246–259.

Tyrer, P., Mulder, R., Kim, Y.-R., & Crawford, M. J. (2019). The Development of the ICD-11 Classification of Personality Disorders: An Amalgam of Science, Pragmatism, and Politics. *Annual Review of Clinical Psychology, 15*(1), 481–502.

Weissman, A. N., & Beck, A. T. (1978). *Development and validation of the dysfunctional attitudes scale.* Paper presented at the American Educational Research Association Annual Convention, Toronto, Canada.

Whelton, W. J., & Greenberg, L. S. (2005). Emotion in self-criticism. *Personality and Individual Differences, 38*(7), 1583–1595. https://doi.org/10.1016/j.paid.2004.09.024

Wilson, A. C., Mackintosh, K., Power, K., & Chan, S. W. Y. (2019). Effectiveness of Self-Compassion Related Therapies: a Systematic Review and Meta-analysis. *Mindfulness, 10*, 979–995. https://doi.org/10.1007/s12671-018-1037-6

World Health Organization(WHO). (1993). *The ICD-10 classification of mental and behavioural disorders.* Geneva, Switzerland: World Health Organization.

Zimmermann, J., Kerber, A., Rek, K., Hopwood, C., & Krueger, R. (2019). A Brief but Comprehensive Review of Research on the Alternative DSM-5 Model for Personality Disorders. *Current Psychiatry Reports, 21*, 92. https://doi.org/10.1007/s11920-019-1079-z

Zuroff, D. C., Blatt, S. J., Sanislow, C. A., III, Bondi, C. M., & Pilkonis, P. A. (1999). Vulnerability to depression: Reexamining state dependence and relative stability. *Journal of Abnormal Psychology, 108*(1), 76–89. https://doi.org/10.1037/0021-843X.108.1.76

Zuroff, D. C., Blatt, S. J., Sotsky, S. M., Krupnick, J. L., Martin, D. J., Sanislow, C. A., 3rd, & Simmens, S. (2000). Relation of therapeutic alliance and perfectionism to outcome in brief outpatient treatment of depression. *Journal of Consulting and Clinical Psychology, 68*(1), 114–124.

Zuroff, D. C., & Duncan, N. (1999). Self-criticism and conflict resolution in romantic couples. *Canadian Journal of Behavioural Science, 31*(3), 137–149. https://doi.org/10.1037/h0087082

Zuroff, D. C., & Fitzpatrick, D. K. (1995). Depressive personality styles: Implications for adult attachment. *Personality and Individual Differences, 18*(2), 253–265. https://doi.org/10.1016/0191-8869(94)00136-G

Zuroff, D. C., Mongrain, M., & Santor, D. A. (2004). Conceptualizing and measuring personality vulnerability to depression: Comment on Coyne and Whiffen (1995). *Psychological Bulletin, 130*(3), 489–511. https://doi.org/10.1037/0033-2909.130.3.489

Zuroff, D. C., Sadikaj, G., Kelly, A. C., & Leybman, M. J. (2016). Conceptualizing and measuring self-criticism as both a personality trait and a personality state. *Journal of Personality Assessment, 98*(1), 14–21. https://doi.org/10.1080/00223891.2015.1044604

Zuroff, D. C., Santor, D., & Mongrain, M. (2005). Dependency, self-criticism, and maladjustment. In J. S. Auerbach, K. N. Levy, & C. E. Schaffer (Eds.), *Relatedness, self-definition and mental representation. Essays in honor of Sidney J. Blatt* (pp. 75–90). New York, NY: Routledge/Taylor & Francis Group.

Part II
Integrative Models of Depression and Personality Dysfunction: Implications for Diagnosis and Treatment

Chapter 8
Complex Depression and Early Adverse Stress: A Domain-Based Diagnostic Approach

Paul A. Vöhringer, Pablo Martinez, and Sergio Gloger

Abstract Complex versus noncomplex depression is a clinically meaningful distinction that should be made in clinical practice. We propose that treatment outcomes might be improved by this clinical differentiation by means of predicting clinical trajectories and, accordingly, defining at earliest opportunity individually tailored therapeutic approaches. Clinical presentation, course, family history, treatment response, and, to some extent, physical and psychiatric comorbidities have been recognized as critical dimensions in the differentiation between complex versus noncomplex depression. Herein we suggest that the addition of early adverse stress, an often-neglected dimension, should also be made, further enriching thoughtful clinical practice. In this regard, we present evidence that early adverse stress is linked to several dimensions of complex depression and that an important proportion of health-damaging and behavioral outcomes might be attributed to early adverse stress, highlighting the need for earlier detection and tailored treatment.

Keywords Complex depression · Critical dimensions · Early adverse stress · Depression prognosis

---

P. A. Vöhringer (✉)
Departamento Psiquiatría Hospital Clínico, Universidad de Chile, Santiago, Chile

Tufts University, Boston, MA, USA

Millennium Institute for Research in Depression and Personality (MIDAP), Santiago, Chile

Hospital Clínico de la Universidad de Chile, Universidad de Chile, Santiago, Chile

Psicomédica Clinical & Research Group, Santiago, Chile

P. Martinez
Millennium Institute for Research in Depression and Personality (MIDAP), Santiago, Chile

Hospital Clínico de la Universidad de Chile, Universidad de Chile, Santiago, Chile

S. Gloger
Psicomédica Clinical & Research Group, Santiago, Chile

Departamento de Psiquiatría y Salud Mental Oriente, Facultad de Medicina, Universidad de Chile, Santiago, Chile

G. de la Parra et al. (eds.), *Depression and Personality Dysfunction*, Depression and Personality, https://doi.org/10.1007/978-3-030-70699-9_8

8.1 Depression: A Global Public Mental Health Threat

Depression is a common yet disabling psychiatric disorder. The global prevalence of depressive disorders has been estimated to be 4.4%, currently being listed as one of the leading causes of disability worldwide, with Latin America being among the most affected globally by these psychiatric disorders (World Health Organization, 2017). Furthermore, depression substantially contributes to the burden of suicide and self-harm worldwide (Vigo, Thornicroft, & Atun, 2016), with nearly 800,000 people dying due to suicide every year (World Health Organization, 2017). Complementarily, a meta-analysis on mortality in mental disorders and global disease burden implications reported that nearly 3 million deaths worldwide are attributable to mood disorders each year, demonstrating the important association of depression with excess mortality (Walker, McGee, & Druss, 2015). The weak global response to mental disorders in general, and particularly in the case of depression, expressed in the scarcity of resources for mental illness and disparities in the allocation of resources (Vigo et al., 2016) and inconsistencies in the management of depressed patients in real-world settings (Pence, O'Donnell, & Gaynes, 2012), adds up to define a major, challenging, and urgent public health problem.

8.2 Depression: A Troublesome Disorder

Depression has an intricate nature. Although it has been labeled as a common mental disorder, with most care for depression being delivered at primary health-care settings, routine diagnosis of depression remains particularly challenging for first-line health-care providers, with important difficulties in the accurate identification of cases (Mitchell & Kakkadasam, 2011; Mitchell, Vaze, & Rao, 2009). As the first step in the depression care continuum, a troublesome scenario arises when diagnosis fails, leading to prolonged duration of untreated depressive episodes and worse clinical outcomes for patients. In this regard, a systematic review and meta-analysis noted that shorter duration of untreated illness exerted positive effects on patient's treatment response and remission, while reductions in delays in the treatment of depression might prevent chronicity (Ghio, Gotelli, Marcenaro, Amore, & Natta, 2014). In a more recent study, Hung, Liu, and Yang (2017) found that longer duration of untreated depression was significantly associated with a greater severity and lower improvement of depression at 2-year follow-up.

An additional layer of complexity is that depression is a highly recurrent disorder, with figures up to 85% after 15 years and the number of previous episodes and subthreshold residual depressive symptoms being the main predictors of recurrence (Hardeveld, Spikjer, De Graaf, Nolen, & Beekman, 2010). The aforementioned suggests that in spite of long-term treatments (e.g., sustained antidepressants and psychotherapy), a high proportion of patients in different clinical settings – from primary health care to specialized mental health care – continue to experience burdening depressive symptoms over the course of their life, affecting functional outcomes (e.g., employment) (Uher & Pavlova, 2016). Besides, well-developed clinical trials, such as the Sequenced Treatment Alternatives to Relieve Depression (STAR*D) study, have reported low rates of sustained remission (30%) after four attempts with different antidepressant agents (Rush et al., 2006), shedding light on to the relative failure of first-line, "one size fits all" treatment strategies for the management of highly heterogeneous phenotypic depressive profiles (Ghaemi & Vöhringer, 2011; Ostergaard, Jensen, & Bech, 2011).

Furthermore, a number of factors have been described to complicate the prognosis of depression. For instance, in a meta-analysis of 34 published studies on personality disorders and the outcome of depression, the chance of response to treatment for depression was doubled in the absence of a personality disorder (Newton-Howes, Tyrer, & Johnson, 2006). Moreover, different treatment modalities (i.e., pharmacotherapy alone, psychotherapy alone, or combination treatment) resulted in poorer outcomes for those patients with personality disorder with depression (Newton-Howes et al., 2006). More recently, an analysis of inpatient treatment for major depressive disorder in a large data sample from 2013 of nearly 60,000 cases from hospitals throughout Germany concluded that, compared with patients with major depressive disorders alone, those with comorbid personality disorders required more complex treatments, had higher rates of recurrent episodes, and nearly doubled hospital readmissions within 1 year (Wiegand & Godemann, 2017).

Medical and/or psychiatric comorbidities also confer an increased likelihood of poor prognosis. In a WHO World Health Survey study, which included 245,404 participants from 60 countries in all regions of the world, comorbid depression and chronic physical diseases were associated with incremental decrements in health compared with depression alone, any chronic disease alone, and any combination of chronic diseases without depression (Moussavi et al., 2007). Deschênes, Burns, and Schmitz (2015), using data from the Epidemiological Catchment Area of Montreal South-West Study, deepened into the link between depression and chronic physical health conditions by examining the effects of persistent and transient depression on disability, finding that persistent major depressive disorder was most strongly associated with functional disability, increasing the likelihood of concurrent disability in the presence of physical health conditions. Furthermore, a systematic review of 52 studies showed that patients with comorbid depression represented a higher economic burden than those with medical conditions alone, having increased length of stay and rehospitalization (Jansen, van Schijndel, van Waarde, & van Busschbach, 2018). Finally, according to systematic reviews and meta-analyses, depression is related to increased risk of mortality in people with chronic diseases, such as heart failure (specifically in older adults) and diabetes, possibly serving as a marker for higher physical disease severity (Gathright, Goldstein, Josephson, & Hughes, 2017; van Dooren et al., 2013).

Regarding mental health comorbidities, analyses of the 2012–2013 National Epidemiologic Survey on Alcohol and Related Conditions III (NESARC-III), which conducted in-person interviews in a United States nationally representative sample (n = 36,309), noted that depression and comorbid psychiatric disorders were fairly common, particularly anxiety and substance use disorders, and that depression with anxious or mixed features represented roughly 90% of all depressed cases, being associated with early onset, poor course and functioning, and suicidality (Hasin et al., 2018).

8.3 The Concept of Complex Depression

As described before, complexity of depression is usually linked to worse clinical outcomes, and one of the most notable effects is a sharp increase in human resources and costs for the health-care system. The clinical guideline for depression in adults of the National Institute for Health and Care Excellence (NICE, 2009), United Kingdom, has grounded its clinical guideline criteria in the aforementioned relationship between increasing complexity of depression and the incremental use of mental health-care services. The NICE clinical guideline proposes a stepped-care model for the management of depression, in which patients are stepped up to more complex interventions if they do not respond to initial, low-intensity interventions. Thus, this model starts with basic support techniques and monitoring (e.g., psychoeducation and "wait and see") to more active primary health-care psychosocial interventions and medication, through referral to a mental health professional, and ends with inpatient multiprofessional mental health services (NICE, 2009). Symptom count and associated functional impairment are the basis for clinical judgment, distinguishing between mild, moderate, and severe depression according to the Diagnostic and Statistical Manual of Mental Disorders, fourth edition (DSM-IV). Complementally, a comprehensive assessment of comorbidities, history of mood elevation, previous treatment experiences and response, and psychosocial factors (i.e., interpersonal relationships, living conditions, and social isolation) should be paramount in deciding treatment complexity (NICE, 2009).

Notably, the NICE clinical guideline describes another severity level, that of "complex and severe" depression. From a system-level perspective, complex and severe depression, owing to its associated complicated problems, is positioned at the top of the stepped-care model, demanding urgent referral to specialist mental health services to receive the most intrusive and complex interventions, such as combined treatments (i.e., medications, with high-intensity psychological interventions), crisis resolution and home treatment services, and multiprofessional and inpatient care (NICE, 2009). According to the NICE clinical guideline definition, people affected with complex and severe depression may present actively suicidal ideas or plans (i.e., with significant risk of suicide or self-harm), endure severe self-neglect, might have psychotic symptoms or severe agitation, or have a history of inadequate response to multiple treatments. Therefore suffering with significant psychiatric comorbidity (particularly, alcohol and substance misuse and personality disorders) or physical conditions. The already described patients, have more need of complex multiprofessional care (NICE, 2009). In practice, the management of complex and severe depression seems to be hard to implement, as multiprofessional collaboration remains an important challenge in real health-care settings (Hermens, Mintingh, Franx, van Splunteren, & Nuyen, 2014). Moreover, a study on socioeconomic status and treatment of depression during pregnancy in British Columbia, Canada, has left in evidence the additional layers of difficulties endured by patients with severe and complex depression in receiving the required specialized treatment, as there are important socioeconomic barriers to access needed and timely care for this condition (Hanley, Park, & Oberlander, 2018).

8.4 Dimensional Markers of Complex Depression

Complex and severe depression entails important individual, familial, and societal costs that are attributed to the significant risk of life-threatening behaviors and self-neglect, atypical symptom presentation, poor treatment response, and multiple health and social problems suffered by patients. In this regard, we consider that an adaptation of the early and groundbreaking work of Robins and Guze (1970) might be a useful means to make a comprehensive distinction between patients with complex versus noncomplex depression.

In their 1970 paper "Establishment of Diagnostic Validity in Psychiatric Illness: Its Application to Schizophrenia," Robins and Guze (1970) provide one of the first applied examples to gain diagnostic validity in psychiatry. Aiming to differentiate between poor and good prognosis "schizophrenia," they relied upon clinical follow-up and family studies, suggesting that clinical features (e.g., symptom profile), the course of the original clinical picture, and evidence of a familial clustering of the same type of behavioral disorders might lead to more refined and homogeneous diagnostic groupings. In our own approach, we have here decided to include the presence of early adverse stress, which will be explained in further detail in the next section, and the occurrence of clinical comorbidities (personality or anxious conditions).

We may claim that complex versus noncomplex depressive episodes differ by:

- Clinical features: Depressive symptoms are present in both categories, but complex depression tends to present psychotic features and higher suicidal risk. Additional severe symptoms, such as marked irritability, agitation or pronounced withdrawal, almost no reactivity to environmental positive stimulation, and mixed features, are more common compared to noncomplex presentations (Goodwin, Jamison, & Ghaemi, 2007).
- Course: Patients are younger at the onset of complex depression (around age 20) and older in the noncomplex group (around age 30) (Goodwin et al., 2007). Complex depression episodes usually present with phasic, seasonal, and recurrent episodes, less associated with environmental stressors; in contrast, noncomplex depression episodes are more frequently associated with stressors, each episode shorter in duration with a more insidious general course (Goodwin et al., 2007).

- Family history: The proportion of ancestors suffering from depression in the complex depression group is consistently higher. Furthermore, genetic studies suggest that complex depressions have a much stronger biological-genetic background than noncomplex ones (Goodwin et al., 2007).
- Treatment response: Noncomplex subjects tend to respond to the first line of treatment (i.e., SSRIs), whereas complex depression responded better to second-line antidepressants (i.e., SNRIs) or third-line treatments (more energetic association treatment schemes, such as antidepressants plus mood stabilizers, or plus novel antipsychotics or lithium).
- Early adverse stressors are more likely to be present in complex presentations of depression, including both physical and emotional abuse and neglect (Nelson, Klumparendt, Doebler, & Ehring, 2017). The same occurs for comorbidities (i.e., dysfunctional personality traits, anxiety and panic disorders, and physical illnesses), which are more likely to be found in complex presentations (Goodwin et al., 2007).

Classifications of mental health conditions currently in use (i.e., CIE-11 and DSM-5) are based on categorical approach. In spite of self-evident progress compared to classifications used before the 1980s, there are notorious voids and unmet needs both in clinical and research grounds. The intention to migrate – or include – a dimensional approach has stumbled with many difficulties meeting consensus. DSM-5 has made valuable but limited progress, adding specifiers and severity indexes (e.g., anxious distress), to any depression diagnosis.

Dealing with everyday challenges, clinicians must rely on diagnostic systems that are short to include the many differences and complexities between two subjects with the same diagnosis (i.e., major depressive disorder) and the often-huge implications for treatment strategies and prognosis. We propose that the inclusion of a complexity dimension to the assessment of individuals suffering from depression adds value to clinical practice, prompting the assessment of predictors of outcome and tailor-made treatments. Additionally, the systematic exploration of early adverse stress, a critical contributor to complexity but often neglected in health assessments, might further enrich a thoughtful clinical practice.

8.5 Early Adverse Stress as a Prognostic Dimension in Depressive Disorders

During the last decades, a robust body of epidemiological and neurobiological research has accumulated evidencing that exposure to early adverse stress has long-lasting negative neurobiological and clinical consequences (Anda et al., 2006; Nemeroff, 2016; Shonkoff, Boyce, & McEwen, 2009), increasing substantially the risk of medical and psychiatric disorders (Hughes et al., 2017; Teicher & Samson, 2013) and of economically burdensome behaviors in adulthood (Caspi et al., 2016; Schickedanz, Escarce, Halfon, Sastry, & Chung, 2019). Early adverse stress, an array of negative and meaningful experiences, such as maltreatment, neglect, separation, or severe household dysfunction (e.g., witnessing physical violence between caregiving figures), occurring during critical periods of childhood and adolescence, are of such health and societal impact that have been found to be consistently related to many of the leading causes of death and disability in adults in Europe and North America (Bellis et al., 2019; Felitti et al., 1998; Merrick et al., 2019; Waehrer, Miller, Silverio Marques, Oh, & Harris, 2020). Although a diverse terminology has been used in the literature for the study of early adverse stress, such as adverse childhood experiences (Anda et al., 1999; Anda et al., 2006; Felitti et al., 1998), childhood trauma (Heim & Nemeroff, 2001; Perry & Pollard, 1998; Teicher, Andersen, Polcari, Anderson, & Navalta, 2002), early life stress or adversity (Nemeroff, 2016; Turecki, Ota, Belangero, Jackowski, & Kaufman, 2014), or toxic stress (Shonkoff 2006), all of these concepts share the common ground of referring to strong, stressful, and disruptive experiences during the early years of life, with long-lasting sequelae.

One of the epidemiological studies that launched the field on the topic of early adverse stress was the Adverse Childhood Experiences (ACEs) study (Anda et al., 1999; Anda et al., 2006; Felitti et al., 1998). The ACEs study was carried out at one of the largest health maintenance organizations of the United States, based in San Diego, California, with a total of 17,337 participants passing a thorough health appraisal and responding to the ACEs survey, which registered exposure to emotional, physical, sexual contact abuse, and household dysfunction (e.g., exposure to alcohol/substance abuse, mental illness, or criminal behavior) during the first 18 years of life (Anda et al., 2006). This study found that 64% of the participants had at least one ACE and that exposure to four or more ACEs was a major contributing factor for mental and somatic health disturbances (e.g., depression, anxiety, sleep disturbance, and severe obesity), substance abuse and sexual risk behaviors (i.e., early intercourse and promiscuity), memory impairment, violent behavior, and comorbidities (Anda et al., 2006).

Two decades later, research is still confirming the burdening consequences of ACEs, as the original ACEs study did. A recent systematic review and meta-analysis aimed to combine studies from Europe and North America to calculate the proportion of adverse health outcomes in the adult population that are attributable to ACEs (i.e., population-attributable fraction [PAF]) and the disability-adjusted life-years (DALYs) and financial costs associated with ACEs (Bellis et al., 2019). The study findings revealed that ACEs might be responsible for a total of 37.5 million DALYs and an estimated $1.3 trillion per year in both regions for harmful alcohol use, illicit drug use, smoking, obesity, anxiety, depression, cancer, cardiovascular disease, diabetes, and respiratory disease. Notably, mental disorders and substance abuse had the highest PAFs associated with ACEs, with about 30 to 40% of these conditions associated with ACEs in both regions (Bellis et al., 2019). Complementarily, the results of a 2015–2017, 25 United States state-based, telephone survey of noninstitutionalized 63,365 adults estimated 23.9%, 27.0%, and 44.1% potential percentage reductions in the number of observed cases (i.e., PAFs) of heavy drinking, chronic obstructive pulmonary disease, and depression attributable to ACEs (Merrick et al., 2019).

As explicitly stated, an important proportion of depressed cases in the general population may be attributable to ACEs, highlighting the robust linkage between early adverse stress and depression in adulthood. In this regard, one of the most recent meta-analysis on children maltreatment and characteristics of adult depression, conducted by Nelson et al. (2017), concluded that history of exposure to any type of early adverse stress (i.e., childhood sexual, physical or emotional abuse, or childhood emotional or physical neglect) significantly increased by nearly threefold the chance (odds ratio [OR] = 2.81, 95% confidence interval [CI] 2.35 to 3.36) of depression in adulthood and that experiences of childhood emotional abuse (OR = 3.73, 95% CI 2.88 to 4.83) and neglect (OR = 3.54, 95% CI 2.48–5.04) were of particular importance in the development of adult depression. Moreover, studies suggest that depressed adults exposed to early adverse stress also have higher rates of disease burden. Analyses of 10-year longitudinal data obtained from the United States National Comorbidity Survey (N = 5001) determined that depression partially mediated the relationship between ACEs and painful medical conditions (e.g., arthritis/rheumatism), increasing their number (Sachs-Ericsson, Sheffler, Stanley, Piazza, & Preacher, 2017). Furthermore, Putnam, Harris, and Putnam (2013), with data from the United States National Comorbidity Survey-Replication (N = 5692), and Widom, DuMont, and Czaja (2007), in a prospective study of neglected children (N = 1196), found that depressed adults exposed to different forms of child abuse and neglect had higher load of psychiatric comorbidity, particularly anxiety disorders and antisocial personality disorder, thus, having a complex psychopathological profile.

Consistent with a higher disease burden, early adverse stress has been associated with more serious and complex presentations of depression. In the meta-analysis of Nelson et al. (2017), the statistical synthesis of 52 studies showed a significant correlation between childhood maltreatment severity and depression severity, while, in further analysis of 10 studies, it was observed that individuals with a history of childhood maltreatment had a mean depression onset 4 years earlier compared with individuals without such a history. Moreover, the same review, based on 11 studies (N = 6194), estimated that the chance of chronic depression was twice times higher in individuals with a childhood maltreatment history than individuals without such a history (OR = 2.05, 95% CI 1.40 to 3.00) (Nelson et al., 2017). A similar estimate was reported by an earlier meta-analysis of 16 epidemiological studies (Nanni, Uher, & Danese, 2012), totaling 23,544 participants, which found an OR for recurrent and persistent depressive episodes of 2.27 (95% CI 1.80 to 2.87) for depressed adults exposed to early adverse stress (in the form of physical or sexual abuse, neglect, or family conflict or violence) compared to the nonexposed. Importantly, both meta-analyses found evidence for a statistically significant increased risk (OR = 1.43, 95% CI 1.11 to 1.83 in Nanni et al., 2012; and OR = 1.90, 95% CI 1.05 to 3.46 in Nelson et al., 2017) of nonresponse to different types of depression treatments (psychotherapy, pharmacotherapy, or combination therapy) attributed to childhood maltreatment history. The latter finding was also stressed by Tokuda et al.'s study (2018), which identified major depressive disorder subtypes in an unsupervised manner, carrying out a cluster analysis of 134 subjects (67 depressive and 67 controls), to identify child abuse and trauma as a classifier for nonresponse to selective serotonin-reuptake inhibitor (SSRI) treatment at 6 weeks.

The aforementioned evidence of early adverse stress as a marker of clinically complex depression is further compounded by the relationship between childhood trauma and depression with atypical or psychotic features (Gaudiano & Zimmerman, 2010; Withers, Tarasoff, & Stewart, 2013). In a comparative study of 96 atypical depression and 196 non-atypical depression patients as defined by the DSM-IV, patients with atypical features of depression (i.e., mood reactivity, significant weight gain or increased appetite, hypersomnia, leaden paralysis, and/or interpersonal rejection sensitivity) reported a statistically significantly higher proportion of traumatic experiences (52.6%) than patients without atypical depression (30.8%) (Withers et al., 2013). Complementarily, Gaudiano and Zimmerman (2010) compared adult outpatients diagnosed with SCID/DSM-IV major depressive disorder with (n = 32) and without psychotic features (n = 591), finding that the former subgroup of patients had a higher and significant chance of reporting histories of physical (OR = 2.81, 95% CI 1.06 to 4.91) or sexual abuse (OR = 2.75, 95% CI 1.05 to 4.73).

There are additional layers of complexity attributed to early adverse stress that have not been discussed yet. For instance, the landmark ACE study found that, among 17,337 members of a health maintenance organization, those reporting experiences of child abuse and neglect, and/or family and household dysfunction, had two- to fivefold increased risk of lifetime attempted suicide compared to those not reporting such exposures (Dube et al., 2001). These results have been mirrored by studies conducted in samples of patients with clinically ascertained depression, stressing the fact that early adverse stress, under different forms, is a significant risk factor for suicide attempts: childhood trauma differentiated between attempters and non-attempters in a sample of low-income, young, depressed new mothers (Ammerman et al., 2019); depressed outpatients maintaining a stable regime of psychiatric medications classified as severely abused and neglected had an increased chance of suicidality (Brodbeck et al., 2018); similarly, in a sample of depressed outpatients free of medications (Johnstone et al., 2016), maternal neglect was the most strong predictor of suicide attempts; while self-report of childhood sexual abuse was significantly associated with attempted suicide in samples of recently admitted psychiatric inpatients (Andover, Zlotnick, & Miller, 2007) and chronically depressed individuals (Ernst et al., 2019).

Complementarily, it has been stated that individuals with a background of ACEs incur in higher health-care use and costs as a result of their subsequent health and social problems and related health-damaging behavior (Anda, Butchart, Felitti, & Brown, 2010; Bellis, Lowey, Leckenby, Hughes, & Harrison, 2014). Given their clinically complex profile (e.g., increased likelihood of resistance to treatment or having a depression with psychotic symptoms), it might be expected that depressed patients with a history of early adverse stress would require highly specialized, invasive therapeutic interventions (e.g., admission to psychiatric inpatient care). To the best of our knowledge, the only example found in the literature directly linking childhood trauma with higher risk of psychiatric hospitalization was the Rytilä-Manninen et al.'s study (2014), which compared adolescents with severe psychiatric disorders (N = 206, 47.6% with mood conditions) in a psychiatric hospitalization unit with healthy controls of the general population (N = 203) to find that the chance of being in the inpatient group increased as a function of the accumulation of adverse childhood experiences.

In synthesis, early adverse stress has been found to be a consistent risk factor for a clinically complex presentation of depression. The exposure to early adverse stress has been linked to early onset of depression, higher medical and psychiatric comorbidity burden, increased symptom severity, higher recurrence and persistence of depressive episodes, resistance to standard depression treatments (including pharmacotherapy, psychotherapy, and combination therapy), atypical and/or psychotic features of depression, higher risk of lifetime suicide attempts, and greater requirement for inpatient psychiatric care.

8.6 Early Adverse Stress and Complex Depression: Recent Findings from a Large Mental Health-Care Facility in Santiago, Chile

As early adverse stress might be considered a prognostic dimension in depressive disorder, we sought to determine the contribution of early adverse stress to different diagnostic validators of complexity in a large mental health-care institution in Santiago, Chile. PsicoMedica Clinical and Research Group is a clinical and research mental health-care facility located at the capital city of Chile (Santiago), providing comprehensive diagnostic and treatment services to individuals with a low-end middle-income background. PsicoMedica is staffed with a multidisciplinary team, including psychiatrists, mental health trained physicians, psychologists, nurses, and occupational and art therapists, attending an average of three thousand patients per month, most of them presenting with mood disorders (85%). In terms of severity of depression, 60% are mild-moderate, 25% are severe, and 15% are severe with serious/risk features, i.e., psychotic, suicidal, or resistant to treatment.

To our ends, clinical data available for 1016 individuals diagnosed with major depressive disorder registered during the years 2013 and 2014 were used. Diagnosis of ICD-10 major depressive disorder, early adverse stress, and diagnostic validators of clinical complexity were identified through thorough clinical diagnostic assessments carried out by psychiatrists or senior psychiatry residents. Early adverse stress was ascertained through administration of the Brief Physical and Sexual Abuse Questionnaire (BPSAQ) developed by Marshall et al. (2000), screening exposure to the following types of childhood and adolescent traumatic events: traumatic separation, harsh physical punishment, injury from physical punishment, witnessing physical violence between parents/caregivers, substance abuse in the home, and forced sexual contact with a relative/nonrelative. Additionally, clinically complex presentations of depression were defined as follows:

- Complex and severe depression, as proposed by the NICE clinical guidelines for adult depression (NICE, 2009), including depression with psychotic symptoms, high suicide risk, or treatment resistance. According to the Chilean clinical guidelines for depression, patients with these presentations must be referred to specialized mental health care (Ministerio de Salud de Chile, 2013).
- High suicide risk, as determined by the Mini-International Neuropsychiatric Interview (MINI) suicidality module total score (Sheehan et al., 1998), with scores of 9 or more indicating high suicide risk.
- Admissions to psychiatric hospitals or units for inpatient treatment.
- Recurrent depression according to ICD-10 criteria for recurrent depressive disorder (World Health Organization, 2004).

In this patient population, exposure to at least one type of early adverse stress was ascertained in almost seven out of ten depressed individuals (68.9%), 13.3% of the sample had complex and severe depression, 13.5% had high suicide risk, 5.0% had a history of previous psychiatric admissions, and 53.3% met ICD-10 criteria for recurrent depression. Early adverse stress consistently predicted the presence of complex and severe depression in adulthood, with multivariate-adjusted ORs of 1.93 (95% CI 1.23 to 3.04) for exposure to any early adverse stress event, 1.74 (95% CI 1.19 to 2.55) for exposure to two or more types of early adverse stress events, and 1.25 (95% CI 1.10 to 1.41) for the accumulation of early adverse stress events (i.e., a composite score, with a 0–7 possible score range). In the same line, exposure to any early adverse stress event was also a robust predictor of high suicide risk (OR = 2.49, 95% CI 1.55 to 4.01), previous psychiatric admissions (OR = 3.42, 95% CI 1.44 to 8.12), and recurrent depression (OR = 1.55, 95% CI 1.18 to 2.05).

Complementarily, there were specific types of early adverse stress events that significantly predicted complex and severe depression after adjustment for study covariates (i.e., sex, age, and occupation): child and adolescence experiences of harsh physical punishment and forced sexual contact with a nonrelative increased around twofold the chance of having a complex and severe depression in adulthood (OR = 1.95, 95% CI 1.31 to 2.91; and, OR = 2.06, 95% CI 1.10 to 3.84, respectively), compared to those subjects without such background. A similar scenario was found for the risk of having high suicide risk, previous psychiatric admissions, or recurrent depression. Forced sexual contact with a relative (OR = 2.60, 95% CI 1.59 to 4.25) and forced sexual contact with a nonrelative (OR = 2.61, 95% CI 1.44 to 4.72) were significant predictors of high suicide risk in the sample. Meanwhile, the chance of previous psychiatric admissions was significantly increased for depressed subjects exposed to traumatic separation (OR = 2.09, 95% CI 1.17 to 3.75) and forced sexual contact with a nonrelative (OR = 4.05, 95% CI 1.93 to 8.48). Finally, traumatic separation was the only specific type of early adverse stress event consistently predicting recurrent depression (OR = 1.11, 95% CI 1.01 to 1.22).

Furthermore, to explore the proportion of clinically complex presentations of depression in this large mental health-care facility that might be attributable to early adverse stress, we calculated the attributable risks (ARs) of these childhood and adolescent traumatic experiences. These latter findings revealed the high burden of early adverse stress in this patient population, for instance, in the case of complex and severe depression ARs of exposure to any early adverse stress, two or more types of early adverse stress events, and the accumulation of early adverse stress events, were 34.6%, 17.9%, and 24.4%, respectively, meaning that up to a third of cases of complex and severe depression in the sample are attributed to childhood and adolescent traumatic experiences (a graphical representation of this contribution is shown in Fig. 8.1). Regarding other diagnostic validators of complexity, ARs of exposure to any early adverse stress event were 45.4% for high suicide risk, 60.9% for previous psychiatric admissions, and 13.7% for recurrent depression, implying that if we were able to avoid early adverse stress, most of the psychiatric admissions and almost half of the cases of high suicide risk in the sample would not have been occurred.

Using the same clinical database, we took a step further. We empirically built a new variable termed "complex depression," composed of those variables discriminating between different levels of functionality among depressed patients (i.e., DSM-IV Global Assessment Functioning Scale [GAF]). Thus, in our discriminant analysis, this variable was finally composed of depression severity (symptom criterion), high suicide risk (MINI), previous psychiatric hospitalizations, and previous depressive episodes (recurrence) – each one with an assigned weight according to the relative magnitude of the effect size (Cohen's d). As a result of these analyses, higher levels of functionality were statistically significantly associated with a lower

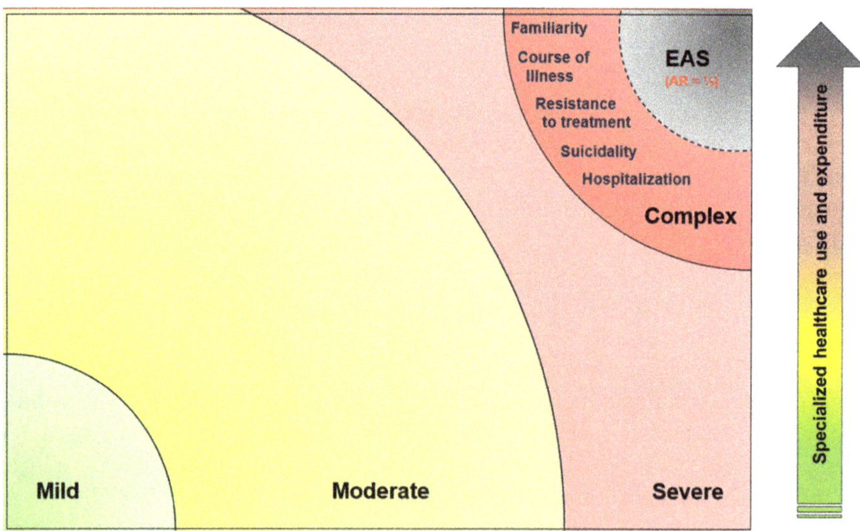

Fig. 8.1 Depression severity, early adverse stress, and other complexity markers
Notes. This is a graphical display for the relationship between depression severity, early adverse stress, and complexity markers, such as familiarity, course of illness, and resistance to treatment. Early adverse stress is attributed up to a third of complex cases of depression (i.e., AR = attributable risk). A higher complexity load is related to a higher use of specialized health-care services and expenditure

Table 8.1 Logistic regression model for prediction of highly complex depressed patients ($n = 514$)

Variable	OR (95% CI)	*p-value*
Sex (male)	1,21 (0,73–2,00)	0,461
Age	0,98 (0,96–0,99)	0,046
Unemployed	4,12 (1,30–13,03)	0,016
Substance abuse in the home	1,75 (1,09–2,80)	0,020
Forced sexual contact (relative/nonrelative)	1,72 (0,96–3,08)	0,070
Previous use of psychotropics	3,50 (2,10–5,80)	0,000
Comorbidity axis II	2,84 (1,70–4,72)	0,000
Constant	0,09 (0,04–0,24)	0,000

Model pseudo-R2 = 14,1% (p < 0,001)
C statistic = 0,76, IC 95% 0,71 a 0,81
Hosmer-Lemeshow goodness of fit test $\chi^2(8) = 7{,}43$, $p = 0{,}4910$

"complexity" score, suggesting a proportionally inverse relationship (β = −0,16; SE = 0,01; $p < 0{,}001$; IC 95% −0,19 a −0,13). Moreover, we classified a "highly complex" subgroup of patients (200 patients from a total sample of 932, 21.46%), i.e., those in the highest quartile of the "complexity" score distribution. Through predictive modeling techniques we seek for predictors of "highly complex" patients. The best fitting model is shown in Table 8.1, where it is observed the important contribution of some early adverse stress events to the "highly complex" subgroup of depressed patients.

8.7 Concluding Remarks

Depression is a serious global public health threat. As a heterogeneous psychiatric disorder, the course of depression might be affected by several contributing factors, such as personality disorders or chronic physical diseases, among others. Importantly, in this chapter we have delved into the concept of complex and severe depression, in accordance with the NICE clinical guidelines. Recognized as the costliest and most disabling entity in the spectrum of depressive disorders, complex and severe depression might be characterized by a grave clinical presentation (e.g., high suicide risk or psychotic features), earlier onset and recurrent course, a family history suggestive of a strong biological background, and poor treatment response, usually demanding multidisciplinary, highly intensive, specialist mental health care. Furthermore, we have presented supporting evidence from our own studies that early adverse stress (i.e., maltreatment, neglect, separation, or severe household dysfunction) might be considered an important marker of complex and severe depression. In this regard, along with the deleterious and long-standing impact of early adverse stress upon several health and behavioral outcomes, a vast amount of literature seems to robustly and conclusively suggest that these early, negative, and meaningful experiences are linked with depression severity, atypical or psychotic features, and lifetime attempted suicide; earlier onset; recurrent, persistent, and/or chronic course; and nonresponse to first-line treatments, incurring in highly specialized and complex mental health care. Moreover, based on our own analyses of a large patient population, we observed that early adverse stress is a statistically significant predictor of complex and severe depression in adulthood and that such types of child abuse and neglect were strongly associated with high suicide risk, previous psychiatric admissions, and recurrent depression. Complementarily, our analyses revealed that an important proportion of these outcomes might be attributed to early adverse stress. Finally, we found that experiences of childhood abuse and severe household dysfunction were among the most significant predictors of a group of highly complex and low-functioning depressed patients. We would like to conclude this chapter by stressing the need and relevance of considering early adverse stress as a fundamental dimension in the comprehensive assessment of complex and severe depression. Thus, along with the clinical presentation, course of depression, family history, and treatment response, clinicians must readily incorporate the screening of early adverse stress in depressed patients to tailor treatment alternatives and intensity. We believe that such an approach may help avoid unnecessary individual suffering of patients and mental health-care costs. Trauma-focused models of psychotherapies are available and have proved their effectiveness in the management of trauma-related psychopathology (Duberstein et al., 2018; Vitriol, Ballesteros, Florenzano, Weil, & Benadof, 2009).

References

Ammerman, R. T., Scheiber, F. A., Peugh, J. L., Messer, E. P., Van Ginkel, J. B., & Putnam, F. W. (2019). Interpersonal trauma and suicide attempts in low-income depressed mothers in home visiting. *Child Abuse & Neglect, 97*, 104126.

Anda, R. F., Butchart, A., Felitti, V. J., & Brown, D. W. (2010). Building a framework for global surveillance of the public health implications of adverse childhood experiences. *The American Journal of Preventive Medicine, 39*, 93–98.

Anda, R. F., Croft, J. B., Felitti, V. J., Nordenberg, D., Giles, W. H., Williamson, D. F., et al. (1999). Adverse childhood experiences and smoking during adolescence and adulthood. *JAMA, 282*, 1652–1658.

Anda, R. F., Felitti, V. J., Bremner, J. D., Walker, J. D., Whitfield, C., Perry, B. D., et al. (2006). The enduring effects of abuse and related adverse experiences in childhood. A convergence of evidence from neurobiology and epidemiology. *European Archives of Psychiatry and Clinical Neuroscience, 256*, 174–186.

Andover, M. S., Zlotnick, C., & Miller, I. W. (2007). Childhood physical and sexual abuse in depressed patients with single and multiple suicide attempts. *Suicide and Life-threatening Behavior, 37*, 467–474.

Bellis, M. A., Hughes, K., Ford, K., Ramos Rodríguez, G., Sethi, D., & Passmore, J. (2019). Life course health consequences and associated annual costs of adverse childhood experiences across Europe and North America: A systematic review and meta-analysis. *The Lancet Public Health, 4*, e517–e528.

Bellis, M. A., Lowey, H., Leckenby, N., Hughes, K., & Harrison, D. (2014). Adverse childhood experiences: Retrospective study to determine their impact on adult health behaviours and health outcomes in a UK population. *Journal of Public Health, 36*, 81–91.

Brodbeck, J., Fassbinder, E., Schweiger, U., Fehr, A., Späth, C., & Klein, J. P. (2018). Differential associations between patterns of child maltreatment and comorbidity in adult depressed patients. *Journal of Affective Disorders, 230*, 34–41.

Caspi, A., Houts, R. M., Belsky, D. W., Harrington, H., Hogan, S., Ramrakha, S., et al. (2016). Childhood forecasting of a small segment of the population with large economic burden. *Nature Human Behaviour, 1*, 0005.

Deschênes, S. S., Burns, R. J., & Schmitz, N. (2015). Associations between depression, chronic physical health conditions, and disability in a community sample: A focus on the persistence of depression. *Journal of Affective Disorders, 179*, 6–13.

Dube, S. R., Anda, R. F., Felitti, V. J., Chapman, D. P., Williamson, D. F., & Giles, W. H. (2001). Childhood abuse, household dysfunction, and the risk of attempted suicide throughout the life span: Findings from the adverse childhood experiences study. *JAMA, 286*, 3089–3096.

Duberstein, P. R., Ward, E. A., Chaudron, L. H., He, H., Toth, S. L., Wang, W., et al. (2018). Effectiveness of interpersonal psychotherapy-trauma for depressed women with childhood abuse histories. *Journal of Consulting and Clinical Psychology, 86*, 868–878.

Ernst, M., Kallenbach-Kaminski, L., Kaufhold, J., Negele, A., Bahrke, U., Hautzinger, M., … Leuzinger-Bohleber, M. (2019). Suicide attempts in chronically depressed individuals: What are the risk factors? *Psychiatry Research*, 112481.

Felitti, V. J., Anda, R. F., Nordenberg, D., Williamson, D. F., Spitz, A. M., Edwards, V., et al. (1998). Relationship of childhood abuse and household dysfunction to many of the leading causes of death in adults. The Adverse Childhood Experiences Study. *American Journal of Preventive Medicine, 14*, 245–258.

Gathright, E. C., Goldstein, C. M., Josephson, R. A., & Hughes, J. W. (2017). Depression increases the risk of mortality in patients with heart failure: A meta-analysis. *Journal of Psychosomatic Research, 94*, 82–89.

Gaudiano, B. A., & Zimmerman, M. (2010). The relationship between childhood trauma history and the psychotic subtype of major depression. *Acta Psychiatrica Scandinavica, 121*, 462–470.

Ghaemi, S. N., & Vöhringer, P. A. (2011). The heterogeneity of depression: An old debate renewed. *Acta Psychiatrica Scandinavica, 124*, 497.

Ghio, L., Gotelli, S., Marcenaro, M., Amore, M., & Natta, W. (2014). Duration of untreated illness and outcomes in unipolar depression: A systematic review and meta-analysis. *Journal of Affective Disorders, 152–154*, 45–51.

Goodwin, F. K., Jamison, K. R., & Ghaemi, S. N. (2007). *Manic-depressive illness: Bipolar disorders and recurrent depression*. New York, NY: Oxford University Press.

Hanley, G. E., Park, M., & Oberlander, T. F. (2018). Socioeconomic status and treatment of depression during pregnancy: A retrospective population-based cohort study in British Columbia, Canada. *Archives of Women's Mental Health, 21*, 765–775.

Hardeveld, F., Spikjer, J., De Graaf, R., Nolen, W. A., & Beekman, A. T. F. (2010). Prevalence and predictors of recurrence of major depressive disorder in the adult population. *Acta Psychiatrica Scandinavica, 122*, 184–191.

Hasin, D. S., Sarvet, A. L., Meyers, J. L., Saha, T. D., Ruan, W. J., Stohl, M., & Grant, B. F. (2018). Epidemiology of adult DSM-5 major depressive disorder and its Specifiers in the United States. *JAMA Psychiatry, 75*, 336–346.

Heim, C., & Nemeroff, C. B. (2001). The role of childhood trauma in the neurobiology of mood and anxiety disorders: Preclinical and clinical studies. *Biological Psychiatry, 49*, 1023–1039.

Hermens, M. L. M., Mintingh, A., Franx, G., van Splunteren, P. T., & Nuyen, J. (2014). Stepped care is easy to recommend, but harder to implement: Results of an explorative study within primary care in the Netherlands. *BMC Family Practice, 15*, 5.

Hughes, K., Bellis, M. A., Hardcastle, K. A., Sethi, D., Butchart, A., Mikton, C., et al. (2017). The effects of multiple adverse childhood experiences on health: A systematic review and meta-analysis. *The Lancet Public Health, 2*, e356–e366.

Hung, C. I., Liu, C. Y., & Yang, C. H. (2017). Untreated duration predicted the severity of depression at the two-year follow-up point. *PLoS One, 12*, e0185119.

Jansen, L., van Schijndel, M., van Waarde, J., & van Busschbach, J. (2018). Health-economic outcomes in hospital patients with medical-psychiatric comorbidity: A systematic review and meta-analysis. *PLoS One, 13*, e0194029.
Johnstone, J. M., Carter, J. D., Luty, S. E., Mulder, R. T., Frampton, C. M., & Joyce, P. R. (2016). Childhood predictors of lifetime suicide attempts and non-suicidal self-injury in depressed adults. *Australian & New Zealand journal of psychiatry, 50*, 135–144.
Marshall, R. D., Schneier, F. R., Lin, S. H., Simpson, H. B., Vermes, D., & Liebowitz, M. (2000). Childhood trauma and dissociative symptoms in panic disorder. *The American Journal of Psychiatry, 157*, 451–453.
Merrick, M. T., Ford, D. C., Ports, K. A., Guinn, A. S., Chen, J., Klevens, J., et al. (2019). Vital signs: estimated proportion of adult health problems attributable to adverse childhood experiences and implications for prevention – 25 states, 2015–2017. *Morbidity and Mortality Weekly Report, 68*, 999–1005.
Ministerio de Salud de Chile. (2013). *Guía Clínica Depresión en personas de 15 años y más.* Santiago, Chile: Ministerio de Salud de Chile.
Mitchell, A. J., & Kakkadasam, V. (2011). Ability of nurses to identify depression in primary care, secondary care and nursing homes - a meta-analysis of routine clinical accuracy. *International Journal of Nursing Studies, 48*, 359–368.
Mitchell, A. J., Vaze, A., & Rao, S. (2009). Clinical diagnosis of depression in primary care: A meta-analysis. *The Lancet, 374*, 22–28.
Moussavi, S., Chatterji, S., Verdes, E., Tandon, A., Patel, V., & Ustun, B. (2007). Depression, chronic diseases, and decrements in health: Results from the world health surveys. *The Lancet, 370*, 851–858.
Nanni, V., Uher, R., & Danese, A. (2012). Childhood maltreatment predicts unfavorable course of illness and treatment outcome in depression: A meta-analysis. *The American Journal of Psychiatry, 169*, 141–151.
National Institute for Health and Care Excellence (NICE). (2009). *Depression in adults: recognition and management.* NICE, London. Available from: https://www.nice.org.uk/guidance/cg90 [updated 2016 Apr].
Nelson, J., Klumparendt, A., Doebler, P., & Ehring, T. (2017). Childhood maltreatment and characteristics of adult depression: Meta-analysis. *The British Journal of Psychiatry, 210*, 96–104.
Nemeroff, C. B. (2016). Paradise lost: The neurobiological and clinical consequences of child abuse and neglect. *Neuron, 89*, 892–909.
Newton-Howes, G., Tyrer, P., & Johnson, T. (2006). Personality disorder and the outcome of depression: Meta-analysis of published studies. *British Journal of Psychiatry, 188*, 13–20.
Ostergaard, S. D., Jensen, S. O., & Bech, P. (2011). The heterogeneity of the depressive syndrome: When number get serious. *Acta Psychiatrica Scandinavica, 124*, 495–496.
Pence, B. W., O'Donnell, J. K., & Gaynes, B. N. (2012). The depression treatment cascade in primary care: A public health perspective. *Current Psychiatry Reports, 14*, 328–335.
Perry, B. D., & Pollard, R. (1998). Homeostasis, stress, trauma, and adaptation. A neurodevelopment view of childhood trauma. *Child and Adolescent Psychiatric Clinics of North America, 7*, 33–51.
Putnam, K. T., Harris, W. W., & Putnam, F. W. (2013). Synergistic childhood adversities and complex adult psychopathology. *Journal of Traumatic Stress, 26*, 435–442.
Robins, E., & Guze, S. B. (1970). Establishment of diagnostic validity in psychiatric illness: Its application to schizophrenia. *The American Journal of Psychiatry, 126*, 107–111.
Rush, A. J., Trivedi, M. H., Wisniewski, S. R., Nierenberg, A. A., Stewart, J. W., Warden, D., et al. (2006). Acute and longer-term outcomes in depressed outpatients requiring one or several treatment steps: A STAR*D report. *The American Journal of Psychiatry, 163*, 1905–1917.
Rytilä-Manninen, M., Lindberg, N., Haravuori, H., Kettunen, K., Marttunen, M., Joukamaa, M., … Fröjd, S. (2014). Adverse childhood experiences as risk factors for serious mental disorders and inpatient hospitalization among adolescents. *Child Abuse & Neglect, 38*, 2021–2032.
Sachs-Ericsson, N. J., Sheffler, J. L., Stanley, I. H., Piazza, J. R., & Preacher, K. J. (2017). When emotional pain becomes physical: Adverse childhood experiences, pain, and the role of mood and anxiety disorders. *Journal of Clinical Psychology, 73*, 1403–1428.

Schickedanz, A. B., Escarce, J. J., Halfon, N., Sastry, N., & Chung, P. J. (2019). Adverse childhood experiences and household out-of-pocket healthcare costs. *American Journal of Preventive Medicine, 56*, 698–707.
Sheehan, D. V., Lecrubier, Y., Sheehan, K. H., Amorim, P., Janavs, J., Weiller, E., ... Dunbar, G. C. (1998). The Mini-International Neuropsychiatric Interview (M.I.N.I): The development and validation of a structured diagnostic psychiatric interview for DSM-IV and ICD-10. *The Journal of Clinical Psychiatry, 59*, 22–33.
Shonkoff, J. P. (2006). A promising opportunity for developmental and behavioral pediatrics at the interface of neuroscience, psychology, and social policy: Remarks on receiving the 2005 C. Anderson Aldrich Award. *Pediatrics, 118*(5), 2187–2191. https://doi.org/10.1542/peds.2006-1728
Shonkoff, J. P., Boyce, W. T., & McEwen, B. S. (2009). Neuroscience, molecular biology, and the childhood roots of health disparities: Building a new framework for health promotion and disease prevention. *JAMA, 301*, 2252–2259.
Teicher, M. H., Andersen, S. L., Polcari, A., Anderson, C. M., & Navalta, C. P. (2002). Developmental neurobiology of childhood stress and trauma. *The Psychiatric Clinics of North America, 25*, 397–426.
Teicher, M. H., & Samson, J. A. (2013). Childhood maltreatment and psychopathology: A case for ecophenotypic variants as clinically and neurobiologically distinct subtypes. *The American Journal of Psychiatry, 170*, 11143–11133.
Tokuda, T., Yoshumoto, J., Shimizu, Y., Okada, G., Takamura, M., Okamoto, Y., ... Doya, K. (2018). Identification of depression subtypes and relevant brain regions using a data-driven approach. *Scientific Reports, 8*, 14082.
Turecki, G., Ota, V. K., Belangero, S. I., Jackowski, A., & Kaufman, J. (2014). Early life adversity, genomic plasticity, and psychopathology. *The Lancet Psychiatry, 1*, 461–466.
Uher, R., & Pavlova, B. (2016). Long-term effects of depression treatment. *The Lancet Psychiatry, 3*, 95–96.
Van Dooren, F. E., Nefs, G., Schram, M. T., Verhey, F. R., Denollet, J., & Pouwer, F. (2013). Depression and risk of mortality in people with diabetes mellitus: A systematic review and meta-analysis. *PLoS One, 8*, e57058.
Vigo, D., Thornicroft, G., & Atun, R. (2016). Estimating the true global burden of mental illness. *The Lancet Psychiatry, 3*, 171–178.
Vitriol, V. G., Ballesteros, S. T., Florenzano, R. U., Weil, K. P., & Benadof, D. F. (2009). Evaluation of an outpatient intervention for women with severe depression and a history of childhood trauma. *Psychiatric Services, 60*, 936–942.
Waehrer, G. M., Miller, T. R., Silverio Marques, S. C., Oh, D. L., & Harris, N. B. (2020). Disease burden of adverse childhood experiences across 14 states. *PLoS One, 15*, e0226134.
Walker, E. R., McGee, R. E., & Druss, B. G. (2015). Mortality in mental disorders and global disease burden implications: A systematic review and meta-analysis. *JAMA Psychiatry, 72*, 334–341.
Widom, C. S., DuMont, K., & Czaja, S. J. (2007). A prospective investigation of major depressive disorder and comorbidity in abused and neglected children grown up. *Archives of General Psychiatry, 64*, 49–56.
Wiegand, H. F., & Godemann, F. (2017). Increased treatment complexity for major depressive disorder for inpatients with comorbid personality disorder. *Psychiatric Services, 68*, 524–527.
Withers, A. C., Tarasoff, J. M., & Stewart, J. W. (2013). Is depression with atypical features associated with trauma history? *The Journal of Clinical Psychiatry, 74*, 500–506.
World Health Organization. (2004). *ICD-10: International statistical classification of diseases and related health problems: Tenth revision* (2nd ed.). Geneva, Switzerland: World Health Organization. https://apps.who.int/iris/handle/10665/42980
World Health Organization. (2017). *Depression and other common mental disorders: Global health estimates*. Geneva, Switzerland: World Health Organization.

Chapter 9
Complex Depression in High-Pressure Care Settings: Strategies and Therapeutic Competences

Guillermo de la Parra, Ana Karina Zúñiga, Paula Dagnino, and Elyna Gómez-Barris

Abstract As shown in this volume and others in this series, it is untenable nowadays to regard depression as a unidimensional phenomenon in terms of diagnosis and treatment. The notion of *complex depression* is closer to the clinical-etiological reality of the disorder and also provides a clearer impression of what professionals must deal with in highly demanding settings, including primary care (PC). This is especially true in low-medium-income countries (LMICs), where patients with complex depression are often likened to those who mental health practitioners call "difficult patients." From this perspective, the present chapter addresses complex depression and highlights its heterogeneous nature, marked by the functioning of patients' personality structure, depressive experience style, suicide risk, contextual factors, and medical comorbidities that have an impact on their response to treatment. After discussing how the treatment context and the characteristics of the professionals who treat these patients interact with the aforementioned factors, we present a model for the psychotherapeutic management of complex depression in high-demand settings, with an emphasis on the handling of personality dysfunctions.

Keywords Complex depression · Psychotherapy · Strategies · Competences · Institutional settings · Primary care

G. de la Parra (✉) · E. Gómez-Barris
Department of Psychiatry, School of Medicine, Pontificia Universidad Católica de Chile, Santiago, Chile

Millennium Institute for Research in Depression and Personality (MIDAP), Santiago, Chile
e-mail: gdelaparra@uc.cl

A. K. Zúñiga
Millennium Institute for Research in Depression and Personality (MIDAP), Santiago, Chile

Programa de Doctorado en Psicoterapia, Pontificia Universidad Católica de Chile y Universidad de Chile, Santiago, Chile

P. Dagnino
Millennium Institute for Research in Depression and Personality (MIDAP), Santiago, Chile

Faculty of Psychology, Universidad Alberto Hurtado, Santiago, Chile

G. de la Parra et al. (eds.), *Depression and Personality Dysfunction*, Depression and Personality, https://doi.org/10.1007/978-3-030-70699-9_9

9.1 Complex Depression

9.1.1 "Complexity" in Healthcare: Towards Personalized Treatment

The Cambridge English Dictionary (n.d.) defines complexity as "the state of having many parts and being difficult to understand or find an answer to," which applies to the multiple factors that influence depression in terms of its etiology, evolution, clinical manifestations, prognosis, and differential responses to treatment. In medicine in general and mental health in particular, the issue of complexity has been hard to define, conceptualize, operationalize, and study. Complexity and its effects on outcomes have posed a challenge to medicine (Safford, Allison, & Kiefe, 2007) inasmuch as clinical guidelines, for instance, guidelines for diabetes, hypertension, or depression, mention diagnoses but tend to exclude factors that "increase patient complexity." These factors include comorbidities, patient preferences, or value systems that may influence treatment adherence, barriers preventing access to treatment, socioeconomic contexts keeping patients from following medical suggestions (e.g., more expensive diets), and obstacles put in place by the medical institutions and practitioners in charge of these patients. Several authors have advanced models of complexity that extend beyond "comorbidity" and mere descriptions, such as the cumulative complexity model (Shippeea, Shaha, Mayc, Maird, & Montori, 2012) or the vector model put forward by Safford et al. (2007), who assert that determinants of health such as socioeconomics, culture, biology/genes, environment/ecology, and behavior have a differential "weight" (vectors) in the determination of the outcome of each case. Since these vectors are interrelated, much like a network, a factor influencing one of them will have an impact on the rest of the vectors and ultimately on the outcome. Thus, regarding the complex determinants of depression, psychotherapy – by influencing internal constructs and/or behavior – can have a positive effect despite the burden that other determinants may be exerting. We agree with the latter authors when they state: "Whether the provider and healthcare system prove helpful or effective depends upon both (1) the complete assessment of the patient's complexity, and (2) the provider and healthcare system being equipped to respond" (Safford et al., 2007, p. 383). This is an interesting point given that, as we will discuss in a later section, providers must possess the necessary competences to address patients' requirements. The authors also note that "an important goal of the medical encounter is for the doctor and patient to develop 'congruence,' or a shared view of realistically attainable health care goals" (p. 384). This notion, taken to the domain of psychotherapy, is consistent with evidence-based psychotherapy practice (APA, 2006; Mulder, Murray, & Rucklidge, 2017), which requires taking into account the patient's preferences and background in every indication process. An inevitable conclusion of this perspective is what the authors refer to as "trade-offs" in the indication process; in other words, they suggest that it is advisable to include not only the patient's factors, preferences, and culture but also the conditions that the institution and the practitioner can realistically offer. This is relevant in high-pressure care settings (HPCS), especially in low- and middle-income countries (LMICs), where the treatments offered must often be adapted to the socioeconomic reality of both patients and healthcare institutions. In mental healthcare, trade-off indication is related to the concepts of "adaptive indication" (Thomä & Kächele, 1987), responsiveness in psychotherapy (Stiles, Honos-Webb, & Surko, 1998; Stiles & Horvath, 2017), and responsiveness in treatments for depression (Hardy, Stiles, Barkham, & Startup, 1998). These approaches converge in the concept of personalized medicine (Hassler, 2010), and, in the psychotherapy field, they are associated with a treatment that is tailored to the patient and his/her depressive style, for instance (Blatt & Luyten, 2009; Luyten & Blatt, 2007, 2011; Luyten, Fonagy, Lemma, & Target, 2012), or, more specifically, adapted to his/her dysfunctions. One such approach is exemplified by the contemporary perspectives of the NIH Research Domain Criteria, which refer to functional domains to be studied (and eventually treated). The psychotherapeutic perspective adopted in this chapter is specifically this adaptive, negotiated trade-off indication, which attempts to focus on the specific dysfunctions of each depressive patient in a given context.

9.1.2 Complex Depression and Its Determinants

Complex-depression patients who seek mental health treatment in HPCS, especially in LMICs, can be likened to those who clinicians and the literature refer to as "difficult patients" (Koekkoek, van Meijel, & Hutschemaekers, 2006; Moukaddam, Flores, Matorin, Hayden, & Tucci, 2017; Ruscio & Holohan, 2006). The determinants of complexity identified in the literature are ascribed to a) the patient and his/her context, b) the healthcare institution where the patient is treated, and c) the mental health professionals in charge of the treatment.

9.1.2.1 Patient Determinants

Personality: Disorders, Dysfunctions, Styles

The complexities derived from the clinical presentation of depression (e.g., recurrent depression, dual depression: dysthymia + major depressive disorder) are covered in other chapters and/or books of this series. However, depressive disorders are among the most frequent comorbidities in patients with borderline personality disorder (BPD, Leichsenring, Leibning, Kruse, New, & Leweke, 2011). This is not only due to their etiological risk factors, but is also a consequence of the overlap of symptoms in both disorders, for instance, affectivity alterations (dysregulation) or suicidal ideation (Behn, Herpertz, & Krause, 2018; Köhling et al., 2015; Leichsenring et al., 2011). The prevalence of these symptoms is such that some authors have advanced the concept of "bipolar depression," a specific phenomenology of depression in borderline personality disorder (BPD) (e.g., Gunderson & Phillips, 1991;

Paris, 2010; Silk, 2010). To date, the categorical view of personality disorders (PD) has facilitated clinicians' communication about patients while also simplifying research and treatment recommendations; however, this approach has several disadvantages such as not considering the high (pseudo) comorbidity observed, the excessive heterogeneity of its categories, the lack of a clear delimitation between what is normal and what constitutes a personality disorder, and clinicians' dissatisfaction with its usage (Clark, 2007; Trull & Durrett, 2005; Widiger & Samuel, 2005). Based on these limitations, there is consensus among authors regarding the need to generate dimensional models focused on identifying the dysfunctions that underlie categorical diagnoses, as this approach should provide a clearer picture of the phenomenon of comorbidity (Safford et al., 2007). This type of diagnosis makes it possible to identify functioning profiles and better reflect the heterogeneous presentation of the symptoms, in this case, those of patients with complex depression. Section III of the DSM-5 (American Psychiatric Association, 2013) and the chapter on PD and related traits in the recent version of the ICD-11 (World Health Organization, 2018) have furthered this dimensional perspective. Both models make it possible to identify generic traits, establish the severity of personality disorders, and study maladaptive functioning. Diagnosis makes it possible to establish deficiencies in both self-functioning and interpersonal relationships (Zimmermann, Kerber, Rek, Hopwood, & Krueger, 2019). A similar diagnostic approach was advanced in the 1990s in Germany: the Operationalized Psychodynamic Diagnosis (OPD Task Force, 2008), which enables practitioners to perform a thorough dimensional diagnosis of the affected functions. The functions evaluated are grouped into four domains: perception/cognition (self-perception and object-perception), regulation (self-regulation and regulation of relationships), communication (internal and external), and attachment (to internal objects and to external objects). Each of these functions has subfunctions that can be measured (see table 1). The separate diagnosis of these functions, which will be described in a later section, makes it possible to estimate an overall level of personality functioning (high integration, moderate integration, low integration, and disintegration). From the perspective of the OPD, patients previously described as "difficult" are those who, apart from having depressive symptoms, have a personality functioning that only allows them to access limited or reduced psychic capabilities or functions to maintain or recover their functional balance in response to internal or external stressors of everyday life, especially those of an interpersonal nature. These people have been unable to develop these functions because they have lived in extremely adverse environments, especially in early childhood, or have grown up in settings marked by conflicts that affect later phases of development, limiting the availability of these functions (OPD Task Force, 2008; Rudolf , 2013).

Clinically, these patients have limited or nonexistent psychic space for self-reflection, being affected by an unstable and shifting self-image or even identity diffusion. Furthermore, the topics of their internal conflicts take on a destructive character or become unrecognizable, becoming permanent conflicts with the outside world. These patients may also have permanent impulse regulation deficits or constrictions with intermittent regulation failures. Their main anxieties revolve around losing meaningful relationships or being hurt by the loss of strongly idealized or strongly devalued people. Affective contact may be either limited and flat or easily overwhelmed and barely tolerant of negative effects. Apart from the complexity that these patient features impose on therapeutic strategies, they activate strong experiences in the therapists that are hardly understandable from the patients' perspective; rather, they generate astonishment or even violence in the therapists (OPD Task Force, 2008).

The concepts of dependence and self-criticism, which constitute another perspective on personality functioning, have also come to be regarded as a vulnerability factor for depression (e.g., Blatt, 2004; Mandel, Dunkley, & Moroz, 2015). These styles were covered in the previous chapter; however, it is worth remembering how they determine different levels of susceptibility to stressors (e.g., abandonment in dependent style, failure in self-critical style) as well as differential responses to treatment: self-critical patients, for instance, display more depressive symptoms at the start of treatment than dependent ones (e.g., Dagnino, Pérez, Gómez, Gloger, & Krause, 2017; de la Parra, Dagnino, Valdés, & Krause, 2017) and show poor response to cognitive behavioral therapy (CBT), interpersonal therapy (IPT), medication, and placebo pill (Blatt, Quinlan, Pilkonis, & Shea, 1995; Chui, Zilcha-Mano, Dinger, Barrett, & Barber, 2016; Marshall, Zuroff, McBride, & Bagby, 2008). Studies conducted by the Chilean Millennium Institute for Research in Depression and Personality (MIDAP) indicate that more self-critical subjects show greater reactivity to stress, less subjective awareness of stress, and reduced performance in general tasks, as well as higher dropout rates (Mellado et al., 2018) and a poorer response to various psychosocial interventions compared to highly dependent patients. Regarding these patients' personality functioning, it was observed that more self-critical ones displayed lower levels of personality functioning integration; specifically, they showed more vulnerabilities in attachment to internal objects (see later section) compared to more dependent patients, who displayed self-perception and relationship regulation vulnerabilities (Dagnino et al., 2018).

Socioeconomic and Gender Determinants

Well-known studies (Hidaka, 2012; Moyano & Barría, 2006) have shown a link between GDP per capita and depression and suicide risk: wealthier countries tend to display higher depression prevalence. As economic growth causes formerly traditional, community-centric societies to become individualistic and competitive, depression seems to increase (Kato & Kanba, 2017; Krause et al., 2015; Orchard & Jimenez, 2016; Patel et al., 2018), especially when perceived inequity is heightened (Jiménez, 2020). Chile, a LMIC that has gradually shifted towards individualism, is a case in point (Jiménez, 2020; Krause et al., 2015). Like the per capita income, perceived inequality and subjective and social distress have increased (PNUD, 1998, 2017). Depression has also risen, reaching 6.2% of the population and surpassing the global rate (4.4%; WHO, 2017). The prevalence of depression in Chilean women is five times higher than in men (10.1% vs. 2.1%), with low-income women displaying the highest depression indexes (ELSOC, 2018; Patel et al., 2018). Thus, in LMICs, it is these women – who are more likely to have complex depression and be difficult patients – who will seek help in HPCS and primary care (Levy & O'Hara, 2010). To get there, they will need to overcome barriers to access determined by their context, such as difficulties finding someone within their support network to care for their children, problems obtaining work leaves, insufficient funds for transportation, and sometimes the inability to pay for their treatment. Furthermore, patients may also be affected by institutional barriers, as will be shown in the next section. Barriers to access are also a result of the patients' value system or bad therapeutic experiences that cause them to expect little from psychosocial treatments (Krause, 2005; Rojas et al., 2015; Zúñiga, 2019).

9.1.2.2 Other Factors That Add Complexity to Depressive Patients Seeking Help in High-Pressure Care Settings: Comorbidities, Suicidality, and Adverse Childhood Experiences

The relation between somatic comorbidities and depression is complex and bidirectional. According to the 2007 World Survey conducted by the World Health Organization (WHO, 2007), 9.3% to 23% of the respondents with one or more chronic diseases also had depression, a significant difference compared to the percentage of subjects who did not suffer from a chronic physical disease. The survey, which covered 245,404 people in 60 countries, also demonstrated that subjects with depression plus a chronic physical disease had the poorest health indexes in relation to those with other morbid states or depression alone. This association between chronic disease and depression is observable across different cultures and primary care levels (Kilzieh, Rastam, Maziak, & Ward, 2008; Martínez et al., 2017). In patients with multiple comorbidities, depression appears to be the most common pathology (Sinnige et al., 2013). Similarly, patients treated and diagnosed with depression in high-pressure care settings, such as primary care centers, display high comorbidity levels (Martín-Merino, Ruigómez, Johansson, Wallander, & García-Rodriguez, 2010). This is exemplified by Martínez et al. (2017), who examined a sample of 256 patients diagnosed with depression and found that 78.13% of them had one or more comorbidities: physical (29%), psychiatric (46%), or physical and psychiatric (25%). In primary care, one of the most common psychic comorbidities is anxiety disorder (Martín-Merino et al., 2010; Olfson et al., 2000), which hinders the prognosis of these patients. In brief, the high prevalence of comorbidities, especially in high demand settings such as primary care, makes it necessary to integrate physical and mental health effectively (Martínez et al., 2017).

Suicidal behavior, in its multiple manifestations, is a multifactor phenomenon that combines common factors and singularities. It tends to appear alongside psychiatric pathology and symptomatology, especially alcohol consumption disorders and depression (Bostwick & Pankratz, 2000; Schneider, 2009), significantly increasing suicide risk when accompanied by comorbidity (Cavanagh, Carson, Sharpe, & Lawrie, 2003). The multiple risk factors affecting people, from the social to the individual, interact in complex and unique ways, progressively affecting them until suicide ideation and/or a suicide attempt occur. Suicide attempt survivors report a trajectory of harmful experiences throughout their lives (Morales, Echávarri, Barros, Zuloaga, & Taylor, 2016). These accumulated experiences are triggered by an event that leads the subject to a categorical confirmation, of a depressive nature, that there is no way out. The person, unable to cope with this situation, attempts suicide. The suicide attempt generally has an underlying intention that may be ambivalent (e.g., seeking help, making a statement, and, at the same time, running the risk of dying); alternatively, the person may be determined to die, expecting the attempt to result in his/her own death (Morales et al., 2016). It is not possible to predict suicide attempts: they are contingent on a temporal condition that can flare up at any given time, being highly sensitive to a person's current state of mind (Fowler, 2012). However, clinical experience and research show that it is possible to prevent states of distress prior to a suicide attempt (Barros et al., 2020). In this regard, psychotherapeutic interventions aimed at preventing suicide attempts are largely focused on detecting depressive states and emotional dysregulation, emphasizing the strengthening of protective factors and the recovery of weakened aspects that could be worked on and trained through psychotherapy. This approach, depending on each individual case, focuses on self-knowledge, emotional regulation, and the development of skills for life, especially regarding the person's relationship with him/herself and others (CONADIC, 2010).

With respect to early adversity, available evidence indicates that it is linked to various mental pathologies in adulthood (Fernandez et al., 2018; Gilbert et al., 2009; Li, D'arcy, & Meng, 2016), including personality disorders, depression, anxiety disorders, and post-traumatic stress disorder, among others (e.g., Adams, Mrug, & Knight, 2018; Comijs et al., 2013; Cougle, Timpano, Sachs-Ericsson, Keough, & Riccardi, 2010; Pajer et al., 2014; White, 2011). It has also been demonstrated that the course of depression, as well as its clinical presentation and treatment response, differs among depressive patients with and without a history of trauma (Chapman et al., 2004; Martins-Monteverde et al., 2019; Vitriol et al., 2014; Vitriol, Cancino, Ballesteros, Núñez, & Navarrete, 2017). The importance of the relationship between early adversity and depression has been examined in detail elsewhere in this book.

Complex Depression: Empirical Profiles

Some authors have studied complex depression from an empirical perspective. For instance, Ruscio and Holohan (2006) proposed a list of over 40 factors that characterized complex cases, grouped into several topics such as symptoms, security, physical aspects, intellectual aspects, and personality. Employing more complex analyses, in an ongoing investigation conducted by one of the authors of this chapter and colleagues studied 251 patients of outpatient clinics with a depression diagnosis. A machine learning procedure has preliminarily revealed three depression profiles, one of which displayed a high level of depressive symptomatology associated with adverse experiences in childhood, a low level of personality functioning integration, a high level of self-criticism, somatization, and limited social networks and low satisfaction with them. This profile was labeled "complex depression" by the authors, being significantly different from the moderate and mild profiles. The moderate profile is characterized by a significant level of physical negligence in childhood, while the mild profile displays multiple satisfactory social networks. It should be noted that certain elements of personality, empirically verified through complex profiles, can be relevant variables when identifying complex depression. In this case, a higher level of self-criticism and a lower level of personality functioning integration, as shown above, interact in specific ways and lead to relevant therapeutic consequences.

Delgadillo, Huey, Bennett, and McMillan (2017), using a similar approach, examined the clinical records for 1512 patients and reported that complex cases are characterized by the presence of measurable factors in several domains: clinical, demographic, characterological, and attitudinal. This complexity also affects the prognosis, as more complex patients benefit from high-intensity therapies (vs low-intensity ones), especially in terms of depressive and anxious symptomatology. These studies make it possible to promptly identify complex cases and match them with interventions suited to these patients.

Institutional Determinants

High-pressure care settings, including primary care, often have waiting lists, lack professionals, and employ treatment models that do not meet the psychosocial requirements of mental health treatment: patients cannot get weekly sessions, sometimes they are not treated by the same therapist, or the sessions are too brief (de la Parra, Errázuriz, Gómez-Barris, & Zúñiga, 2019; Fischer, Cottin, Behn, Errázuriz, & Díaz, 2019; Koekkoek et al., 2006; Moukaddam et al., 2017; Rojas et al., 2015). Despite having clinical guidelines for depression treatment, these institutions often lack treatment models to deal with complex patients (Fischer et al., 2019; Koekkoek et al., 2006; Martínez et al., 2017; Zúñiga, Núñez, Araya, de la Parra, & Taubner, 2019). Thus, patients describe their psychotherapeutic experience in primary care as "just talking," without reporting a therapeutic effect derived from these sessions with a professional (Koekkoek et al., 2006; Rojas et al., 2015; Zúñiga, 2019; Zúñiga, Balboa & de la Parra, 2018). Therapists in these institutions complain about their working conditions: heavy workloads, productivity pressure, excessive paperwork, insufficient supervision, and a lack of recognition from professionals who do not work in mental health (Fischer et al., 2019; Haas, Leiser, Magill, & Sanyer, 2005; Koekkoek et al., 2006; Zúñiga, Balboa & de la Parra 2018).

Practitioner Determinants in Institutional Contexts

Especially within the context of primary care, depression management tends to be unsatisfactory and ineffective both in industrialized countries and LMICs (Araya, Flynn, Rojas, Fritsch, & Simon, 2006; Neumeyer-Gromen, Lampert, Stark, & Kallischnigg, 2004). One of the possible underlying factors of this situation is the lack of qualified professionals with the necessary competences and training to handle mental health disorders and address these patients' contextual factors (Patel, Chowdhary, Rahman, & Verdeli, 2011). In general, mental health specialists are less integrated in these settings, which forces clinicians (who are not experts) to treat more complex patients unaided (Rubenstein et al., 1999). Authors have shown that physicians (GPs) find it hard to diagnose depression, underestimating its severity and considering that their competences are limited (Acuña et al., 2016; Alvarado & Rojas, 2011; Burroughs et al., 2006; Shah & Harris, 1997). This situation, compounded by a negative attitude towards diagnosing depression, results in unsatisfactory clinical performance (Dowrick, Gask, Perry, Dixon, & Usherwood, 2000; Haddad et al., 2011). Therefore, GPs are more likely to act intuitively and often avoid diagnosing depression, as they feel that they cannot offer their patients anything better due to their limited training in therapeutic interventions, short time per session, and the impossibility of referring them to a psychologist or to secondary level care due to long waiting lists, among other aspects (Burroughs et al., 2006; Chew-Graham, Mullin, May, Hedley, & Cole, 2002).

It has also been observed that depressed patients prefer to be listened to and do not only wish to receive medical treatment for their depression; in this regard, they complain that providers do not listen, lack empathy, or are only interested in filling out their medical records and provide no guidance for their problems (Johnston et al., 2007; Zúñiga, 2019).

Psychological treatments for depression, having been created in high-income countries (HIC) (e.g., cognitive behavioral therapy based (CBT-based) and interpersonal therapy (IPT)), cannot be readily used in LMICs. Although they can be effective after implementing specialized training and supervision for therapists (Patel et al., 2011), it is necessary to adapt them to the contextual factors and characteristics of the community to be treated, considering its expectations and stigmatization regarding the disease (Patel et al., 2011).

In Latin America, most therapists report being psychodynamic (44.8%), followed by cognitive behavioral (31.9%) and integrative or eclectic (20.1%), while a smaller number are systemic (12.7%) and humanist (9.8%) (de la Parra, 2013). This characterization of the theoretical orientation of Latin American professionals will be relevant for the therapeutic model that we will present below.

Although psychologists receive undergraduate-level training in routine practice, authors have stressed that this is insufficient to work as a therapist (Jiménez 1998/2000); also, psychologists working in primary care have noted that undergraduate programs must provide more training in clinical psychology (31.5%), community psychology (16.8%), public policies (15.8%), and primary care management (8.4%) (Scharager & Molina, 2007). In this regard, it has been reported that primary care psychologists' depression management competences are lowest for "treatment" ($Z < 0.10$), followed by "sociocultural approach," "treatment plan," and "clinical diagnosis" (slightly over 0.20) (Bedregal, 2017). Particularly in depressive disorders, psychotherapeutic competences correlate slightly, but positively and significantly, with better treatment outcomes ($r = 0.28$) (Webb, DeRubeis, & Barber, 2010). Therefore, it can be presumed that, if professionals lack the necessary competences to treat the disorder, they are limiting these users' chances of receiving effective treatment. With respect to the management of difficult patients with personality dysfunctions, it has been reported that, when therapists receive training in personality disorders with the aim of improving attitudes and service provision, they can develop competences such as empathy and the ability to provide a suitable diagnosis, thus increasing the likelihood of a successful treatment outcome (Beryl & Völlm, 2017; Shanks, Pfohl, Blum, & Black, 2011). Beyond competence deficits, therapist experience is another determinant: it has been observed that more years of practice correlate with better therapeutic management of complex patients, better communication, and good respectful interaction (Edgoose, 2012; Hinchey & Jackson, 2011). In contrast, younger clinicians tend to report frustrations, especially physicians who treat patients with psychosocial issues (Krebs, Garrett, & Konrad, 2006). Patients' interpersonal functioning, a major determinant in practitioners' performance, is influenced by dysfunctions associated with their personality structure (e.g., personality disorder) and others derived from their interaction with their providers and their own vulnerable background. These issues trigger feelings of rejection, pessimism, fatigue, and unease in professionals, reinforcing their idea that they are dealing with a difficult patient (Fischer et al., 2019; Koekkoek et al., 2006).

In brief, the evidence reviewed thus far shows how the interaction between patients' variables, their socioeconomic context, and therapists' variables, as well as their work context and competences, interact in the definition of a difficult or complex patient. Clinical complexity can thus be said to be a dimensional measure; that is, patients can be placed along a continuum ranging from less to more complexity (Delgadillo et al., 2017) depending on their accumulation of disadvantages in these multiple domains. Patients, apart from bringing their own complexity, may also react to negative attitudes in practitioners (Fischer et al., 2019), which can be triggered by idiosyncratic reasons or poor working conditions and/or a high-pressure job. Thus, in the interactional model proposed by Fischer et al. (2019) to explain "difficult" patients, the negative effect on the therapist's work and competences derives not only from the patient's characteristics and attitudes but also from the practitioner's feeling that he/she is working in a setting perceived as demanding and unsuitable. As these authors suggest (Fischer et al., 2019), a depressive patient with certain personality dysfunctions that color his/her clinical presentation may be regarded as an average patient in a work setting with sufficient resources; however, in a context marked by deficits, he/she may be considered complex or difficult.

9.2 The Treatment of Complex Depression: Towards a Competence-Based Model in High-Pressure Care Settings

9.2.1 Strategies

Although very severe personality disorders require complex, multidisciplinary settings, where patients can be treated in rapid succession by a variety of practitioners using, for instance, dialectical behavior therapy (DBT) (Chapman, 2006; Dimeff & Koerner, 2007; Linehan, 1993), the clinical reality of primary care, especially in LMICs, shows that many patients with a range of personality dysfunctions can benefit from individual treatments (Cuijpers, Quero, Dowrick, & Arroll, 2019; Gunderson & Links, 2014) that meet certain requirements, as we will discuss in a later section. Overall, authors have suggested that these patients be treated using a transdiagnostic perspective, that is, addressing both mood dysfunctions ("depressive mood"; see Cuijpers et al., 2019) and personality dysfunctions or those that characterize the self-critical or dependent styles, taking into account the patient's context and the therapist's work settings.

It has been established that, when personality dysfunctions color a patient's complex depression, therapists should focus on these aspects first (Clarkin, Petrini, & Diamond, 2019; Gunderson et al., 2014; Gunderson, Herpertz, Skodol, Torgersen, & Zanarini, 2018; Gunderson & Links, 2014); therefore, "structure-oriented psychotherapy" for addressing these patients will be discussed in detail. As previously mentioned, the model is based on the assumption that the primary care therapists working in high-pressure settings have a variety of therapeutic orientations, especially in LMICs (de la Parra, 2013); therefore, we have adopted the common factors model (CFM, Laska, Gurman, & Wampold, 2014; Wampold, 2015). This model makes it possible to explain why these different orientations can produce changes (e.g., Lambert, 2013), as any therapy that meets the requirements for a bona fide therapy can be effective.

A bona fide therapy can be defined as a procedure intended to be therapeutic and which includes a psychological theory of disease and healing, a convincing rational framework regarding treatment, therapeutic actions consistent with its underlying theories, and active collaboration between patient and therapist. In addition, the therapist is expected to perform the usual therapeutic actions, be flexible enough to adapt to each individual patient, and align with the treatment that he/she is providing (Wampold et al., 1997, 2010). In this regard, with respect to depression, Cuijpers et al. (2019) note:

> There is no evidence that the effects of different types of therapy significantly differ from each other. Trials directly comparing different types of therapy, as well as network meta-analyses, suggest that all major types of therapy have comparable effects. (p. 2)

Although these authors suggest taking these results cautiously and given that the controversy regarding specific and common factors in psychotherapy is far from being settled (e.g., Cuijpers, Reijnders, & Huibers, 2019; Mulder et al., 2017), selecting the CFM is also a practical, cost-effective decision due to the diversity of the professionals working in PC and HPCS in LMICs.

The next list presents the elements of psychotherapy for complex depression in high-pressure care settings that guide therapeutic strategies from a CFM perspective:

1. Adaptive indication – responsiveness – trade-off indication
2. Brevity:
   A. Frequency and duration
   B. Responsive regulation of treatment duration (Barkham et al., 2006)
   C. One session, one pearl
3. Focus; focusing on structure
4. Therapeutic alliance, patient-therapist relationship

Adaptive Indication The term "adaptive indication" was coined by German psychotherapists in the 1980s (Thomä & Kächele, 1987) and was later rendered into English as "responsiveness" (Kramer & Stiles, 2015; Stiles & Horvath, 2017). Adaptive indication means that the treatment is modified to adapt to the patient in terms of the patient's needs, culture, and context, explanatory models of disease, difficulties in accessing treatment, and the maintenance of the therapeutic process. In addition, the treatment is modified to adapt to institutional conditions and needs. This conceptualization of adaptive indication is fully consistent with the concept of trade-off indication mentioned above: both suggest that the treatment of complex depression should consider not only the patient's clinical, personal, and contextual characteristics, as well as his/her ability to access treatment, but also the actual opportunities that the institution can offer the patient.

Brevity In high-pressure care settings and primary care, especially in LMICs, it is imperative to shorten waiting lists. Reducing waiting lists implies shortening treatments so that professionals can have an adequate patient turnover, which enables them to receive new patients; therefore, in this context, adaptive or trade-off indication means conducting brief treatments. Although authors have questioned the effectiveness of brief therapies for achieving full recovery from depression (Sotsky et al., 1991), several studies such as the meta-analysis performed by Nieuwsma et al. (2012) and the recent study by Cuijpers et al. (2019) indicate that brief therapies, including those for depression delivered in primary care in LIMCs, have positive outcomes. It should be noted that these examples and the literature on depression treatment in PC (Barley et al. 2011) do not refer to complex depression or difficult (depressive) patients as described in this chapter. Thus, when clinical depression takes center stage, sidelining the patient's personality traits, depressive symptoms must be prioritized, following the successful example of behavioral activation in PC in LMICs (Cuijpers, Quero, et al., 2019). Although the term "brief therapy" can refer to a set of 6 to 8 sessions, as in crisis interventions (Jacobson, 1979; Yeager & Roberts, 2015), and despite the fact that psychotherapies of this duration have been given preference in depression treatment (Nieuwsma et al., 2012), the model described in the present chapter stipulates a maximum length of 12 weekly sessions. This decision was made following the revised guidelines issued by the Mental Health Department of the Chilean Ministry of Health (MINSAL 2017), which conclude that "after the 12-session course, each additional psychotherapy session would reduce the patient's score on standardized scales of depressive symptom evaluation by 0.038 points, controlling for time of contact with the therapist, duration in weeks, and psychotherapeutic approach" (p. 21). Twelve sessions also make it possible to cement the therapeutic relationship in patients with personality dysfunctions and/or a background of early adversity. For complex patients with more severe personality dysfunctions, these 12 sessions may be insufficient. In those cases, series of 12 sessions are recommended, after which patients are temporarily discharged until a new set of sessions with the same therapist: the therapy ends, but not the relationship, which can be resumed to establish a corrective emotional experience (Divac-Jovanovic & Svrakic, 2017; Gunderson & Links, 2014), as will be discussed in a later section.[1]

Regarding termination, it has been established that dropout rates range from over 45% to 20% (Swift & Greenberg, 2012; Wierzbicki & Pekarik, 1993). Studies with follow-up components have shown that some patients who interrupt their treatment and do not return felt better and are satisfied with the care received (de la Parra, Gómez-Barris, Zuñiga, Dagnino, & Valdés, 2018; Simon, Imel, Ludman, & Steinfeld, 2012), which means that their gains had reached a good enough level (Barkham et al., 2006; Stiles, Barkham, & Wheeler, 2015). This means that it is necessary to provide therapists with skills to detect these "good enough" gains and thus terminate therapies according to patient response, in other words, a "responsive regulation of treatment duration" (Barkham et al., 2006; Stiles et al., 2015). This would preserve the relationship for future therapeutic contacts, especially in primary care settings, where users must return to the same centers and meet the same practitioners.

Given the limited number of sessions and barriers to access, either due to patient factors or institutional reasons, the model proposed is informed by the notion of "one session, one pearl" (Defey, 2013), which means that each contact between the therapist and the user must be meaningful: the patient must always "take something home," so that a set of meaningful sessions will gradually form the therapy process, "the pearl necklace." This is consistent with patients' expectations of psychological care, a finding we have observed in ongoing research conducted by the first authors of this chapter.

Focus – Focusing on Structure According to the above, focusing makes it possible to abbreviate psychotherapy and contributes to the challenge of implementing brief psychotherapeutic treatments in HPCS. Several models of focal psychotherapy

[1] In the present chapter, we do not cover the psychotherapeutic treatment of the depressive symptoms of noncomplicated depression, since this topic is discussed in other chapters of this book and there is abundant literature on it.

exist in the psychodynamic domain (Messer & Warren, 1995), which are essentially based on addressing conflicts or maladaptive interpersonal patterns that underlie symptoms (Leichsenring & Schauenburg, 2014; OPD Task Force, 2008). Other psychotherapeutic traditions also focus on solving problems, which can involve behavioral patterns, emotional regulation, or dysfunctional cognitive patterns in patients with a personality pathology (Beck, Davis, & Freeman, 2015; Kellogg & Young, 2006; Linehan et al., 2006). In the present chapter, we will not discuss the traditional focal approach mentioned above nor will we cover other perspectives, since other chapters elaborate on these topics and the literature also provides further information about alternative approaches.

In consequence, when symptoms are largely generated and maintained by personality functioning deficits, treatment should address those deficits; in this case, the strategy will consist in focusing on these functional difficulties. In other words, this strategy involves centering psychotherapeutic work on patients' specific deficits, helping them to identify and recognize them in their everyday functioning and then develop self-regulation and adaptation processes in response to these structural limitations. These deficits can be identified following OPD-2 guidelines (OPD Task Force, 2008), which distinguish four domains defined earlier and detailed in the following table (see Table 9.1).

Table 9.1 Structural personality functions according to Axis IV of OPD-2

[1] Domain	Function	Sub-function
Perception/cognition	Self-perception	Self-reflection
		Affect differentiation
		Identity
	Object perception	Self-object differentiation
		Whole object perception
		Realistic object perception
Regulation	Self-regulation	Impulse control
		Affect tolerance
		Regulation of self-esteem
	Regulation of relationships	Protecting relationships
		Balancing interests
		Anticipation
Communication	Internal communication	Experiencing affect
		Use of fantasies
		Bodily self
	External communication	Making contact
		Communicating affect
		Empathy
Attachment	Attachment to internal objects	Internalization
		Utilizing introjects
		Variability of attachment
	Attachment to external objects	Capacity for attachment
		Accepting help
		Detaching from relationships

Structure-focused therapy (SFT) (Rudolf, 2013) is a therapeutic proposal that complements the OPD system (OPD Task Force, 2008), providing general recommendations about strategic decisions for planning therapy and specific therapeutic work techniques for difficult patients due to structural deficits or vulnerabilities. In SFT, the patient's difficulties are largely understood to be an expression of his/her deficits, with the therapist attempting to place in the field of observation (focus) those functions whose development was probably hindered by deficiencies in early emotional support. In this proposal for personality structure-oriented psychotherapy, apart from focusing on specific functions depending on each patient's profile, we suggest general work strategies adapted to the overall functioning characteristics of these patients. Some of the main strategies are presented in Table 9.2.

Table 9.2 General characteristics of therapeutic work in SFT

Therapist Attitude	
Emphasis on an enabling therapeutic attitude	1. The therapist is fully oriented towards the construction of the relationship
	2. Prepare yourself to connect with a "less than pleasant" patient
	3. Be a stable therapist, who strives to avoid feeling threatened, discouraged, or irritated
	4. Have a flexible stance in your reactions to the patient; that is, answer questions, display willingness to react to the patient's need for help and share your views on situations experienced by the patient
	5. Be respectful of the patient's coping attempts
	6. Empathize with the patient's experiences of adversity and precariousness
	7. Be available as a mentor-therapist, as a parental figure that encourages development
Therapeutic Relationship	
Prepare yourself for an intense countertransference	1. The patient's relational offer is characterized by intense needs and demands and little tolerance to frustration
	2. Relational needs are understood to be real and not unconscious instinctive desires
	3. The therapist does not interpret the patient's behavior as an offer necessarily directed to him/her
	4. Together, they seek to identify problematic patterns and learn to deal with them more effectively, gradually becoming more accountable
	5. The therapist pays attention to qualities, talents, and interests
	6. Therapist together with patient does not lose hope

(continued)

Table 9.2 (continued)

Focus selection and goal-setting (together with the patient)	1. Exploring and evaluating the structural functions that require more support
	2. Transforming them into focal points and goals of the therapy
	3. Including the patient's gradual increase in accountability as a therapeutic goal
Therapeutic Techniques and Interventions	
General techniques and interventions	1. Interpretations of meaning become secondary: focusing on "how" and not "why"
	2. Techniques to reinforce the basic stabilization of the self:
	Reflecting
	Asking
	Clarifying to focus the narrative
	Creating distance between the patient and his/her problems (disidentification)
	Stimulating mental production through words and other means
	Structure-generating interventions (helping the patient to plan, take care of him/herself, and set limits)
	Establishing hypotheses and connections
Establishing patterns	1. Learning to see behavior and experiences as patterns
	2. Learning to see behavioral patterns as emotional responses to current external or internal situations
	3. Developing a functional scheme
	4. Accepting that the scheme was biographically mediated and that it contains coping attempts
	5. Studying current functionality/dysfunctionality
	6. Accepting the pattern as part of oneself and taking responsibility
	7. Testing alternative possibilities
	8. Learning to use the therapeutic situation

(continued)

Table 9.2 (continued)

Adopting therapeutic relational "positions" with respect to the patient	1. Therapist positions him/herself behind the patient by:
	Identifying with the patient (sharing his/her perspective)
	Providing emotional support (embracing the pain and working through it)
	Compassion
	Auxiliary self
	Aid (mentor, coach)
	2. Therapist positions himself alongside the patient by:
	Sharing focus on the patient's situation (both look at a third party [the patient and his functioning], *insight* not about the meaning but about the patient's patterns and functioning)
	"Watching from the hill" to look at the patient's situation and functioning and generate affective distance
	Meta-observation
	3. Therapist positions him/herself in front of the patient by:
	Reflecting (therapist's perception is returned to the patient)
	Responding (allowing the therapist's emotional resonance to be seen)
	Highlighting differences with the other, for example, the therapist: alterity
	Confronting (aspects of reality and one's responsibility)
	4. Therapist positions him/herself ahead of the patient
	Foreseeing difficulties, tasks, and development issues and sharing them with the patient
	Avoiding harm by anticipating problems with an attitude of concern and care

(Adapted from Rudolf, 2013)

Box 9.1 Dependent Patients

According to the study cited, dependent patients perform more poorly in self-perception and self-regulation (with the latter including affect tolerance and regulation of self-esteem) as well as in attachment to external objects (as shown in Table 1, it includes the ability to detach from relationships). These structural functions should be proposed as the therapeutic focus and jointly agreed upon with the patient to be prioritized in therapy. In the case of dependent depressive patients, it is precisely dependence that will be used as a therapeutic resource, as their need to establish a bond becomes a chance to generate a therapeutic relationship quickly and thus work with a more permeable patient.

To work on these patients' self-perception deficits, the therapist takes an active interest in their subjective experience. Therapeutic interventions are aimed at supporting patients' self-reflection (see Table 1), helping them to reflect on and differentiate their self-image, improving their ability to connect their affects to events in their lives (affective contextualization of events), and strengthening their ability to construct/produce their identity. The therapist can anticipate reasoning, feelings, and planning (positioning him/herself "ahead of the patient"), operating as an auxiliary self; on other occasions, he/she offers his/her own perception, sharing his/her thoughts and expressing his/her disagreements with the patient (positioning him/herself "in front of the patient"). Here, it is essential to use reflection and clarification techniques through detailed questions that encourage and organize the patient's communication. Work with dysfunctions in attachment to external objects in dependent depressive patients is based on the "parental attitude" proposed by Rudolf (2013). This makes it possible to regulate the distance with a patient who tends to cling on to others. Together with the patient, the therapist explores experiences of pain and anguish due to loss and separation and stimulates the ability to deal with mourning, helping the patient with the affective handling of these situations. Even in brief therapies, the working-through of the topic of separation is highly significant, since it enables the patient to experience separations that do not entail abandonment and boosts his/her ability to accept unfulfilled expectations while tolerating aggression and disillusionment regarding the lost object. Parental attitude, as will be discussed below, means that the therapist becomes a real object for the patient, which the patient is expected to internalize and take home after a series of 12 sessions ends, and they meet again at an unspecified point in the future. Thus, as previously noted, the therapy ends but the relationship remains: internal and external availability of the therapist within the framework of a corrective emotional experience (Alexander & French, 1946; Gunderson & Links, 2014). Dysfunctions in self-regulation require (Rudolf, 2013) therapist work focused on developing strategies for impulse management and integration, affect tolerance and responsibility, and regulation of self-esteem and feelings of humiliation. The aim of these efforts is to prevent an emotional inundation. This involves learning to perceive overwhelming affects quickly, setting up an early warning system to identify affective movements that are becoming stronger, and learning to see the relational context (the situation that triggered the affect) to find out how to overcome it. At the beginning of the therapy, the patient depends on the concrete experience of receiving external comfort from the therapist, who helps him/her to identify the affect and determine how to soothe him/herself. After recovering his/her composure, it is possible to work on the identification of the triggering event. This work entails the construction of an "observing self" encouraged by the "alongside the patient" position, where both participants adopt a "watching from the hill" perspective that allows them to see the patient's functioning from a distance.

In complex depression cases, as defined in this chapter, an approach based on specific structural deficits should focus on the most severely affected functions. As an example, in the box below, we will address the OPD personality functions that are supposed to be most affected in dependent and self-critical patients, according to preliminary results in de la Parra et al. (2017).[2]

Box 9.2 Self-Critical Patients

Constitute a larger challenge, not only due to what has been defined as the pathogenic power of self-critical perfectionism (Blatt, 1995) and associated barriers preventing the establishment of a therapeutic alliance, especially in brief treatments (Blatt, 2004; de la Parra et al., 2017; Mellado et al., 2018; see also the thorough review in the previous chapter), but also in connection with findings that reveal higher levels of self-criticism in patients with more complex profiles in personality structure. According to the preliminary findings cited (de la Parra et al., 2017), patients belonging to this profile find it more difficult to access the OPD functions of object perception and attachment to internal objects. Both dysfunctions are consistent with the clinical theory of the depressive and self-critical patient: inasmuch as he/she is concerned with permanent self-definition and uninterested in his/her ties to others (Blatt & Luyten, 2009), he/she will encounter more difficulties with object perception, while his/her dysfunctional attachment to internal objects will manifest itself through self-criticism and not through internal objects that support and console. Thus, from the perspective of structure-oriented psychotherapy, both self-criticism and its underlying dysfunctions become therapeutic focal points. Since self-criticism appears early on in the therapeutic process, it must be established from the start as a focal point through shared attention. The self-criticism process is observed from the "alongside the patient" relational position (see Table 2 and Kannan & Levitt, 2013); that is, the participants explore when and how it is activated and not why it is activated, since structure-oriented psychotherapy does not concern itself with the underlying meaning of a given functioning but with the actions needed to address it.

Difficulties in the alliance established with these patients can be viewed as a result of issues with object perception and attachment to internal objects. Therefore, it is necessary to construct, care for, and actively monitor the therapeutic alliance (Bateman & Fonagy, 2012; Safran & Muran, 2000). The therapist places him/herself in front of the patient as a real object, revealing his/her own perceptions and emotions in a therapeutic manner, encouraging differentiation, and thus leaving behind (traditional)neutral therapeutic positions.

[2] We reiterate the need to take these illustrations as a clinical exercise how to work structurally oriented, since a later study in another sample (Dagnino et al. 2018) did not replicate the same associations between dependence and self-criticism and specific structural dysfunctions. More research in greater clinical samples is needed.

Work on the object-perception function requires that the therapist foster the patient's ability to differentiate between self and object, that is, to verify what the self wants, thinks, or fears, in contrast to the objects' presumed intentions. In addition, it is essential to be able to perceive the other integrally and produce a realistic image, without idealizing or underestimating him/her, but accepting that the other is different and has experiences and convictions that may be opposed to those of the patient. To do this, the patient and the therapist can analyze the external situation that the patient has described, probing its affective meaning.

Deficits in attachment to internal objects functions must be addressed directly. Supporting oneself and using positive introjects to soothe oneself must be actively pointed out to be a necessity of life and should be rehearsed in some way. The therapist helps the patient to identify positive internal objects (internal aids) such as positive childhood figures or positive aspects of these figures, friends, teachers, and pets, among others, as well as experiences with a positive connotation (e.g., sports, hobbies, places). Once these objects have been identified, the participants can seek ways of using them for the patient to soothe him/herself. In addition to this explicit work, the therapist has an effect on implicit memory to support the operation of internal bonds: through the strategy of becoming a real object "to be internalized," by interacting with the patient, taking care of him/her, and offering him/her emotional support (similar to maternal holding and baby manipulation).

Therapeutic Alliance, Patient-Therapist Relationship We will not discuss here the extensive literature on the therapeutic alliance (Flückiger, Del Re, Wampold, & Horvath, 2018; Klein et al., 2003); however, what has been presented thus far has clearly illustrated the major importance of the therapeutic relationship. This relationship often moderates change; that is, psychosocial interventions, regardless of their theoretical perspective, will only be effective if they take place in a favorable relational climate. In other cases, as in complex depression with personality dysfunctions and/or a history of trauma, the relationship will mediate change, operating like a repairing relationship (Gunderson & Links, 2014). This means that the therapist must purposively conduct the relationship as described below, taking into account the relevant competences.

9.2.2 *Competences for Addressing Complex Depression*

Competences have been defined as the knowledge, skills, and attitudes – as well as the integration of these components – that enable therapists to fulfill various functions in healthcare centers, regardless of the therapeutic orientation of these professionals (Kaslow, Dunn, & Smith, 2008; McDaniel et al., 2014). As has been shown in this chapter, it is a challenge for therapists to treat patients with complex depression in precarious and high-pressure care settings; however, from the patients' perspective, during in-depth interviews, psychologists can become facilitators who will enable them to access satisfactory treatment if they offer a helping relationship informed by the patients' expectations of change and bonding (ongoing research, Zúñiga & de la Parra,).

Considering that responsive competences are contextually dependent (Barber, Sharpless, Klostermann, & McCarthy, 2007; Stiles et al., 1998), the first authors of this chapter have conducted research aimed at generating a model of psychotherapeutic competences for treating complex depression in primary care centers that takes into account the users' views, the experience of the psychologists who work in these contexts, and the insights of academic experts (Zúñiga, 2019; Zúñiga, Balboa, & de la Parra, 2018). The preliminary results of this study, which refer to the source of depressive patients seeking help in high-pressure settings, are summarized in Fig. 9.1. The figure shows how institutional limitations and the lack training of therapists can prevent patients treated in PC from meeting their change expectations through psychological care. However, if the patients' expectations

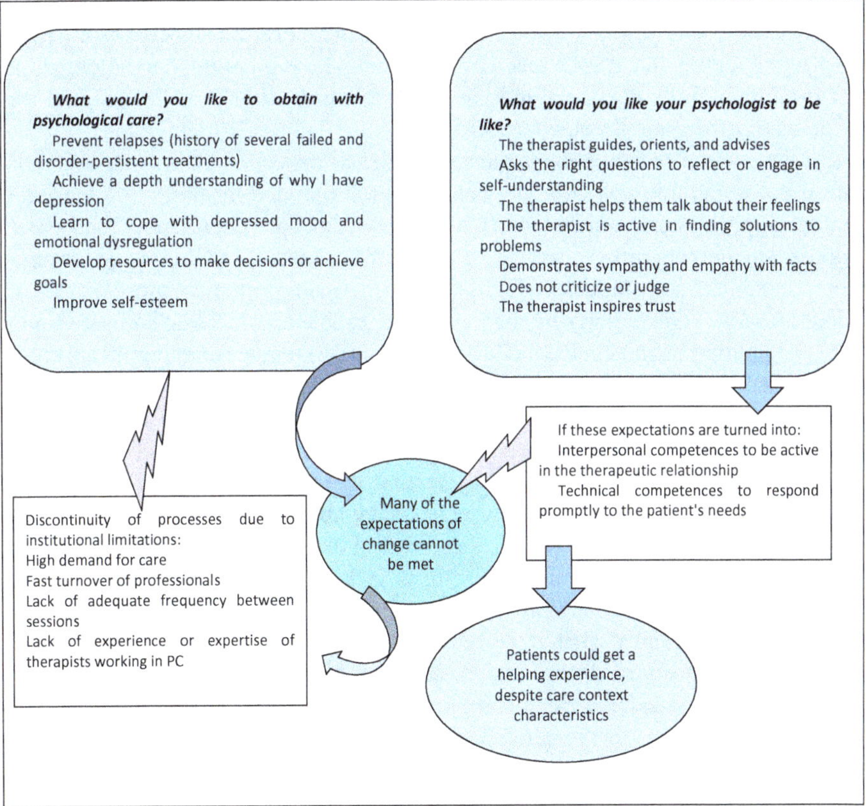

Fig. 9.1 Institutional limitations and the role of therapist competences for patients to meet their expectations in terms of care (Zúñiga et al., 2019)

regarding therapists are transformed into interpersonal competences allowing them to participate actively in the helping relationship and gain technical competences to respond *lively* to their needs, patients could get a helping experience despite of the limitations of the care context (Zúñiga et al., 2019).

According to these preliminary results, there appears to be a convergence between the patients' expectations regarding the therapeutic relationship and the experience of the psychologists working in PC. Both these elements stress the importance of therapists being warm, affectionate, empathetic, charismatic, and friendly when treating their patients. In the words of one patient, therapists should "smile when greeting me," "show interest in treating me," and essentially "keep me on their mind." For patients, it is essential that therapists do not judge them and inspire trust so that they can express what they are experiencing (Zúñiga, 2019; Zúñiga et al., 2018).

An ongoing analysis points out that therapists and experts have stressed the need for therapists to offer a therapeutic relationship based on humility, "acknowledging the mistakes made," "acting quickly in response to conflicts with the patient" (competences to repair alliance ruptures), and "working to prevent patients from slamming the door on their way out," since each and every moment with the patient is relevant in these contexts, where the continuity of the process is never guaranteed ("one session, one pearl," as noted earlier). Furthermore, for experts, if a patient goes home feeling like he/she met a professional who is committed to helping him/her even though the next session is in 1 month's time, it is enough to regard this effort as repairing and therapeutic in itself.

At the level of technical competences, patients' expectations show how important it is for therapists to offer and conduct a relevant and meaningful therapeutic dialog, helping them to understand "why me, why do I have depression?" and assisting them in their attempts to regulate their depressive mood and their negative emotions, thoughts, and impulses (Zúñiga, 2019). Again, therapists are expected to adopt an active role, identifying the *underlying* problem (which the patients cannot see) and guiding them to solve it (Zúñiga et al., 2018). Patients are highly appreciative of therapists' ability to suggest new points of view and listen actively, reminding what therapist worked with the patients in previous sessions and sharing a reflection or impression from the session (Zúñiga, 2019; Zúñiga et al., 2019).

Also, psychologists and experts agree that therapists should be familiar with public health and multiple treatment modes to be able to indicate the most suitable interventions for patients' problems, thus keeping therapists from depriving patients from accessing better treatments due to a lack of knowledge (or dogmatism) (Zúñiga, Balboa & de la Parra 2018). These sources also highlighted the relevance of teamwork, especially when treating complex patients (due to their disorder and/or adverse psychosocial determinants), knowing how to implement specific interventions to address suicide risk, distinguishing and applying interventions for managing depression and personality pathologies, offering psychoeducation, aiding patients when they are confronting their issues, and supporting their functioning (Zúñiga, Balboa & de la Parra, 2018; Zúñiga, 2019).

Lastly, psychologists and experts have stressed the importance of knowing how to adapt psychological techniques (interventions and therapeutic dialog) to patients' needs and their cultural context, bearing in mind gender- and belief-related barriers that may underlie the depressive disorder (Zúñiga, 2019; Zúñiga et al., 2018). This ability, referred to as "cultural competence," has been shown to increase the effectiveness of interventions in both developed countries and LMICs (Griner & Smith, 2006; Levy & O'Hara, 2010). Authors have suggested that, in LMICs, these cultural competences should be called "structural competences" to highlight the need for clinicians to be aware of the sociocultural context of their patients and actively mitigate the determinants of their mental health problems (Patel et al., 2018).

It should be noted that patients' expectations and psychologists' experiences are perfectly consistent with the model proposed above. Thus, when patients expect to "understand themselves," "get to the bottom of the problem," and "just understand," we are talking about focus, that is, the dynamics that underlies their reasons for seeking help. So, when they refer to their expectations regarding the therapist's personal characteristics, they mention relational characteristics like warmth and empathy, and when note that they expect to get insights in each session, they are referring to the pearl metaphor. Likewise, when psychologists mention relational qualities, the ability to adapt, and the need to possess a diverse toolset, they are talking about adaptive indication, that is, having a variety of resources to be able to adapt and respond to the needs of all their patients (de la Parra et al., 2019).

9.3 Conclusions

After reviewing a broad definition of complex depression, which goes far beyond the patient's diagnostic characteristics, we defined possible ways of approaching this disorder, with a special emphasis on structure-oriented therapy and the necessary competences to offer care to these patients. Yet, these descriptions leave out the context: the patients' contextual factors and the practitioners' work settings. These aspects are covered in the "Training Program in Psychotherapy Competences for Depression Treatment," which we developed for primary care and which will be tested in a number of centers in Chile (FONIS Project No. SA1910021). This program comprises six modules. Module I covers the theoretical-empirical basis of the model, including adaptive indication and the desirable competences for professionals, as explained above. Module II is wholly devoted to complex depression, addressing personality dysfunctions, self-critical and dependent functioning, and aspects of trauma. Module III focuses on the therapeutic relationship, laying out how the patient's context and the therapist's work setting influence the latter's emotional functioning. Self-care measures for the therapist are also discussed. Module IV is devoted to brief therapies, structure-focused therapy, and crisis interventions. Module V covers the management of suicide risk. Finally, Module VI discusses culturally informed psychotherapy and therapists' community-related competences, such as patients' community involvement and network activation, among others.

Through the present chapter, we expect to have contributed to the understanding of complex depression and its management in HPCS, especially in LMICs.

Acknowledgments This work was funded by the ANID-Millennium Science Initiative/Millennium Institute for Research on Depression and Personality-MIDAP and by ANIS/FONIS Project N° SA19I0021.

We wish to thank Catalina Aravena for her valuable support in the production of this chapter and Susana Morales for her contribution to several sections of the text.

References

Acuña, J., Rdz-Navarro, K., Huepe, G., Botto, A., Cárcamo, M., & Jiménez, J. P. (2016). Habilidades clínicas para el manejo de Trastornos depresivos en médicos generales en Santiago de Chile. *Revista Médica de Chile, 144*, 47–54. https://doi.org/10.4067/S0034-98872016000100007

Adams, J., Mrug, S., & Knight, D. (2018). Characteristics of child physical and sexual abuse as predictors of psychopathology. *Child Abuse & Neglect, 86*, 167–177. https://doi.org/10.1016/j.chiabu.2018.09.019

Alexander, F., & French, T. M. (1946). *Psychoanalytic therapy; principles and application*. New York: Ronald Press.

Alvarado, R., & Rojas, G. (2011). El programa nacional para el diagnóstico y tratamiento de depresión en atención primaria: una evaluación necesaria. *Revista Médica de Chile, 139*(5), 592–599. https://doi.org/10.4067/S0034-98872011000500005

American Psychiatric Association. (2013). *Diagnostic and statistical manual of mental disorders* (5th ed.). Washington, DC: American Psychiatric Association.

American Psychological Association. (2006). Evidence-based practice in psychology, APA presidential task force on evidence-based practice. *American Psychologist, 61*(4), 271–285. https://doi.org/10.1037/0003-066X.61.4.271

Araya, R., Flynn, T., Rojas, G., Fritsch, R., & Simon, G. (2006). Cost-effectiveness of a primary care treatment program for depression in low-income women in Santiago, Chile. *The American Journal of Psychiatry, 163*(8), 1379–1387. https://doi.org/10.1176/ajp.2006.163.8.1379

Barber, J., Sharpless, B., Klostermann, S., & McCarthy, K. (2007). Assessing intervention competence and its relation to therapy outcome: A selected review derived from the outcome literature. *Professional Psychology: Research and Practice, 38*(5), 493–500. https://doi.org/10.1037/0735-7028.38.5.493

Barley, E., Murray, J., Walters, P., & Tylee, A. (2011). Managing depression in primary care: A metasynthesis of qualitative and quantitative research from the UK to identify barriers and facilitators. BMC Family Practice, 12, 47.

Barkham, M., Connell, J., Stiles, W., Miles, J., Margison, F., Evans, C., & Mellor-Clark, J. (2006). Dose-effect relations and responsive regulation of treatment duration: The good enough level. *Journal of Consulting and Clinical Psychology, 74*(1), 160–167. https://doi.org/10.1037/0022-006X.74.1.160

Barros, J., Morales, S., García, A., Echávarri, O., Fischman, R., Szmulewicz, M., … Tomicic, A. (2020). Recognizing states of psychological vulnerability to suicidal behavior: A Bayesian network of artificial intelligence applied to a clinical sample. *BMC Psychiatry, 20*, 1–40. https://doi.org/10.1186/s12888-020-02535-x

Bateman, A. W., & Fonagy, P. (2012). Handbook of mentalizing in mental health practice. American Psychiatric Publishing, Inc

Beck, A. T., Davis, D. D., & Freeman, A. (Eds.). (2015). *Cognitive therapy of personality disorders* (3rd ed.). New York, NY: Guilford Press.

Bedregal, P. (2017). *Professional competencies of psychologists and physicians working in the GES-depression Program of Primary Care and its relationship with clinical outcomes*. Lecture, General Clinical Meeting of the Department of Psychiatry of the Pontificia Universidad Católica de Chile.

Behn, A., Herpertz, S. C., & Krause, M. (2018). The interaction between depression and personality dysfunction: State of the art, current challenges, and future directions. Introduction to the Special Section. *Psykhe, 27*(2). https://doi.org/10.7764/psykhe.27.2.1501

Beryl, R., & Völlm, B. (2017). Attitudes to personality disorder of staff working in high-security and medium-security hospitals. *Personality and Mental Health, 12*(1), 25–37. https://doi.org/10.1002/pmh.1396

Blatt, S. J. (1995). The destructiveness of perfectionism: Implications for treatment of depression. *American Psychologist, 50*(12), 1003–1020. https://doi.org/10.1037//0003-066x.50.12.1003

Blatt, S. J. (2004). Experiences of depression: Theoretical, clinical, and research perspectives. American Psychological Association Washington, DC: American Psychological Association doi: https://doi.org/10.1037/10749-000.

Blatt, S. J., & Luyten, P. (2009). A structural-developmental psychodynamic approach to psychopathology: Two polarities of experiences across the life span. *Development and Psychopathology, 21*(3), 793–814. https://doi.org/10.1017/S0954579409000431

Blatt, S. J., Quinlan, D. M., Pilkonis, P. A., & Shea, T. (1995). Impact of perfectionism and need for approval on the brief treatment of depression: The national institute of mental health treatment of depression collaborative research program revisited. *Journal of Consulting and Clinical Psychology, 63*(1), 125–132. https://doi.org/10.1037//0022-006x.63.1.125

Bostwick, J. M., & Pankratz, V. S. (2000). Affective disorders and suicide risk: A reexamination. *American Journal of Psychiatry, 157*(12), 1925–1932. https://doi.org/10.1176/appi.ajp.157.12.1925

Burroughs, H., Lovell, K., Morley, M., Baldwin, R., Burns, A., & Chew-Graham, C. (2006). 'Justifiable depression': How primary care professionals and patients view late-life depression? A qualitative study. *Family Practice, 23*(3), 369–377. https://doi.org/10.1093/fampra/cmi115

Cambridge Dictionary. (s.f.). Complexity. In *Cambridge Dictionary*. https://dictionary.cambridge.org/dictionary/english/complexity?q=Complexity. Accessed 9 May 2020.

Cavanagh, J. T., Carson, A. J., Sharpe, M., & Lawrie, S. M. (2003). Psychological autopsy studies of suicide: A systematic review. *Psychological Medicine, 33*(3), 395–405. https://doi.org/10.1017/S0033291702006943

Centro de Estudios de Conflicto y Cohesión Social. (2018). *Resultados Primera Ola, Estudio Longitudinal Social de Chile (ELSOC), Módulo 6: Salud y bienestar*. Salud Mental en el Chile de hoy. https://coes.cl/wp-content/uploads/2018/01/N6.-ELSOC.-Salud-y-bienestar.pdf. Accessed 9 May 2020.

Chapman, A. L. (2006). Dialectical behavior therapy: Current indications and unique elements. *Psychiatry (Edgmont), 3*(9), 62–68.

Chapman, D. P., Whitfield, C. L., Felitti, V. J., Dube, S. R., Edwards, V. J., & Anda, R. F. (2004). Adverse childhood experiences and the risk of depressive disorders in adulthood. *Journal of Affective Disorders, 82*(2), 217–225. https://doi.org/10.1016/j.jad.2003.12.013

Chew-Graham, C. A., Mullin, S., May, C. R., Hedley, S., & Cole, H. (2002). Managing depression in primary care: Another example of the inverse care law? *Family Practice, 19*(6), 632–637.

Chui, H., Zilcha-Mano, S., Dinger, U., Barrett, M. S., & Barber, J. P. (2016). Dependency and self-criticism in treatments for depression. *Journal of Counseling Psychology, 63*(4), 452–459. https://doi.org/10.1037/cou0000142

Clark, L. A. (2007). Assessment and diagnosis of personality disorder: Perennial issues and an emerging reconceptualization. *Annual Review of Psychology, 58*, 227–257. https://doi.org/10.1146/annurev.psych.57.102904.190200

Clarkin, J. F., Petrini, M., & Diamond, D. (2019). Complex depression: The treatment of major depression and severe personality pathology. *Journal of Clinical Psychology, 75*(5), 824–833. https://doi.org/10.1002/jclp.22759
Comijs, H. C., van Exel, E., van der Mast, R. C., Paauw, A., Oude Voshaar, R., & Stek, M. L. (2013). Childhood abuse in late-life depression. *Journal of Affective Disorders, 147*(1–3), 241–246. https://doi.org/10.1016/j.jad.2012.11.010
CONADIC. (2010). *Habilidades para la vida: guía práctica y sencilla para el promotor nueva vida*. CONADIC, Secretaría de Salud. http://www.conadic.salud.gob.mx/pdfs/nueva_vida/nvhabilidades_guiapractica.pdf. Accessed 16 May 2020.
Cougle, J. R., Timpano, K. R., Sachs-Ericsson, N., Keough, M. E., & Riccardi, C. J. (2010). Examining the unique relationships between anxiety disorders and childhood physical and sexual abuse in the National Comorbidity Survey-replication. *Psychiatry Research, 177*(1–2), 150–155. https://doi.org/10.1016/j.psychres.2009.03.008
Cuijpers, P., Quero, S., Dowrick, C., & Arroll, B. (2019). Psychological treatment of depression in primary care: Recent developments. *Current Psychiatry Reports, 21*(129). https://doi.org/10.1007/s11920-019-1117-x
Cuijpers, P., Reijnders, M., & Huibers, M. J. H. (2019). The role of common factors in psychotherapy outcomes. *Annual Review of Clinical Psychology, 15*, 207–231. https://doi.org/10.1146/annurev-clinpsy-050718-095424
Dagnino, P., Pérez, C., Gómez, A., Gloger, S., & Krause, M. (2017). Depression and attachment: How do personality styles and social support influence this relation? *Research in Psychotherapy: Psychopathology, Process and Outcome, 20*, 53–62. https://doi.org/10.4081/ripppo.2017.237
Dagnino, P., Valdés, C., de la Fuente, I., de los Ángeles Harismendy, M., Gallardo, A. M., Gómez-Barris, E., & de la Parra, G. (2018). Impacto de la Personalidad y el Estilo Depresivo en los Resultados Psicoterapéuticos de Pacientes con Depresión. *Psykhe, 27*(2), 1–15. https://doi.org/10.7764/psykhe.27.2.1135. Copyright.
de la Parra, G. (2013). Psychotherapy research in developing countries: The case of Latin America. *Psychotherapy Research, 23*(6), 609–623. https://doi.org/10.1080/10503307.2013.830794
de la Parra, G., Dagnino, P., Valdés, C., & Krause, M. (2017). Beyond self-criticism and dependency: Structural functioning of depressive patients and its treatment. *Research in Psychotherapy: Psychopathology, Process and Outcome, 20*(1), 43–52. https://doi.org/10.4081/ripppo.2017.236
de la Parra, G., Errázuriz, P., Gómez-Barris, E., & Zúñiga, A. K. (2019). Propuesta para una psicoterapia efectiva en atención primaria: un modelo basado en la experiencia y la evidencia empírica. *Temas de la Agenda Pública, 14*(113), 1–20. Centro de Políticas Públicas UC.
de la Parra, G., Gómez-Barris, E., Zuñiga, A. K., Dagnino, P., & Valdés, C. (2018). From the "couch" to the outpatient clinic: A model of psychotherapy for institutions. Learning from (empirical) experience. *Revista Argentina de Clínica Psicológica, 27*(2), 182–202. https://doi.org/10.24205/03276716.2018.1057
Defey, D. (2013). Adecuación de la psicoterapia a la realidad de las instituciones de salud. *Jornada Psicoterapia en Instituciones de Salud. Conferencia llevada a cabo en Unidad de Psicoterapia Adultos, Departamento de Psiquiatría, Pontificia Universidad Católica, Santiago de Chile.*
Delgadillo, J., Huey, D., Bennett, H., & McMillan, D. (2017). Case complexity as a guide for psychological treatment selection. *Journal of Consulting and Clinical Psychology, 85*(9), 835–853. https://doi.org/10.1037/ccp0000231
Dimeff, L. A., & Koerner, K. (2007). *Dialectical behavior therapy in clinical practice*. New York, NY: Guilford Press.
Divac-Jovanovic, M., & Svrakic, D. (2017). Integrative treatment of personality disorder. Part I: Psychotherapy. *Psychiatria Danubina, 29*(1), 2–13. https://doi.org/10.24869/psyd.2017.2
Dowrick, C., Gask, L., Perry, R. E., Dixon, C., & Usherwood, T. (2000). Do general practitioners' attitudes towards depression predict their clinical behaviour? *Psychological Medicine, 30*(2), 413–419. https://doi.org/10.1017/s0033291799001531

Edgoose, J. Y. (2012). Rethinking the difficult patient encounter. *Family Practice Management, 19*(4), 17–20.

Fernandez, R., Kokoulina, E., Campos, X., Carballido, E., García, I., Rey, A., & Vázquez, P. (2018). Ecofenotipos en la depresión mayor: el papel del maltrato físico en la infancia. *Revista de la Asociación Española de Neuropsiquiatría, 38*(133), 75–97. https://doi.org/10.4321/S0211-57352018000100004

Fischer, C., Cottin, M., Behn, A., Errázuriz, P., & Díaz, R. (2019). What makes a difficult patient so difficult? Examining the therapist's experience beyond patient characteristics. *Journal of Clinical Psychology, 75*, 898–911. https://doi.org/10.1002/jclp.22765

Flückiger, C., Del Re, A. C., Wampold, B. E., & Horvath, A. O. (2018). The alliance in adult psychotherapy: A meta-analytic synthesis. *Psychotherapy: Theory, Research, Practice, Training, 55*(4), 316–340. https://doi.org/10.1037/pst0000172

Fowler, J. C. (2012). Suicide risk assessment in clinical practice: Pragmatic guidelines for imperfect assessments. *Psychotherapy, 49*(1), 81–90. https://doi.org/10.1037/a0026148

Gilbert, R., Widom, C. S., Browne, K., Fergusson, D., Webb, E., & Janson, S. (2009). Burden and consequences of child maltreatment in high-income countries. *Lancet, 373*(9657), 68–81. https://doi.org/10.1016/S0140-6736(08)61706-7

Griner, D., & Smith, T. B. (2006). Culturally adapted mental health intervention: A meta-analytic review. *Psychotherapy: Theory, Research, Practice, Training, 43*(4), 531–548. https://doi.org/10.1037/0033-3204.43.4.531

Gunderson, J., Herpertz, S., Skodol, A., Torgersen, S., & Zanarini, M. (2018). Borderline personality disorder. *National Library of Medicine, 4*, 18029. https://doi.org/10.1038/nrdp.2018.29

Gunderson, J. G., & Links, P. (2014). *Handbook of good psychiatric management for borderline personality disorder*. Arlington, TX: American Psychiatric Publishing.

Gunderson, J. G., & Phillips, K. A. (1991). A current view of the interface between borderline personality disorder and depression. *The American Journal Psychiatry, 148*(8), 967–975. https://doi.org/10.1176/ajp.148.8.967

Gunderson, J. G., Stout, R. L., Shea, M. T., Grilo, C. M., Markowitz, J. C., Morey, L. C., … Skodol, A. E. (2014). Interactions of borderline personality disorder and mood disorders over 10 years. *Journal of Clinical Psychiatry, 75*(8), 829–834. https://doi.org/10.4088/JCP.13m08972

Haas, L. J., Leiser, J. P., Magill, M. K., & Sanyer, O. N. (2005). Management of the difficult patient. *American Family Physician, 72*(10), 2063–2068.

Haddad, M., Menchetti, M., Walters, P., Norton, J., Tylee, A., & Mann, A. (2011). Clinicians' attitudes to depression in Europe: A pooled analysis of depression attitude questionnaire findings. *Family Practice, 29*(2), 121–130. https://doi.org/10.1093/fampra/cmr070

Hardy, G., Stiles, W., Barkham, M., & Startup, M. (1998). Therapist responsiveness to client interpersonal styles during time-limited treatments for depression. *Journal of Consulting and Clinical Psychology, 66*(2), 304–312. https://doi.org/10.1037//0022-006x.66.2.304

Hassler, G. (2010). Fisiopatología de la Depresión: ¿Tenemos alguna evidencia sólida de interés para los clínicos? *World Psychiatry, 9*, 155–161.

Hidaka, B. H. (2012). Depression as a disease of modernity: Explanations for increasing prevalence. *Journal of Affective Disorders, 140*(3), 205–214. https://doi.org/10.1016/j.jad.2011.12.036

Hinchey, S. A., & Jackson, J. L. (2011). A cohort study assessing difficult patient encounters in a walk-in primary care clinic, predictors and outcomes. *Journal of General Internal Medicine, 26*(6), 588–594.

Jacobson, G. (1979). Crisis-oriented therapy. *Psychiatric Clinics of North America, 2*(1), 39–54. https://doi.org/10.1016/S0193-953X(18)31023-2

Jiménez, J. P. (2020). *Chile en el diván: de la depresión al estallido social*. https://psiconecta-web.s3.amazonaws.com/chile_en_el_diván.pdf. Accessed 9 May 2020.

Johnston, O., Kumar, S., Kendall, K., Peveler, R., Gabbay, J., & Kendrick, T. (2007). Qualitative study of depression management in primary care: GP and patient goals, and the value of listening. *British Journal of General Practice, 57*(544), 872–879. https://doi.org/10.3399/096016407782318026

Kannan, D., & Levitt, H. M. (2013). A review of client self-criticism in psychotherapy. *Journal of Psychotherapy Integration, 23*(2), 166–178.

Kaslow, N., Dunn, S., & Smith, C. (2008). Competencies for psychologists in academic health centers (AHCs). *Journal of Clinical Psychology in Medical Settings, 15*(1), 18–27. https://doi.org/10.1007/s10880-008-9094-y

Kato, A., & Kanba, S. (2017). Modern-type depression as an "adjustment" disorder in Japan: The intersection of collectivistic society encountering an individualistic performance-based system. *American Journal of Psychiatry, 174*(11), 1051–1053. https://doi.org/10.1176/appi.ajp.2017.17010059

Kellogg, S. H., & Young, J. E. (2006). Schema therapy for borderline personality disorder. *Journal of Clinical Psychology, 62*(4), 445–458. https://doi.org/10.1002/jclp.20240

Kilzieh, N., Rastam, S., Maziak, W., & Ward, K. D. (2008). Comorbidity of depression with chronic diseases: A population-based study in Aleppo, Syria. *The International Journal of Psychiatry in Medicine, 38*(2), 169–184. https://doi.org/10.2190/PM.38.2.d

Klein, D. N., Schwartz, J. E., Santiago, N. J., Vivian, D., Vocisano, C., Castonguay, L. G., ... Keller, M. B. (2003). Therapeutic alliance in depression treatment: Controlling for prior change and patient characteristics. *Journal of Consulting and Clinical Psychology, 71*(6), 997–1006. https://doi.org/10.1037/0022-006X.71.6.997

Koekkoek, B., van Meijel, B., & Hutschemaekers, G. (2006). "Difficult patients" in mental health care: A review. *Psychiatric Services, 57*(6), 795–802. https://doi.org/10.1176/ps.2006.57.6.795

Köhling, J., Moessner, M., Ehrenthal, J. C., Bauer, S., Cierpka, M., Kämmerer, A., ... Dinger, U. (2015). Affective instability and reactivity in depressed patients with and without borderline pathology. *Journal of Personality Disorders, 5*(2), 1–20. https://doi.org/10.1521/pedi_2015_29_230

Kramer, U., & Stiles, W. B. (2015). The responsiveness problem in psychotherapy: A review of proposed solutions. *Clinical Psychology: Science and Practice, 22*(3), 277–295. https://doi.org/10.1111/cpsp.12107

Krause, M. (2005). *Psicoterapia y Cambio. Una Mirada desde la subjetividad [Psychotherapy and change. A look from the subjectivized]*. Santiago, Chile: Ediciones Universidad Católica de Chile.

Krause, M., Güell, P., Jaramillo, A., Zilveti, M., Jiménez, J. P., & Luyten, P. (2015). Changing communities and increases in the prevalence of depression: Is there a relationship? *Universitas Psychologica, 14*(4), 1259–1268. https://doi.org/10.11144/javeriana.upsy14-4.ccip

Krebs, E. E., Garrett, J. M., & Konrad, T. R. (2006). The difficult doctor? Characteristics of physicians who report frustration with patients: An analysis of survey data. *BMC Health Services Research, 6*(1), 128. https://doi.org/10.1186/1472-6963-6-128

Lambert, M. J. (2013). The efficacy and effectiveness of psychotherapy. In M. J. Lambert (Ed.), *Bergin and Garfield's handbook of psychotherapy and behavior change* (6th ed., pp. 139–193). New York, NY: Wiley.

Laska, K. M., Gurman, A. S., & Wampold, B. E. (2014). Expanding the lens of evidence-based practice in psychotherapy: A common factors perspective. *Psychotherapy, 51*(4), 467. https://doi.org/10.1037/a0034332

Leichsenring, F., Leibning, E., Kruse, J., New, A. S., & Leweke, F. (2011). Borderline personality disorder. *The Lancet, 377*(9759), 74–84. https://doi.org/10.1016/S0140-6736(10)61422-5

Leichsenring, F., & Schauenburg, H. (2014). Empirically supported methods of short-term psychodynamic therapy in depression – Towards an evidence-based unified protocol. *Journal of Affective Disorders, 169*, 128–143. https://doi.org/10.1016/j.jad.2014.08.007

Levy, L. B., & O'Hara, M. W. (2010). Psychotherapeutic interventions for depressed, low-income women: A review of the literature. *Clinical Psychology Review, 30*(8), 934–950. https://doi.org/10.1016/j.cpr.2010.06.006

Li, M., D'arcy, C., & Meng, X. (2016). Maltreatment in childhood substantially increases the risk of adult depression and anxiety in prospective cohort studies: Systematic review, meta-

analysis, and proportional attributable fractions. *Psychological Medicine, 46*(4), 717–730. https://doi.org/10.1017/S0033291715002743
Linehan, M. (1993). *Skills training manual for treating borderline personality disorder*. New York, NY: Guilford Press.
Linehan, M. M., Comtois, K. A., Murray, A. M., Brown, M. Z., Gallop, R. J., Heard, H. L., … Lindenboim, N. (2006). Two-year randomized controlled trial and follow-up of dialectical behavior therapy vs therapy by experts for suicidal behaviors and borderline personality disorder. *Archives of General Psychiatry, 63*(7), 757–766. https://doi.org/10.1001/archpsyc.63.7.757
Luyten, P., & Blatt, S. J. (2007). Looking back towards the future: Is it time to change the DSM approach to psychiatric disorders? The case of depression. *Psychiatry, 70*(2), 85–99. https://doi.org/10.1521/psyc.2007.70.2.85
Luyten, P., & Blatt, S. J. (2011). Psychodynamic approaches of depression: Whither shall we go? *Psychiatry, 74*, 1–3. https://doi.org/10.1521/psyc.2011.74.1.1
Luyten, P., Fonagy, P., Lemma, A., & Target, M. (2012). Depression. In A. Bateman & P. Fonagy (Eds.), *Handbook of mentalizing in mental health practice* (pp. 385–417). Washington, DC: American Psychiatric Publishing.
Mandel, T., Dunkley, D. M., & Moroz, M. (2015). Self-critical perfection- ism and depressive and anxious symptoms over 4 years: The mediating role of daily stress reactivity. *Journal of Counseling Psychology, 62*, 703–717. https://doi.org/10.1037/cou0000101
Marshall, M. B., Zuroff, D. C., McBride, C., & Bagby, R. M. (2008). Self-criticism predicts differential response to treatment for major depression. *Journal of Clinical Psychology, 64*, 231–244. https://doi.org/10.1002/jclp.20438
Martínez, P., Rojas, G., Fritsch, R., Martínez, V., Vöhringer, P., & Castro, A. (2017). Comorbidity in people with depression seeking help at primary health care centers in Santiago, Chile. *Revista Médica de Chile, 145*, 25–32. https://doi.org/10.4067/S0034-98872017000100004
Martín-Merino, E., Ruigómez, A., Johansson, S., Wallander, M., & García-Rodriguez, L. (2010). Study of a cohort of patients newly diagnosed with depression in general practice: Prevalence, incidence, comorbidity, and treatment patterns. *The Primary Care Companion to the Journal of Clinical Psychiatry, 12*(1), e1–e8. https://doi.org/10.4088/pcc.08m00764blu
Martins-Monteverde, C., Von Werne Baes, C., Reisdorfer, E., Padovan, T., De Carvalho, S., & Juruena, M. (2019). Relationship between depression and subtypes of early life stress in adult psychiatric patients. *Frontiers in Psychiatry, 10*(19). https://doi.org/10.3389/fpsyt.2019.00019
McDaniel, S. H., Grus, C. L., Cubic, B. A., Hunter, C. L., Kearney, L. K., Schuman, C. C., … Johnson, S. B. (2014). Competencies for psychology practice in primary care. *American Psychologist, 69*(4), 409–429. https://doi.org/10.1037/a0036072
Mellado, A., Pérez, C., Suarez, N., Dagnino, P., Gloger, S., & Krause, M. (2018). Self-criticism in patients with depression and its impact on dropout in short-term psychotherapies: Exploring the mediator role of the therapeutic alliance and the moderator role of patients' age. *Psykhe, 27*(2), 1–18. https://doi.org/10.7764/psykhe.27.2.1137
Messer, S. B., & Warren, S. C. (1995). *Models of brief psychotherapy*. New York, NY: Guilford Press.
Ministerio de Salud de Chile. (2017). *Guía Clínica: Para el tratamiento de la Depresión en personas mayores de 15 años: Actualización en Psicoterapia*. https://diprece.minsal.cl/wrdprss_minsal/wp-content/uploads/2017/07/GPC_depresion_psicoterapia.pdf. Accessed 9 May 2020.
Morales, S., Echávarri, O., Barros, J., Zuloaga, F., & Taylor, T. (2016). Percepción del propio riesgo suicida: estudio cualitativo con pacientes hospitalizados por intento o ideación suicida. *Revista Argentina de Clínica Psicológica, 25*(3), 245–258.
Moukaddam, N., Flores, A., Matorin, A., Hayden, N., & Tucci, V. T. (2017). Difficult patients in the emergency department: Personality disorders and beyond. *The Psychiatric Clinics of North America, 40*(3), 379–395. https://doi.org/10.1016/j.psc.2017.05.005
Moyano, E., & Barría, R. (2006). Suicidio y Producto Interno Bruto (PIB) en Chile. *Revista Latinoamericana de Psicología, 38*(2), 343–359.

Mulder, R., Murray, G., & Rucklidge, J. (2017). Common versus specific factors in psychotherapy: Opening the black box. *Lancet Psychiatry, 4*(12), 953–962. https://doi.org/10.1016/S2215-0366(17)30100-1

Neumeyer-Gromen, A., Lampert, T., Stark, K., & Kallischnigg, G. (2004). Disease management programs for depression: A systematic review and meta-analysis randomized controlled trials. *Medical Care, 42*(12), 1211–1221. https://doi.org/10.1097/00005650-200412000-00008

Nieuwsma, J. A., Trivedi, R. B., McDuffie, J., Kronish, I., Benjamin, D., & Williams, J. W. (2012). Brief psychotherapy for depression: A systematic review and meta-analysis. *International Journal of Psychiatry in Medicine, 43*(2), 129–151. https://doi.org/10.2190/PM.43.2.c

Olfson, M., Shea, S., Feder, A., Fuentes, M., Nomura, Y., Gameroff, M., & Weissman, M. M. (2000). Prevalence of anxiety, depression, and substance use disorders in an urban general medicine practice. *Archives Family Medicine, 9*(9), 876–883. https://doi.org/10.1001/archfami.9.9.876

OPD Task Force (Ed.). (2008). *Operationalized psychodynamic diagnosis OPD-2: Manual of diagnosis and treatment planning*. Cambridge, MA: Hogrefe Publishing.

Orchard y Jimenez. (2016). ¿Malestar de qué? A propósito de ciertos malentendidos entre malestar y sufrimiento psíquico en Chile. In E. Radiszcz (Ed.), *Malestar y destinos del malestar, Políticas de la desdicha Volumen 1* (pp. 71–95). Santiago, Chile: Social-Ediciones.

Pajer, K., Gardner, W., Lourie, A., Chang, C., Wang, W., & Currie, L. (2014). Physical child abuse potential in adolescent girls: Associations with psychopathology, maltreatment, and attitudes toward child-bearing. *The Canadian Journal of Psychiatry, 59*(2), 98–106. https://doi.org/10.1177/070674371405900205

Paris, J. (2010). Personality disorders and mood disorders: Phenomenological resemblances vs. pathogenetic pathways. *Journal of Personality Disorders, 24*(1), 3–13. https://doi.org/10.1521/pedi.2010.24.1.3

Patel, V., Burns, J. K., Dhingra, M., Tarver, L., Kohrt, B. A., & Lund, C. (2018). Income inequality and depression: A systematic review and meta-analysis of the association and a scoping review of mechanisms. *World Psychiatry, 17*(1), 76–89. https://doi.org/10.1002/wps.20492

Patel, V., Chowdhary, N., Rahman, A., & Verdeli, H. (2011). Improving access to psychological treatments: Lessons from developing countries. *Behaviour Research and Therapy, 49*(9), 523–528. https://doi.org/10.1016/j.brat.2011.06.012

Programa de las Naciones Unidas para el Desarrollo. (1998). *Desarrollo Humano en Chile. Las paradojas de la modernización*. Santiago, Chile: PNUD.

Programa de las Naciones Unidas para el Desarrollo. (2017). *Desiguales. Orígenes, cambios y desafíos de la brecha social en Chile*. Santiago, Chile: PNUD.

Rojas, G., Santelices, M. P., Martínez, P., Tomicic, A., Reinel, M., Olhaberry, M., & Krause, M. (2015). Barriers restricting postpartum depression treatment in Chile. *Revista Médica de Chile, 143*(4), 424–432. https://doi.org/10.4067/S0034-98872015000400002

Rubenstein, L. V., Jackson-Triche, M., Unützer, J., Miranda, J., Minnium, K., Pearson, M. L., & Wells, K. B. (1999). Evidence-based care for depression in managed primary care practices: A collaborative approach shows promise in improving care of depression in a variety of sites. *Health Affairs, 18*(5), 89–105.

Rudolf, G. (2013). *Strukturbezogene Psychotherapie* (3ª ed.). Stuttgart, Germany: Schattauer.

Ruscio, A. M., & Holohan, D. R. (2006). Applying empirically supported treatments to complex cases: Ethical, empirical, and practical considerations. *Clinical Psychology: Science and Practice, 13*(2), 146–162. https://doi.org/10.1111/j.1468-2850.2006.00017.x

Safford, M. M., Allison, J. J., & Kiefe, C. I. (2007). Patient complexity: More than comorbidity. The vector model of complexity. *Journal of General Internal Medicine, 22*(3), 381–390. https://doi.org/10.1007/s11606-007-0307-0

Safran, J. D., & Muran, J. C. (2000). *Negotiating the therapeutic alliance: A relational treatment guide*. New York: Guilford Press.

Scharager, J., & Molina, M. L. (2007). El trabajo de los psicólogos en los centros de atención primaria del sistema público de salud en Chile. *Revista Panamericana de Salud Pública, 22*(3), 149–159.

Schneider, B. (2009). Substance use disorders and risk for completed suicide. *Archives of Suicide Research, 13*(4), 303–316. https://doi.org/10.1080/13811110903263191

Shah, S., & Harris, M. (1997). A survey of general practitioners' confidence in their management of elderly patients. *Australian Family Physician, 26*(suppl 1), S12–S17.
Shanks, C., Pfohl, B., Blum, N., & Black, D. W. (2011). Can negative attitudes toward patients with borderline personality disorder be changed? The effect of attending a STEPPS workshop. *Journal of Personality Disorders, 25*(6), 806–812.
Shippeea, N., Shaha, N., Mayc, C., Maird, F., & Montori, V. (2012). Cumulative complexity: A functional, patient-centered model of patient complexity can improve research and practice. *Journal of Clinical Epidemiology, 65*(10), 1041–1051. https://doi.org/10.1016/j.jclinepi.2012.05.005
Silk, K. R. (2010). The quality of depression in borderline personality disorder and the diagnostic process. *Journal of Personality Disorders, 24*(1), 25–37. https://doi.org/10.1521/pedi.2010.24.1.25
Simon, G., Imel, Z., Ludman, E., & Steinfeld, B. (2012). Is dropout after a first psychotherapy visit always a bad outcome? *Psychiatric Services, 63*(7), 705–707. https://doi.org/10.1176/appi.ps.201100309
Sinnige, J., Braspenning, J., Schellevis, F., Stirbu-Wagner, I., Westert, G., & Korevaar, J. (2013). The prevalence of disease clusters in older adults with multiple chronic diseases – A systematic literature review. *PLoS One, 8*(11), e79641. https://doi.org/10.1371/journal.pone.0079641
Sotsky, S. M., Glass, D. R., Shea, M. T., Pilkonis, P. A., Collins, J. F., Elkin, I., … Moyer, J. (1991). Patient predictors of response to psychotherapy and pharmacotherapy: Findings in the NIMH treatment of depression collaborative research program. *American Journal of Psychiatry, 148*(8), 997–1008. https://doi.org/10.1176/ajp.148.8.997
Stiles, W., Barkham, M., & Wheeler, S. (2015). Duration of psychological therapy: Relation to recovery and improvement rates in uK routine practice. *The British Journal of Psychiatry, 207*(2), 115–122. https://doi.org/10.1192/bjp.bp.114.145565
Stiles, W. B., Honos-Webb, L., & Surko, M. (1998). Responsiveness in psychotherapy. *Clinical Psychology: Science and Practice, 5*(4), 439–458. https://doi.org/10.1111/j.1468-2850.2009.01148.x
Stiles, W. B., & Horvath, A. O. (2017). Appropriate responsiveness as a contribution to therapist effects. In L. G. Castonguay & C. E. Hill (Eds.), *How and why are some therapists better than others?: Understanding therapist effects* (pp. 71–84). Washington, DC: American Psychological Association. https://doi.org/10.1037/0000034-005
Swift, J. K., & Greenberg, R. P. (2012). Premature discontinuation in adult psychotherapy: A meta-analysis. *Journal of Consulting and Clinical Psychology, 80*(4), 547–559. https://doi.org/10.1037/a0028226
Thomä, H., & Kächele, H. (1987). *Psychoanalytic practice: Vol. 1. Principles*. New York, NY: Springer.
Trull, T. J., & Durrett, C. A. (2005). Categorical and dimensional models of personality disorder. *Annual Review of Clinical Psychology, 1*, 355–380. https://doi.org/10.1146/annurev.clinpsy.1.102803.144009
Vitriol, V., Cancino, A., Ballesteros, S., Núñez, C., & Navarrete, A. (2017). Depresión y trauma temprano: hacia una caracterización clínica de perfiles de consulta en un servicio de salud secundario. *Revista Chilena de Neuro-Psiquiatría, 55*(2), 123–134. https://doi.org/10.4067/S0717-92272017000200007
Vitriol, V., Cancino, A., Weil, K., Salgado, C., Asenjo, M. A., & Potthoff, S. (2014). Depression and psychological trauma: An overview integrating current research and specific evidence of studies in the treatment of depression in public mental health services in Chile. *Depression Research and Treatment, 2014*(6), 1–10. https://doi.org/10.1155/2014/608671
Wampold, B. E. (2015). How important are the common factors in psychotherapy? An update. *World Psychiatry, 14*(3), 270–277. https://doi.org/10.1002/wps.20238
Wampold, B. E., Imel, Z. E., Laska, K. M., Benish, S., Miller, S. D., Flückiger, C., … Budge, S. (2010). Determining what works in the treatment of PTSD. *Clinical Psychology Review, 30*(8), 923–933. https://doi.org/10.1016/j.cpr.2010.06.005

Wampold, B. E., Mondin, G. W., Moody, M., Stich, F., Benson, K., & Ahn, H. (1997). A meta-analysis of outcome studies comparing bona fide psychotherapies: Empirically, “All must have prizes”. *Psychological Bulletin, 122*(3), 203–215. https://doi.org/10.1037//0033-2909.122.3.203

Webb, C. A., DeRubeis, R. J., & Barber, J. P. (2010). Therapist adherence/competence and treatment outcome: A meta-analytic review. *Journal of Consulting and Clinical Psychology, 78*(2), 200–211. https://doi.org/10.1037/a0018912

White, C. (2011). Childhood maltreatment is linked to recurrent depression. *British Medical Journal, 343*, d5246. https://doi.org/10.1136/bmj.d5246

Widiger, T. A., & Samuel, D. B. (2005). Diagnostic categories or dimensions: A question for DSM–V. *Journal of Abnormal Psychology, 114*(4), 494–504. https://doi.org/10.1037/0021-843X.114.4.494

Wierzbicki, M., & Pekarik, G. (1993). A meta-analysis of psychotherapy dropout. *Professional Psychology: Research and Practice, 24*(2), 190–195. https://doi.org/10.1037/0735-7028.24.2.190

World Health Organization. (2007). *World Health Statics*. https://www.who.int/whosis/whostat2007.pdf?ua=1. Accessed 15 May 2020.

World Health Organization. (2017). *Depression and other common mental disorders global health estimates*. Geneva. https://apps.who.int/iris/bitstream/handle/10665/254610/WHO-MSD-MER-2017.2-eng.pdf;jsessionid=638457BC203C0E542D98939AC11BC16F?sequence=1. Accessed 9 May 2020.

World Health Organization. (2018). *ICD-11 for mortality and morbidity statistics (ICD-11 MMS)*. https://icd.who.int. Accessed 9 May 2020.

Yeager, K., & Roberts, A. (2015). *Crisis intervention handbook: Assessment, treatment, and research*. New York, NY: Oxford University Press.

Zimmermann, J., Kerber, A., Rek, K., Hopwood, C. J., & Krueger, R. F. (2019). A brief but comprehensive review of research on the alternative DSM-5 model for personality disorders. *Current Psychiatry Reports, 21*(92). https://doi.org/10.1007/s11920-019-1079-z

Zúñiga, A. K. (2019, July 4–21). *Which Psychotherapeutic Competencies Are Needed to Treat Complex Depression in Institutional Setting? Building Bridges between “Real Practice” and “Empirical Evidence”*. [Conference Presentation] Phd Summer School 2019 Personality functioning in depression and personality disorders, millennium institute for research in depression and personality (MIDAP) and University of Basil, Suiza. Basel, Suiza.

Zúñiga, A. K., Balboa, M., & de la Parra, G. (2018, June 27–30). *Brief paper: Which psychotherapists competences are important in the Management of Complex Depression in an institutional setting?* Integrating patients expectations and psychologists experience [Conference presentation] SPR 49° annual meeting of Society for Psychotherapy Research. Amsterdam, Netherlands.

Zúñiga, A. K., Núñez, L., Araya, P., de la Parra, G., & Taubner S. (2019, June 6–8). *Developing a transtheoretical model of psychotherapeutic competencies to care depressive patients in primary care (PC)*. [Poster Presentation] SEPI Society for the Exploration of Psychotherapy Integration 2019, 35th Annual Conference Lisbon, Portugal.

Chapter 10
Modular Treatment for Complex Depression According to Metacognitive Interpersonal Therapy

Antonella Centonze, Paolo Ottavi, Angus MacBeth, Raffaele Popolo, and Giancarlo Dimaggio

Abstract Depression in personality disorders come from multiple sources, ranging from poor metacognition to maladaptive interpersonal schemas and dysfunctional coping strategies, such as avoidance or perfectionism. A modular treatment is needed in order to tackle with the different path leading to low mood in this population. Metacognition Interpersonal Therapy (MIT) adopts such a modular strategy. Five modules are adopted: Module 1 aims at forming a shared understanding of intrapersonal and interpersonal functioning that leads to depression. Module 2 aims at reducing interpersonal repetitive thinking (rumination and worry). Module 3 tackles with behavioural coping, such as avoidance or perfectionism. Therapists and patients negotiate behavioural tasks, such as behavioural activation or trying to counteract perfectionistic strategies. Module 4 aims at helping clients to realize their maladaptive schemas about self, and others are mostly ideas and do not necessarily correspond to the truth. Here, therapists try to help them contact alternative and more benevolent views of human relationships they already might have had but did not notice. Module 5 aims at giving room to healthy, positive, and benevolent views of the self and giving them more room in the stream of consciousness and let the person's actions be guided by them. During all modules, therapists use a wide array of experiential techniques ranging from guided imagery and rescripting, bodily work, role-play, two chairs and attention training. In order to illustrate how this modular treatment works, we describe the case of a 62-year-old woman with major depression comorbid with paranoid PD with passive-aggressive and avoidant personality traits.

A. Centonze (✉) · P. Ottavi · R. Popolo · G. Dimaggio
Center for Metacognitive Interpersonal Therapy, Rome, Italy

A. MacBeth
Department of Clinical and Health Psychology, School of Health in Social Science, University of Edinburgh, Edinburgh, Scotland

G. de la Parra et al. (eds.), *Depression and Personality Dysfunction*, Depression and Personality, https://doi.org/10.1007/978-3-030-70699-9_10

Keywords Complex depression · Personality disorders · Maladaptive interpersonal schemas · Metacognition · Guided imagery and rescripting · Worry and rumination

10.1 Understanding Complex Depression

Personality disorders (PDs) frequently constitute maintaining factors in depression. The relationship between PD and depression is strengthened by evidence that individuals with depression, where the comorbid PD is left unaddressed by psychological treatments, have greater odds of responding poorly to treatment than individuals without PD (Newton-Howes, Tyrer, & Johnson, 2006). Depressive symptoms in persons with comorbid PD are more persistent than in individuals with no such comorbidity, supporting the idea that the first group's depression was mostly personality-related (Bateman & Fonagy, 2015; Morey et al., 2010). As a consequence, when persons have both depression and PD, both need to be treated in order to achieve optimal likelihood of depression remission.

Historically, it was presumed that during a depressive episode, it is difficult to distinguish state-dependent features from stable personality traits (Zimmerman, 1994). More recently, it has been suggested that a PD diagnosis made during a depressive episode actually reflects underlying presence of PD, independent of current mood (Morey et al., 2010). Therefore, any improvement in personality functioning observed in the course of treatment for depression can also be taken as evidence of change at personality level and not merely the effect of mood improvement. In short, as the presence of PD complicates treatment of depression (Reich, 2003), clinicians need to consider and target the underlying PD within treatment.

Looking at the interaction between PD and depression from the angle of PD treatments, therapies are effective in reducing depression in clients primarily treated for their PD. Among patients with borderline PD (BPD), 71% treated with a combination of dialectical behaviour therapy (DBT) and medication reported remission of depression, unlike 47% of patients treated with medication only (Lynch et al., 2007). Similar results have been obtained with mentalization-based therapy for BPD (Bateman & Fonagy, 2015; Jørgensen et al., 2013; Rossouw & Fonagy, 2012), with schema therapy for a wide range of PDs (Bamelis, Evers, Spinhoven, & Arntz, 2014; Carter et al., 2013; Körük & Özabacı, 2018), and with metacognitive interpersonal therapy (MIT) for overcontrolled PD (Gordon-King, Schweitzer, & Dimaggio, 2018). Relatedly, interventions addressing interpersonal problems, itself a hallmark of PD, such as interpersonal therapy (IPT; Klerman, Weissman, Rounsaville, & Chevron, 1984; Weissman, Markowitz, & Klerman, 2000) can also be effective in addressing depression.

10.2 Treating Comorbid Depression and PD

Depression includes painful emotions, ranging from sadness to guilt and shame, and ideas of failure or loss and tendencies to self-blame. In PD, these aspects of subjective experience are triggered and sustained by (a) maladaptive interpersonal schemas, (b) impaired metacognition, and (c) dysfunctional coping. Finally, the combination of schemas, poor capacity to understand mental states underlying social interactions, and tendency to enact dysfunctional copings pave the way for problematic interpersonal cycles, which further deteriorates interpersonal relationships, so making depression more likely to take place.

As a reaction to predictions that core wishes, such as attachment, social rank, autonomy and exploration, etc., will be chronically frustrated, patients with PD enact dysfunctional coping strategies, using both cognitive (e.g. repetitive thinking) and behavioural (e.g. avoidance, overcompliance) approaches which in turn sustain depression.

Targeting depression comorbid with PD requires the adjustment of treatment to pivot towards the latter's psychopathological mechanisms. We now briefly describe the core features of PD as considered by MIT (Dimaggio, Montano, Popolo, & Salvatore, 2015; Dimaggio, Ottavi, Popolo, & Salvatore, 2020) – the psychotherapy approach we adopt here – and in particular how they sustain depression in this population. We then explain how these problems can lead to depression onset and maintenance. Each element of psychopathology is the target of a specific intervention module, consisting with the idea that psychotherapy for complex disorders needs to be modular (Livesley, Dimaggio, & Clarkin, 2016). Our final step is to describe the treatment procedures that MIT adopts so as to be a modular and structured approach for depression comorbid with PD. MIT has been tailored in order to treat PD and their co-occurrent symptoms.

Maladaptive interpersonal schemas. Depression in PD is most often the outcome of problematic expectations about interpersonal relationships, whereby patients predict that others will frustrate their core wishes. Schemas (Dimaggio, Montano et al., 2015; Dimaggio, Ottavi et al., 2020; Luborsky & Crits-Christoph, 1998) serve to make meaning out of interpersonal exchanges and to predict if others will fulfil the individuals' core wishes, for example, whether then other will provide the desired outcome of approval or instead will harshly criticize the individual. Schemas emerge as a function of one's developmental history and act as heuristic mechanisms to decode communicative signals, particularly those that function as road maps towards social action (Dimaggio, Montano et al., 2015; Dimaggio, Ottavi et al., 2020). Interpersonal schemas are built around a series of core evolutionary-selected motives (Gilbert, 1989; Lichtenberg, 1989; Liotti & Gilbert, 2011; Panksepp, 1998):

(a) Attachment – the need to be protected and cared for and to feel safe and nurtured (Bowlby, 1969)
(b) Social rank – defining order of access to limited resources within a group
(c) Autonomy-independence and exploration – the drive to act according to one's own preferences and interests (Panksepp & Biven, 2012) and to explore one's

environment, both physical and intellectual, in order to find resources and new solutions to problems

(d) Caregiving – providing care to those in suffering or distress
(e) Group inclusion – the need to belong (Baumeister & Leary, 1995; Lichtenberg, 1989)
(f) Sexuality – mating in the service of forming long-term sensual, reciprocally committed relationships
(g) Cooperation – reaching shared goals once having defined each individual's role and tasks (Tomasello, Carpenter, Call, Behne, & Moll, 2005)

Core elements of schemas are:

(a) Nuclear self-images underlying every specific wish/motive. For example, when social rank is active, the person may hold a dominant idea of self as *unworthy*, which parallels the idea of self as *worthy*, the latter being over-modulated and with no easy conscious access.
(b) The response of the other, which is also multifaceted. The dominant representation in PD is negative, for example, *harshly critical* in the domain of social rank. Again, an alternative, benevolent, representation is present, e.g. being *accepting and valuing* in the social rank area. Even if these benevolent representations are present, the person is less likely to note them, to interpret communicative behaviours as manifestations of their existence, and to consider them true.
(c) The self-response to the others' response. These include cognitions, affects, and somatic reactions and usually include a confirmation of the core self-idea.

As an example, a patient driven by social rank hopes to be appreciated but expects that the other will criticize her or ignore her if she shows her "true" qualities in certain situations. In her mind, distressing representational memories may appear, in which she recalls her father harshly criticizing her, making her feel incapable in the current moment. These memories trigger distress, which is sustained in one's mind by a core idea of self as unworthy and unable to react. Under the influence of these ideas about self and others, the individual enters into a state of mind of sadness, loneliness, shame, and low self-worth – constituting a depressive mood. In parallel, she feels deprived of energy, agency declines, and anhedonia emerges as a function of the difficulty in engaging with herself in pleasant or creative activities. The individual predicts that it is unlikely that the other will appreciate her, and so she withdraws, thus remaining emotionally and socially alone.

In summary, schemas include negative expectations about how others will respond to one's core wishes. This coupling of core negative images of both self, e.g. *unworthy*, and others (SINGULAR), *critical and spiteful*, is in itself a path to depression.

Another problem that sustains depression in PD is poor metacognition (Dimaggio & Lysaker, 2015; Semerari, Carcione, Dimaggio, Falcone et al., 2003; Semerari, Colle et al., 2014). Metacognition includes skills with which people (a) recognize mental states and ascribe them to themselves or others; (b) think, reflect, and reason about their own mental states (self-reflectivity) and others' (understanding other's mind); and (c) use this knowledge, reflecting to take decisions, solve psychological and interpersonal problems, and master subjective suffering (mastery, Carcione et al., 2011).

Self-reflective monitoring is the capacity to distinguish and name a series of thoughts and affects and describe with nuances, for example, being able to say: "I'm sad because I feel abandoned" vs. "I'm tense".

Self-reflectivity includes *differentiation*, that is, the capacity to consider one's ideas as hypotheses and not objective descriptions of the external reality, in particular in the relational domain. It includes understanding that our assessments of others' behaviour sometimes depend not on what one really thinks and feels but on our learned tendencies to make sense of relationships. Pragmatically speaking, differentiating means moving from a maladaptive, deterministic prediction to a more nuanced understanding of mental states. For example, adapting from "I think she will belittle me and that is certain" to "I think she will belittle me but I am not sure how likely this is. I realize that in the past I have learned that if I do something my own way, I will likely be criticized and belittled". It is a differentiation of the type "my belief is true" vs. "my belief is learned". In relation to our previous example, the student worries: "My exam will go really bad. There's no hope for me". During the exam she interprets every expression on the professor's face as a criticism. In this case, the patient does not understand that the way to interpret the other and the reality depends on what she has learned in her developmental history, that is, on her father's criticism and not due to an actual, inescapable impending criticism and public humiliation.

Another type of differentiation is the possibility of accessing healthy aspects of schemas (Dimaggio et al., 2015). The patient passes from "it's always true" to "in some cases I see myself and others in a more benevolent way". In a state of no differentiation, a student keeps on repeating to herself: "I'm a disaster. I've always been a failure". Consequently, this sustains depressed mood. Instead, if the same student can retrieve memories of other occasions in which she was successful (e.g. exams, sport), she may be able to think: "I've always thought I'm a person who does everything wrong. Now I realize it's not exactly like this, that I have skills others appreciate, and in some moments I am aware of them". With this more nuanced idea, mood is more likely to improve. A third form of differentiation implies becoming aware of having agency over own mental states. It corresponds to passing from: "I believe my mental state completely depends on others" to "I have power and agency over my mental state". Other forms of differentiation, for example, passing from being fully convinced of own negative belief to having a minor degree of conviction, are also relevant (see Dimaggio et al., 2020).

Empirical evidence supports the position that metacognition is compromised in PD (Semerari, Carcione, Dimaggio, Falcone et al., 2003; Semerari, Carcione, Dimaggio, Nicolo et al., 2005). PD and symptom severity are correlated with each other and with more impaired metacognition. In other words, individuals with more severe PD and less metacognition are more depressed (Semerari et al., 2014), as they have greater difficulties in the following: being aware they have negative beliefs about the self and the others, taking a critical stance (differentiation) towards this belief, and realizing they have power over their depression, which correspondingly leads to poorer metacognitive mastery. The outcome of these metacognitive problems is that patients act with minimal awareness of their wishes and, when they are aware of them, they are unable to imagine the possibility of meeting their goals, remaining stuck rather than committing themselves to adaptive goal-oriented actions, and culminating in depression as the end state.

10.3 Coping

10.3.1 Cognitive Coping

Another construct linked to depression in PD is the tendency to enact maladaptive coping strategies. Dysfunctional coping, both cognitive and behavioural, forms toxic mechanisms that perpetuate depression. Cognitive coping includes various forms of repetitive thinking, e.g. worry and rumination, which, although adaptively aimed at trying to understand the causes of loneliness and generate strategies for repair, has the maladaptive by-product of engaging in endless cognitive effort without action, neither solving the problem nor improving mood, thus reducing self-esteem, cognitive efficiency, and the capacity to experience pleasure and motivation (McLaughlin, Borkovec, & Sibrava, 2007; Nolen-Hoeksema, Wisco, & Lyubomirsky, 2008). Evidence identifies that a number of cognitive coping strategies, particularly rumination (Martin & Tesser, 1989; Nolen-Hoeksema, 2000; Papageorgiou & Wells, 2008), initially adopted with the aim of regulating negative emotions, become toxic proximal antecedents of increased negative affectivity and eventually depressive symptoms (Watkins, Moberly, & Moulds, 2008).

Rumination is a passive and repetitive thought mode, where patients typically focus on what has made them depressed and what the consequences of their depression will be (Nolen-Hoeksema, 2000). Rumination usually revolves around a specific theme, such as failure, loss, or humiliation (Martin & Tesser, 1989; Papageorgiou & Wells, 2008).

Anxious worry is another form of repetitive thinking linked to depression. Worry is about future scenarios, in which the patient is uncertain of the outcome (Robichaud & Dugas, 2006). When worrying, patients try to understand whether and under which conditions negative consequences could occur. Consequently, they hold in mind negative scenarios, strengthening the power of negative images and, by association, increasing negative feelings. Sustained anxiety tends to result in low mood as the person is exhausted by this unproductive engagement with negative ideas about the self and the future.

Both rumination and worry are also present in PD (Dimaggio et al., 2020; Richman, Unoka, Dudas, & Demetrovics, 2018) and also contribute to the maintenance depression in this population. In PD their content is interpersonal. Patients either ruminate or worry about their social relationships in forms such as "What will they think about me?", "Will I be ashamed?", "Why is she not texting me anymore?". Furthermore, worry is often about the social consequences of depression: "What will my colleagues think if they see me lethargic and down?". Although there is agreement that patients with depression resort to repetitive thinking as a response to negative mental states in general (Nolen-Hoeksema, 2000), our observation is that with comorbid PD, worry and rumination often intrude when maladaptive schemas are triggered. For example, a middle-aged man with depression and narcissistic PD, in the context of the break-up of his relationship with his extremely wealthy partner, ruminated about having lost the opportunities to live the grand life he had always envisaged. Or, after an argument with her boss, a woman in her 40s with depression and dependent PD worried she could not live up to her boss's expectations of her.

10.3.2 Behavioural Coping

At the same time as using maladaptive cognitive coping, a patient may also implement dysfunctional coping strategies on a behavioural level. For example, he might avoid relationships with others and refrain from working activities and from emotional relationships. Addictive behaviours can be understood as highly dysfunctional coping strategies, such as alcohol or substance abuse, Internet and cell phone dependency, and so forth. Coping may also merge cognitive and behavioural aspects. For instance, perfectionism is another path to depression in patients with PD. For example, when a student is about to take a university exam, social rank is active and she becomes prey of the core self-image of *self as unworthy* and of the other as *critical and spiteful*. As a result, she resorts to perfectionism, which likely leads to her feeling overwhelmed, as she thinks nothing she does will be sufficient enough, making her feel low and lacking in self-efficacy. Perfectionism may then also end up in behavioural avoidance when the exam is near. This may ultimately result in her giving up, which, although bringing momentary relief from performance-based anxiety, then triggers depression via confirmation of the belief in her own chronic failure. Alternatively, if the student decides to face the exam and her professor critiques her answers, she may then feel worthless and unable to respond. In response to this, she may then cope via withdrawal – hardly speaking in class – which may reinforce her prediction that the professor believes she is inadequate. The end result is likely further perceived failure, which eventually will sustain her depression.

The interaction of maladaptive expectations about how others will respond and the dysfunctional coping strategies the person enacts to deal with these ideas, e.g. "the other will humiliate me", are likely to evoke negative reactions in the "real" others, which foster a vicious interpersonal cycles where negative ideas are sustained (Safran & Muran, 2000) and drop down the odds that anything good will happen, again a source for sustained depression.

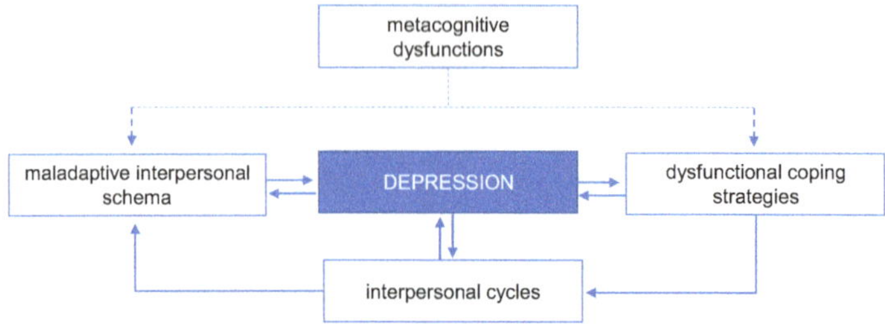

Fig. 10.1 Interaction of elements triggering and sustaining depression

In Figure 10.1, we illustrate how these elements interact in triggering and sustaining depression in PD.

10.4 Modular Treatment of Complex Depression

MIT has been manualized and is based around a decision-making procedure (Dimaggio, Montano et al., 2015; Dimaggio, Ottavi et al., 2020) with two macro-sections: *shared formulation of functioning* and *change promoting.*

The *shared formulation* is aimed at helping patients understate their inner world to the point of realizing they are guided by maladaptive interpersonal schemas, which are the primary cause for suffering and interpersonal problems. Once clients reach this awareness, they are ready for the *change-promoting phase*, whereby clinicians help them take a critical distance from their ideas about self and others, access and sustain more benevolent and healthier self and other representations, and experiment with new behaviours. The goal here is to nurture the emerging and adaptive patterns of thoughts and affects whilst trying to live a life richer in opportunities and where they can hope their core wishes will be fulfilled (Fig. 10.2).

Our framework for a modular (Livesley et al., 2016) treatment of complex depression is centred around the above procedures. We anticipate that the different modules can be used in parallel or sequentially, depending on the moment-to-moment shared formulation. We now describe each specific module:

10.4.1 Module 1: Shared Formulation of Functioning

This module is aimed at forming a shared understanding of how maladaptive interpersonal patterns form the roots of personal suffering and maladaptive behaviours. In doing so, we help patients to understand that they frequently predict that their core interpersonal wishes will remain unmet.

The first step is to collect specific narrative episodes about interpersonal exchanges, thus developing a clearer understanding of the nuances of subjective

SHARED CASE FORMULATION

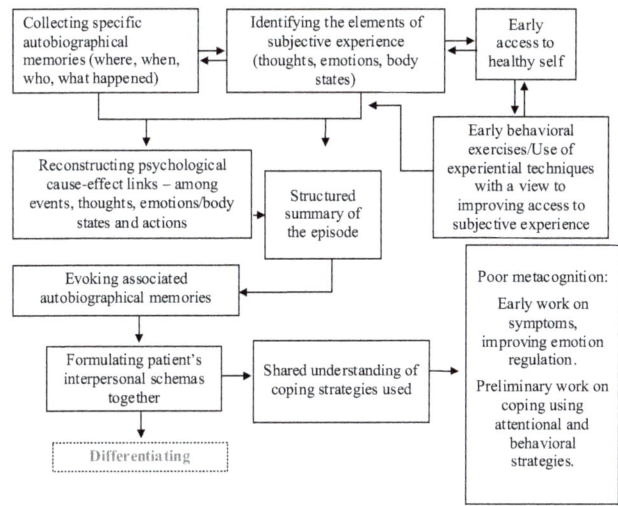

CHANGE PROMOTING

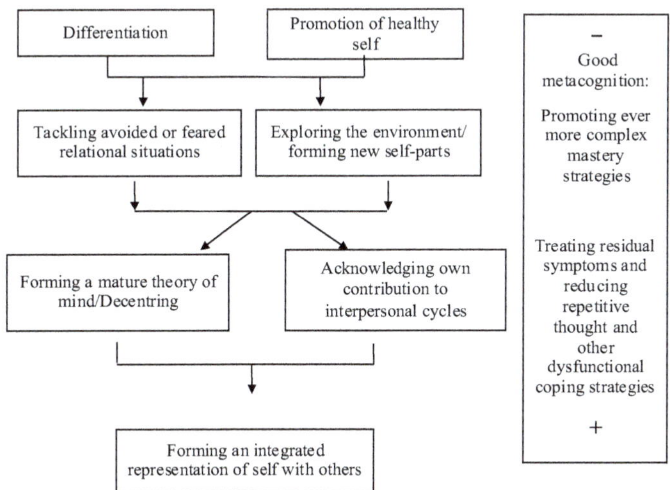

Fig. 10.2 Decision-making procedure

experiences. Relying on specific narratives to make meaning out of one's own problems, instead of relying upon intellectualizing, abstract theories, or generalized memories (e.g. "I have been the kind of person that…", "My husband never delivers the promise he holds"), forms a much stronger, more detailed basis for the clinician to attend to the nuances of patients' inner experience, from which the schema formulation will be built. Consequently, it is necessary to take some time over this stage, in order to collect sufficient, specific details about interpersonal episodes, including the cognitive-affective antecedents of low mood.

With some patients, obtaining specific narratives is quite difficult. For example, a woman may only report that her husband did not deliver the promises he made her, without elaborating or providing specific examples. In this instance, whilst discussing the issue, the therapist can ask her to say what she thinks and feels in the moment. If emotion-laden material appears, this can offer leverage for a deeper understanding of thoughts and potential psychological cause-effect associations.

Another pathway to a richer understanding of inner states from a narrative episode is the use of experiential techniques. For example, using guided imagery, the therapist can invite the client to re-experience the episode or to role-play part of it, in order to identify or draw attention to aspects of mental states the patient did not notice in the first retelling. In the previous, a specific episode may have been related where the woman could only say she was upset. Replaying using guided imagery enables a scanning of the episode, in which the woman discovers a more nuanced interpretation, discovering that just before becoming upset, she felt sad at the idea of being neglected and not listened to.

A further technique to increase the patients' awareness of the thoughts and affects antecedent to depression is to agree upon between-session behavioural exercises. The therapist first needs to identify the habitual coping strategies that the patient enacts when in a "trigger" situation. For example, in the previous scenario, the woman may tend to either rapidly overreact or withdraw into a hostile silence. Therefore, therapist may ask her to abstain from either behaviour, in order to attend to and understand what is passing through her mind "in the moment". For instance, the woman may discover that she does not remain silent out of sheer hostility but rather out of fear of further neglect, which would correspondingly increase her sadness. Alternatively, she may realize that she is afraid of the potential of her own anger to destroy her relationships, and thus she prefers to withdraw, avoiding the perceived risk of relationship breakdown and ultimately ending up alone.

We underscore that these initial behavioural experiments are not primarily aimed at promoting change. They are instead part of what we call *dynamic assessment* (Dimaggio et al., 2020). Here, we ask the patient to do something, with a view to identifying and observing the contents of inner experience "in the moment". In doing so, the patient also suspends his or her automatic coping procedures, which have hitherto served to reduce awareness of the "what and why" of what he or she is thinking and feeling.

The above techniques are all aimed at understanding psychological cause-effect links between environmental triggers, thoughts, affects, and behaviours. Through this understanding of psychological processes, the therapist summarizes events according to the schema structure. In doing so, the therapist orientates the patients' attention towards their core wishes, their core self-images, their expectations of the others would respond, how they react when their wishes are frustrated, and what types of coping strategies they enact to deal with the distress of thinking their wishes will remain unmet.

Using the structured summary, the therapist also asks for associated memories, for example: "Does this remind you of other situations in which you longed for attention but you perceived others neglected you, leaving you feeling alone, sad or angry?". Following the previous example, memories where the woman was neglected by her depressed mother may have appeared. By building these associated memories, a joint formulation of the schema becomes possible, strengthened though memories that patients themselves have provided in connection with the original episode. Therefore, it is highly likely that there is reciprocity between the clinician's interpretation and the patients actual functioning. Once the schema formulation has been clarified and shared, modular therapy can move towards the introduction of change-promoting techniques.

10.4.2 Module 2: Treating Cognitive Coping

Treating cognitive coping can start very early in the therapeutic process, with a focus on enabling patients to become aware of maladaptive aspects of cognitive coping how they can purposefully adapt it. Addressing these strategies often comprises one of the first elements of treatment, regardless of specifics, as patients usually enter therapy reporting chronic preoccupation about their interpersonal relationships. Addressing this highly problematic thinking pattern helps the patient to feel understood by the therapist and also gives them a sense that the therapy is active, consistent with the shared goal that the patient's distress will be alleviated. In short, addressing cognitive coping helps in forming and sustaining the therapeutic alliance.

The first part in the treatment of rumination and worry is to help patients identify when they are adopting these strategies when they try to describe their experience to the therapist. The clinician gently observes how the individuals appears to be running around in circles, repeating the same ideas with no apparent exit. In doing so, the clinician tries to avoid entering into this spiral, by trying to offer a solution which the client would not accept, as this could then be included in cycle. For example: a woman is worried that her friends will criticize her about the posts she wrote in a WhatsApp group. She rapidly proceeds to worrying that her colleagues will also criticize her for her perceived mistakes, and then her parents will be disappointed in her. Her worry leads to snowballing anxiety and the catastrophic cognition that she will become crazy. There is little gain in focusing in on and deconstructing each of the former episodes in a search for counterevidence, as the woman will soon jump to another "failure/criticism scenario". It is instead important to let the client discover that the cognitive process of engaging in repetitive thinking is fruitless and eventually deteriorates her mood.

It is also important to help patients note that the more they adopt this repetitive thinking style in search of a solution, the more likely it is to be counterproductive, reinforcing anxiety and ultimately lowering mood. Therapists can help patients note non-verbal markers to let them note how their negative affects increase when they engage themselves in repetitive thinking and contrastingly become less pronounced when they stop worrying and ruminating. Once the presence and role of cognitive coping has been jointly observed, therapy moves to adopting techniques aimed at reducing it. MIT has many experiential techniques for this purpose (Dimaggio et al., 2020; Ottavi et al., 2019).

The first of these is "splitting attentional space" (Dimaggio et al., 2020). It is a mixed imagery and sensory awareness technique. We ask the patient to close their eyes and visualize a painful scene, which is the focus of repetitive thinking – e.g. a Facebook post in which hid ex-partner is with a new boyfriend or a situation where his boss criticized him in front of his colleagues. We then we ask the patient to attend to both external stimuli, i.e. sounds, and interoceptive signals, such as breathing, and sensations from hands and feet. Attention is sustained on these stimuli until the painful image recedes. The therapist then asks the patient to focus on the painful image again, but this time asking him to observe it from the outside, as a spectator.

The goal of the technique is to experientially help patients realize the following:

(a) They can remember something painful with different degrees of involvement, and they can experience intense feelings whilst also observing them in a more detached way. This enables the connection to be made between degree of involvement and modulation of distress.
(b) The trigger for rumination is the negative affect associated with memory. Patients discover that, through rumination, they try to cope with distress through a process of evaluation, reasoning, and judgment, but this leads to a ruminative, ineffectual mental state.
(c) They have power and agency over their mental states. They can engage themselves in repetitive thinking, as they usual do once a distressing image intrudes into their mind, but they have power over their level of involvement. They can divert attention and discover that thoughts and feelings are less intense, which often fade away leaving room for other non-depressogenic thoughts and feelings.

Specifically for worry, we often use "dynamic attentional regulation" (Dimaggio et al., 2020). This consists of guiding patients to note the process by which the way they describe situations that worry them leads to an increase in sadness and anxiety, which builds towards a sense of hopelessness, desperation, and lack of energy. We invite patients to continue to talk about their worry, the feared consequences, and the actions they imagine they would do (or avoid doing) in order to manage the problem (e.g. humiliation or abandonment) but at the same time develop a dual attentional focus on somatic signals, for example, sensations from the hands or the feet. With repeated practice, patients discover they can think about negatively charged situations without anxiety snowballing and impacting on mood.

Another technique we use is *non-directive regulation and interoceptive refocusing* (Dimaggio et al., 2020), inspired by *Focusing* (Gendlin, 1981; Price & Hooven, 2018). When patients are recounting their experience, we invite them to focus their attention on somatic sensations connected to their story and to track the way these change as the story unfolds. After a while, we ask patients to shift focus away from cognition and instead increase their focus on somatic sensations. Usually with this sustained focus on bodily signals, patients discover they achieve a degree of emotion regulation, which is more effective than previous cognitive strategies such as worry and rumination. MIT also adopts a wide array of mindfulness-based techniques to promote emotion regulation and reduce reliance upon cognitive coping (e.g. metacognitive interpersonal-based mindfulness training, MIMBT; Ottavi, Passarella, Pasinetti, Salvatore, & Dimaggio, 2015; Ottavi et al., 2019).

10.4.3 Module 3: Treatment of Behavioural Coping

From the outset of therapy, MIT utilizes many types of behavioural experiments in order to counteract maladaptive behavioural coping. At therapy onset, the aim is to try and counteract maladaptive coping, with the goal of increasing awareness of the patient's own functioning. For clients with complex depression, trying to resist the urge to avoid, to enact perfectionism, and to comply with the other's expectations leads to increased arousal, with thoughts and affects underlying maladaptive behaviours coming to the fore, informing more nuance and detailed case formulation. At the same time, the client, as in behavioural activation for depression (Lewinsohn, 1974), should be aware from the start of therapy that activity and the pursuit of salutogenic goals are essential elements of treatment success.

In later points in therapy, once the client has become aware of how behavioural coping strategies are responses to their own maladaptive schemas, the focus of behavioural experiments becomes different: the therapist invites the client to pursue their deep-seated wishes, thus fostering contact with the healthy self. The intention here is to develop optimism and stimulate the belief that one has self-worth, which can be nurtured towards positive experiences, such as joy, self-efficacy, fulfilment, relaxation, control, and so forth. It is important that experiments are tailored around core wishes – e.g. to be loved and cared for, achieve status-related goals, be autonomous, and explore the environment – or around personal preferences, such as engaging in leisure activities and learning a skill.

Patients with depression comorbid with PD are driven by maladaptive schemas, which may create obstacles in the therapeutic alliance, preventing commitment to behavioural tasks. Other problems stem from poor metacognition, as patients may experience difficulties in identifying goals they wish to pursue. In order to maximize the likelihood that patients will focus their energies on behavioural tasks, some adjustment in task assignment may be necessary. Therapist and client review the conditions that decrease mood, e.g. spending time on the sofa, spending time browsing social media, or giving up positive activities for fear of the others' reactions. They then note activities that could potentially make them feel better: e.g. going out with friends.

Module 3 is largely based on connecting with healthy self-aspects. These include positive, more benevolent views of self and others and connecting with deep-seated aspirations and desires that could, if enacted, improve the individual's mood. When therapists, in cooperation with their patients, design a behavioural experiment, the aim is to ensure the planned activity is consistent with the individuals core motives. For example, is the patient planning a task to fulfil social rank, which if unsuccessful will reinforce perfectionistic tendencies, or is the task aimed to fulfil curiosity and exploration? The goal here is design tasks consistent with an individual's positive preferences, such as travelling, playing an instrument, or doing sports, rather than to please others.

Specificity is also important to the activity. What is the activity? Which point in the day/week does the patient chooses to try the activity? Where will it take place? For example, if the task is calling a friend the patient has not seen for a while, the task should include the following: What the patient hopes to do with her friend: Having a drink? Seeing a movie? Going to a restaurant? Having a ride with their bikes? Timing and planning are also crucial: When will she text her friend? The night after the session? The following day? These elements are important in modelling change as in negotiating the "why", "how", "when", and "where" of the task current coping comes to the fore and can be addressed. If the task is left generic, the patient may be more likely to use existing suboptimal coping strategies, such as avoidance, procrastination, and compulsive caregiving.

During planning of the task, and once it has been agreed, the therapy should assess the immediate impact on the patients' subjective experience. Does she feel curious and motivated or anxious and despondent? What is the balance of positive and negative emotions? It may be useful to rehearse the task using guided imagery to address potential problems in the safe space of the therapy room, making in vivo exposure less distressing. Some tasks may be enacted with the therapist present, counteracting avoidance and allowing monitoring of "in the moment" thoughts. Typically, a patient might write the text of a message in session, and either thinking about or actually sending the text, whilst the therapist monitors changes in thoughts and feelings during the exercise.

Given that patients with depression and PD are prone to interpretation of events via maladaptive schemas, it is likely they will interpret the task as something they must perform in order to please the therapist or to avoid her criticism. Therefore, the therapist should emphasize that success is not the goal, and she will not be disappointed if the patient does not perform the task. Instead, the goal of any task is to increase the awareness of one's own experience, gradually discovering agency over mental states. If the patient experiences negative affect before or during the task and then gives up, the therapist can review progress by encouraging reflection on the thoughts passing through the patient's mind at the point of abandoning the task. In the following session, the task can be jointly reviewed and a revised or alterative task co-created.

The cycle here is one of experiment planning-implementation-feedback-new planning. However, the clinician must be alert to signals over several task cycles that the patient is struggling, even in the context of a shared understanding of the potential for mental states underlying resignation and avoidance. In this case, the clinicians may need to recognize a problem in the task component of therapeutic alliance (Bordin, 1979; Safran & Muran, 2000), requiring revision of the therapeutic contract. The therapist therefore may need to gently enable the patient to become aware of the need for commitment to between session tasks. We label this as "active impotence" (Dimaggio et al., 2020) – the therapist says his input is unlikely to be effective without corresponding commitment from the patient, but when explaining this tension, he remains calm, compassionate, and well-regulated. In doing so, the therapist conveys a sense of openness, trust, and curiosity, letting the patient know he is there for her and will be supportive regardless of the patients' decisions. He can then invite the patient to reflect upon whether she is engaging with therapy in order to overcome depression or whether the motivation for therapy is simply the need for human company and connection. If the latter, the therapist may choose to continue to offer this, albeit without any promise of stable symptom change. It is only when the patient has realized that commitment is necessary for improvement that the clinician can then start engaging or engaging her in the process of behavioural experiment planning.

10.4.4 Module 4: Promoting Differentiation

Differentiation begins in Module 1 but takes a more prominent role as therapy deepens. To a certain extent, the last steps of a shared formulation of functioning are also the beginning of differentiation. Patients discover the extent to which they are driven by stereotyped biased in meaning-making, linked to recurring patterns of emotions and bodily states. This often promotes insight: "So it's me *seeing* things this way!".

Once a patient's interpersonal functioning has been jointly formulated, the next goal is to guide patients to understand that their ideas about interpersonal relationships do not necessarily mirror reality and instead represent firmly held, often rigid beliefs. There are various ways to promote differentiation. The first focuses on promoting the *true* vs. *learned* type. This requires the patient to become aware that she interprets reality according to developmentally acquired patterns.

A 35-year-old woman, a scientific researcher, presented as depressed, with the interpersonal components comprising a sense of social alienation and loneliness. She gradually comes to understand that she uses social (and relational) avoidance as a coping strategy for managing her underlying sense of unworthiness and her fear of criticism. During a session, she related how anxious and ashamed she felt during a dinner with friends and the accompanying perception of her own inferiority: "My usual reaction... there it is... the usual sense of emptiness... I always think that people are uninterested in me because I am worth nothing". The therapist asks her for related memories – a core step in the *shared formulation of functioning*. The therapist asked her to recall autobiographical memories, where she found herself in similar situations, i.e. when she would have liked to belong to a group but felt rejected and ridiculed. She remembered that in the past she had been repeatedly excluded and ridiculed by her classmates and older sisters. From this association with distal memories, she realized that her current fears of rejection and social exclusion were learned responses: "I longed for connection but it always ended up the same way; they said I could not play with them because I was clumsy". Thanks to this understanding, she also realized that in the present there are times in which she feels welcome and accepted, but she tends to discount and not attend to these instances, instead remaining focused on her ingrained expectation of rejection.

Usually, the therapist also tries to promote a second type of differentiation – *differentiation* via *access to healthy self-aspects* (Dimaggio et al., 2020), such as the one "*my negative idea of myself is always true*" vs. "*in some cases I see myself and others differently, in a more benevolent way*". Instead, the strategy is to let the patient note instances in which she recognizes a more benevolent, positive self-image, but does not note it, or rapidly switched to the habitual negative self-image. In the former example, the young woman with depression and social avoidance may focus on memories where others neglected her, interpreted by her as a sign of lack of interest. However, on questioning, she reported memories of receiving positive feedback.

Here, the MIT therapist does not dispute the patients' beliefs or try to convince them that the others' behaviour can be interpreted in a different way. Instead, he lets the patient note that when she reports a positive reaction from others, she displays clear non-verbal signs. In the moment, she appreciates this reaction and looks happy. The clinician may ask: "What do you think and feel about yourself right now?". Through this form of inquiry, healthy self-representations the patient already possessed are noticed and brought to the centre of consciousness. The therapist then helps the patient connect herself with bodily and emotional correlates of this positive beliefs, and with repetition she is able to realize that she can endorse these positive, healthy self-representations. Together with the previous modules, the therapist is vigilant for moments in which the patient switches to the habitual dominant negative idea about self and others. The therapist then helps the patient recognize the switch: "I notice that until a few seconds ago you were happy about feeling accepted, having been invited by friend. You noticed they were cheerful, and you felt confident and happy about the idea of spending Friday night together with them. But now your face has changed, and you are no longer in touch with the thoughts and feelings you had a few seconds ago. It looks like, though you're aware it's there, it is really difficult for you to hold in your mind ideas in which you think you are worthy and can feel appreciated by others".

Experiential techniques are also very useful in promoting this kind of differentiation, such as guided imagery with rescripting. For example, during imagery, the woman may re-experience the dinner, where she felt inferior and rejected, whilst everyone else was happy, superior to her, and getting along with each other. In the first part of the imagery, the therapist asks her to focus on the feelings and bodily sensations associated with ideas of inferiority and exclusion. She notes that her body is bent and slumped and her shoulders are low and her forehead points towards the ground. The therapist asks her to adopt a so-called power pose (Cesario, Jonas, & Carney, 2017), standing up, clenching her fists, raising up her shoulders and head, and looking straight in front of her. As soon as she adopts the new pose, her self-representations change and she feels more self-confident, energetic, and connected to the others. The therapist lets her note that she has changed her mind, using a simple change in posture. Therefore, her idea of being unworthy and disconnected from others is not a factual certainty but just a perspective, which she has power over. This is exactly the second type of differentiation we advocate: *always true (and negative)* vs. *sometimes, it sounds true but at other times I see things from a different (and more benevolent) angle*.

In this case, differentiation was not approached top-down – we did not ask the client to refute her negative beliefs. Change proceeded from the bottom-up: we let the patient change her body posture and attitude and then observed how ideas changed as a consequence. With these techniques, we target the embodied component of maladaptive schemas, proposing that cognitive change will follow (Centonze, Inchausti, MacBeth, & Dimaggio, 2020). In a second phase, imagery may have full rescripting, that is, the therapist invites the woman to respond differently – to try to join the conversation and say the jokes she had imagined telling but had suppressed because she had thought she would have sounded ridiculous. During rescripting, the woman gave clear non-verbal signs that she found the joke amusing, which was shared by the therapist.

A third form of differentiation is of the type *I believe my mental state completely depends on others* vs. *I have power and agency over my mental state*.

Continuing with the example of the young woman, during a conversation with friends, she may think others are judging her and excluding her. She feels dejected and inferior, so she remains silent for the rest of the night. Here, the therapist may help understand that, whether or not others are really devaluing her or not, she may feel sad and inferior, but she has power and agency over this mental state. She can act on her inner world in order to find an exit out from that mental state without having to address the context. For example, the therapist may help her note, with attentional techniques (see above), that when she does not ruminate on the attitudes of the others, she may feel better. The therapist can also ask her to return to the conversation within guided imagery and invite her to retrieve the negative self-image and to explore its bodily correlates, e.g. weakness, tension, and heaviness in the chest. Then, the therapist can use a short mindful breathing exercise to explore if the negative self-image stays (see Matos & Steidl, 2020 for a similar intervention with compassion-focused therapy). The therapist may then invite her to retrieving a moment of playfulness, observing what self-image is endorsed. Alternating between these different images a few times is usually sufficient to help a patient realize that the negative state is not a matter of fact (she *is* inferior) but is instead a subjective mental state, which changes according to different perspectives and connections to other more benevolent and positive self-states.

10.4.5 Module 5: Promoting the Healthy Self

This module aims to identify and strengthen positive images of self and others, in the service of sustaining the healthy self. Multiple sources, including psychotraumatology (Fosha, 2000; Leeds, 2009) and positive psychology (Seligman & Csikszentmihalyi, 2014), note that enhancing the capacity to experience positive affect is crucial to successful therapy. Strategies from positive psychology, such as developing personal strengths, seeking direction and meaning, and engagement in daily life, offer tools for the prevention and treatment of depression whilst also aiding staying well and relapse prevention (Santos et al., 2013). MIT adopts the same approach in treating PD and the process of connection with inner wishes, promotion of representational change, and associated enactment of change serves to increase a positive sense of agency: both over one's own distress and over one's own choices. There are therefore many elements through which MIT fosters the healthy self in patients with depression comorbid with PD.

(a) *Increasing experiential access to positive* states. During sessions, the therapist invites clients to retrieve instances in which they felt positive, satisfied, hopeful, being nurtured, curious, and strong and had some self-efficacy. This is in the service of helping the patient realize that in these moments, they were guided by representation of self and others more positively, discrepant from previous negative representations that reinforce maladaptive interpersonal schemas.

For example, David was a 28-year-old teacher, presenting with covert narcissistic PD. During his first session, he reports that he feels anxious before playing tennis. He thought he was inferior and would lose to his opponent, who at the end of the game would sneer at him, making David feel ashamed. He experienced bodily tension, as the image of himself as a loser was activated in him, whilst another part of himself hoped to be skilled enough to play a good tennis match. Guided by the negative self-image, he imagined the opponent will consider him to be inept and he accordingly he felt ashamed. The therapist asked him to contact and explore experiences in which he played well and felt positive, regardless of outcome. David remembered a number of episodes – both wins and some of losses. The therapist explored commonalities between these episodes: David felt calm and steady and his body was relaxed; he was not concerned about his opponent's appraisals, and David was guided by a self-image of adequacy. David understood that he holds more benevolent images of himself and others, which surface when he focuses on the activity in questions and not on social rank issues.

(b) The second approach to accessing positive self-aspects is through discussion. The therapist lets the therapeutic discourse include topics, such as patient's interests or things they are curious about, not limiting the dialogue to symptoms and problems. The therapist tries to be as spontaneous as she can, expressing, where appropriate to do so, personal preferences, knowledge, and experience she has about the topic, e.g. sport, leisure activities, computer gaming, a TV series, or painting. The therapist attends closely non-verbal markers, bringing the patients' attention towards instances in which expression shifts towards the positive, which may signal the emergence *innovative* (Gonçalves et al., 2017) or *sparkling* moments (White & Epston, 1990).

For example, the therapist may observe: "While you were telling me about your biking tour, your face was more relaxed, your voice brighter, and your shoulders opened up. You also seemed to talk confidently, like you were proud of the distance you covered and enjoyed the landscapes you saw. It is very different from when you talked to me about your boss, where you considered yourself flawed and unable to do anything. Does it make sense to you?".

The therapist helps the patient to hold these positive states in mind for as long as possible during the session. The therapist may suggest the use of reminders to support patients in connecting themselves to the positive state between sessions. For example, the therapist can ask the patient to write down a few lines, or a voice memo, describing the sensations, or to label the part of the self-identified in the positive state. With these aide-mémoires, the patient is more likely to remember the positive state when home and re-experience it. Then, when connected to the positive state, they have the possibility of exiting from the negative mood state and in doing so interrupt the maintenance of depression.

(c) A further way to foster contact with the healthy self is through the therapeutic relationship. When the therapist succeeds in validating and supporting patients' wishes and experiences, the latter is likely to show changes in the facial expression and feelings, such as shifting from anxious and sad states to relaxed and relieved. This pivot offers the therapist an opportunity to entrench the connection with positive states, as in the following example. A man in his 20s with avoidant PD presents as depressed, anhedonic, and socially isolated. He states that he always feels in a bad mood and nothing interests him. During one session, the man seemed to be sitting in an agitated and posture. The therapist asked the patient what had happened, and he replied that the chair (which was newly bought) is very uncomfortable. The therapist replies that she was about to buy a second one, because she liked it. However, as she knows the patient and trusts his judgement, she will not buy it after all. The patient smiles and relaxes: he feels validated, as the therapist has taken his opinion into account.

In doing so, the therapist's response disconfirms the patient's maladaptive schema that others will disagree with him, and therefore the therapeutic relationship passes a relational test (Gazzillo et al., 2019; Weiss, 1993).

(d) Another fundamental way to sustain healthy self-aspects is by validating core wishes and not the ones that patients adopt as coping strategies. As an example: A 40-year-old journalist presents with dependent personality disorder and depression. His complaint is that when he wishes to be free and to explore, he imagines that others will fiercely criticize him. This makes him feel inadequate, signalling a shift into the social rank motive. The therapist intervenes by validating the primary wish for autonomy, whilst simultaneously noting that the rank concern is a secondary mechanism for coping with the primary concern of the underlying negative self-image. The therapist summarizes as follows: "We know that if you act according to your wish to be autonomous, you will be harshly criticized and consequently feel inadequate and a failure. At this point you abandon the outcome that you really long for and become depressed. In contrast, I notice that when you talk about things you do like, you appear energized and alive. It would be great if we could find ways to help you remain in touch with that part of you".

(e) *Using experiential techniques and behavioural experiments in the early sessions.* This is part of what MIT calls *dynamic assessmen*t – improving patients' awareness of their mental processes using experiential techniques and behavioural experiments. Clinicians know that the goal here is not to change anything but instead increase metacognition (i.e. helping clients become aware that their range of experiences is greater than they previously thought and that they can hold positive ideas and feelings about themselves than they did not previously notice). For example, asking a client to abstain from avoidance may help him recognize that he experiences a degree of self-efficacy he did anticipate. Adopting power poses or using grounding may generate an untapped sense of strength. This way, early in therapy, patients are able to discover that they have resources they can draw upon interpersonally, changing their relationship with their depression to something that they have control over. This improves motivation for treatment and instils hope.

(f) *Using experiential techniques to increase confidence in healthy states and adopt behaviours driven by more benevolent ideas of self and others.* Once patients have understood that, in parallel to their familiar negative schema, they also hold positive beliefs about self and others, there is a scope to promote sustaining these positive beliefs in mind and enabling a greater sense of control over conscious thoughts and behaviour. Experiential techniques are crucial in promoting this step.

For example, a depressed woman is diagnosed with comorbid obsessive-compulsive PD. She reports that whenever she wishes to act autonomously according to her own preferences, she predicts that others will not support her and will instead create obstacles and criticize her. In these moments, she shifts into the social rank motive, becoming vulnerable to a self-image of inferiority and inadequacy, accompanied by emotional-behavioural sequelae of loneliness, sadness, and avolition. The therapist can adopt bodily exercises to break this cycle. For example, she can invite the patient to imagine that the block is a pillow she holds in her hands. She can then push the pillow away saying something like: "I am free. I won't let myself be trapped by this obstacle". Very often, these experiences foster agency, alongside, and the idea that one is able to act according to their innermost wishes and preferences, weakening the vulnerability to negative schema-driven ideas and behaviours. Experiential techniques aimed at sustaining the healthy self need to be followed by behavioural experiments, as we described above.

10.5 Using Experiential Techniques in MIT

In its most recent manualized form (Dimaggio et al., 2020), MIT adopts a wide array of experiential techniques, including guided imagery and rescripting (Hackmann, Bennett-Levy, & Holmes, 2011), role-play and two-chair approaches (Greenberg, 2002; Moreno, 1975; Perls, Hefferline, & Goodman, 1951), bodily exercises (Lowen, 1971; Ogden & Fisher, 2015) behavioural experiments, and mindfulness attention regulation. Deciding which technique to use and when is guided by shared decision-making in therapy, with the goal of techniques changing over therapy through an ongoing re-evaluation of the case formulation.

1. *Improving knowledge of own inner states* – or metacognitive monitoring (Semerari et al., 2003). For example, these techniques can increase awareness of affective experiences and then help patients label them.
2. *Fostering agency.* Through experiential techniques, patients are guided to discover that they have power and control (agency) over their own mental states. This aids them to discard maladaptive self-images, such as “I’m passively responding to others”, and embody more adaptive self-images, such as “I have power over my experiences, and am not simply hostage to my thoughts and feelings. I want to act according to my own view and I have the power to do so”.
3. *To face symptoms and emotional regulation.* If the patient has pervasive symptoms and emotional distress, these block or slow down the necessary exploration of psychological functioning. Body techniques can help regulate these states, for example through breathing or grounding (Lowen, 1971). A meditation session promotes the transition from one state of intense emotional reactivity to another, in which the emotion persists but does not spiral out of control and translate into dysfunctional behaviour.
4. *Promoting differentiation.* Of note, the second step, promoting agency, includes the first element of differentiation, in the process of moving from “I cannot control my reactions” to “I believed that I was a passive recipient of others’ intentions, but now I realize that this is not true as I have power over myself”. Furthermore, as we will see in the clinical case, through the experiential techniques the patient discovers that she holds more benevolent self-images, and she understands that her way of looking at reality depends on her past and does not necessarily correspond to the truth.
5. *Accessing healthy self.* This relates to helping individuals to gain awareness of positions imbued with positive qualities such as “lovable”, “worthy”, “strong”, “energy-driven”, and so forth. The techniques are effective in facilitating access to healthy positions, as we discussed in the earlier part of the chapter.
6. *Improving mastery* (Semerari et al., 2003). This relates to acquiring and honing the skills with which it is possible to intentionally and fully consciously use metacognitive knowledge to take decisions, solve problems, and master subjective suffering. During role-play, guided imagery, and behavioural experiments, the patient discovers new ways of dealing with events, learning to respond differently, for example, to a jealous partner or a mother who blocks autonomy.

7. *Facilitate understanding of the other's mind.* To foster better interpersonal relationships, MIT also promotes a richer, more nuanced, and decentralized understanding of the other. However, in MIT, therapists do not attempt to improve patients' theory of mind unless differentiation and access to healthy parts of the self have already been consolidated. Once these conditions have been met, experiential techniques, in particular role-play and two chairs, are particularly useful for this purpose. We now describe a case example, demonstrating a modular approach to implementing these techniques. The client was a 62-old-year woman presenting with major depression and paranoid PD with passive-aggressive and avoidant personality traits. She was treated by the first author.

10.6 Clinical Case

Isabel is a lecturer and is married to a doctor with whom she has a conflictual and difficult relationship. She has two adult sons. Isabel asked for therapy due to a major depressive episode of 1-month duration. She was on sick leave from work, stating that she felt deprived of both energy and motivation. Isabel spent her days at home, doing nothing and constantly ruminating about the idea that her husband was cheating on her. Over the past 2 years, she had developed morbid jealousy towards him, becoming suspicious and starting to obsessively control him. As an example, her husband habitually talks to himself when alone. Isabel bugged the house with micro recorders, hoping to uncover clues about his infidelity. Hearing tapes, she captures passages where, more than once, he speaks about being torn between Isabel and "Diana". Isabel considers this as incontrovertible evidence that he is cheating on her.

Isabel had entrenched, chronic rumination and was convinced that she could not recover her mental state, was "crazy", and subsequently fell into depression. Her husband initially denied her accusations, stating that she was crazy and needed treatment, thus reinforcing her belief. A few months later, when Isabel was already in the psychotherapy we are describing here, he disclosed that he was having an affair. She asked for therapy on her own. Her son, concerned about seeing her depressed and always in bed, encourages her to seek therapy.

Isabel reported that she was familiar with depressive states, having had "breakdowns" in the past. She said she often felt neglected and sad, because she always fought with her husband. In the past, her depression emerged after long periods in which she felt unimportant in the eyes of her husband, who was instead focused on his job and hobbies. He also used to mock her job and he would criticize her if she was down.

10.6.1 Module 1 (Early Therapy Step): Shared Formulation of Functioning

Isabel entered therapy amotivated, anhedonic and hopeless. Her arousal increased only when talking about her husband's infidelity. She became angry, rapidly followed by sadness, tearfulness, and desperation. Isabel recalled an episode in which she yelled at her husband after she had listened to one of his "solitary monologues", where he mentioned his feelings for Diana. He denied that Diana was real and Isabel became even angrier.

The therapist asks her to replay the episode using guided imagery, with the goal of exploring Isabel's inner state and developing a richer sense of the underlying affect, as Isabel could only identify and recognize anger. In the scene, the therapist asked Isabel to focus on her husband's face, and she described it as spiteful and cold. He said she was mad and has become obsessed. The therapist asks what Isabel's thought and feelings are in connection to her husband's expression and words. Isabel first notices that she is angry as she deserves more respect but then discovers that she quickly falls into a state of dejection and humiliation – "like an empty bag falling to the floor". Though the imagery exercise had already met its goal (improving enriching awareness of self-states), Isabel was distressed by recalling the dejected state. The therapist first helped her regulate it with mindful breathing and grounding and then helped her to connect with her core wish – to be appreciated and valued, alongside the associated positive idea of deserving appreciation.

Once guided imagery ended, Isabel and the therapist co-constructed a preliminary formulation of the psychological processes underlying the episode. This enables further exploration of associations and then deepens understanding of the maladaptive interpersonal schema. In the above episode, Isabel was driven by the social rank domain and the wish to be appreciated by her husband, which met a response from the other as spiteful and cheating. The corresponding response of the self is to think that she is unworthy and deserving of maltreatment, paving the way to dejection, shame, and depression. In parallel, the response of the spiteful/cheating other matches with a core idea of being worthy, so she thinks she is being treated unfairly, thus also triggering anger. A series of these episodes were collected during the early sessions, all of similar structure, enabling this formulation to be with Isabel. In doing so, Isabel could identify herself within the formulation.

10.6.2 Module 2: Treating Cognitive Coping

On the occasions when Isabel became absorbed into her negative schema (feeling that she was despised and deserved to be cheated on), her main coping strategy was rumination. She would spend hours thinking she was the cause of her husband looking for a lover and analysing what she could have done to prevent it. Rumination had the dual, toxic effects of increasing her depression and her passivity. Simultaneously, Isabel was haunted by images of her husband together with his lover. These images would intrude into her mind and become chronically active, precipitating increasing waves of anxiety and reinforcing her negative cognitive schema.

To tackle rumination, the therapist used the *splitting attentional space* technique described above. She asks Isabel to focus on the most emotionally intense episode she could recall. Isabel imagines her husband being with "Diana". Isabel experiences growing tension and stomach ache; her legs shake and her heart pounds; she frowns and her shoulders are contracted. She realizes that that she feels a combination of jealousy and anger, mixed with sadness. The therapist then asks to split her attention: she devotes part of her focus to the episode, and the other attends to the "here and now" sounds of the office and its surroundings. After a minute, Isabel's emotions are already less intense, her heart beats more regularly, and her legs are no longer shaky, though she still feels a stomach ache and tension.

At this point, the therapist invites her to further split her attention: the first part still focused on the imaginal episode, the second part to the sounds in the "here and now", and the third on her breathing. At a certain point, she exclaims: "I can't hold the image back!", at which point her negative affect and muscle tension fade away. Next, the therapist explains the power of attention in letting negative emotions grow in intensity and maintaining their position in consciousness. The therapist explains that as Isabel is able to let her attention shift away from negative images, she gains control over her mental state, and eventually that impacts on her mood.

As a final step, the therapist asks Isabel to recall the episode again, but this time "as if" she is an outside observer. Isabel performs the task and discovers that she does not experience any painful emotion. After a minute or so, to Isabel's surprise and relief, the image spontaneously fades away. She now understands, for the first time, that distress is something that she has power over and that she can act to soothe her distress rather than ruminate on it.

10.6.3 Module 3: Treating Behavioural Coping

The dominant behavioural coping strategies Isabel used were passivity and resignation. She did not meet with male or female friends and did not make time for things she liked or felt were important, such as her physical appearance and health. Isabel said these things no longer made sense to her anymore. The therapist anticipated that the type of behavioural coping enacted would become clearer after they agreed on a schedule of behavioural tasks. Recall that Isabel's vulnerability schema made her see herself as inferior, inadequate, and unsuccessful. This led her to imagine herself as incapable of doing pleasurable activities, or if she did try, she would be unable to do them well, reinforcing the schema. Resignation and passivity became strategies to alleviate her distress.

As a first step, the therapist asks Isabel to remember past episodes when she cared about herself and her interests, such as trekking, walking, collecting stones, and shopping for clothes. When she recalled these memories, she reported a sense of power, purpose, and higher self-esteem.

As a behavioural exercise, the therapist suggested Isabel went shopping for clothes. Her initial reaction was one of disappointment, as she saw no value in addressing her appearance whilst her marriage was deteriorating. The therapist helped Isabel notice that she had suddenly lost the energy and power she had had only moments previously, when remembering past instances of the same activities. The therapist then explained to Isabel that the goal of the exercise was not to do these things for their own sake but as a way to explore how her mind worked when spending time doing things she once liked, rather than succumbing to passivity.

Isabel agreed, though the therapist noted that she remained somewhat sceptical. In fact, she did not complete the task before the next session. It is important to remember that the actual performance is not the goal of behavioural task assignments in MIT. Often the aim is to help the patient to focus on the mental processes occurring at the very moment they give up on the task. Exploring the moment in which Isabel tried to go out and shop was extremely important. She got dressed and when she thought about seeing the shop fronts, she felt motivated to proceed. However, as she left her house, a thought intruded: if her husband saw her happy and carefree, he would be happy as that would be to him proof his infidelity was unpunished. Isabel then started to ruminate about past betrayals with mounting anger. At that point, she decided to give up shopping, thus not letting her husband "win". In describing this to her therapist, it became clear that the reciprocal of her passivity was vengeance – her stuckness was a form of retaliation against her husband, a way to perhaps worry him and perhaps even confess his infidelity. Isabel's passivity was driven not only by depression and deactivation but also by a maladaptive consequence of a social rank strategy – whereby her husband could not "win" by his indiscretions remaining unpunished. In dialogue Isabel and her therapist reasoned that this was not a fair trade off as Isabel did not get anything from this strategy (in terms of her husband reaction), and the cost was to deprive her of sources of pleasure recreation. The following week, Isabel completed the task. Although she had numerous intrusive thoughts, she used attentional techniques to modulate these and eventually went out on an enjoyable shopping trip.

10.6.4 Module 4: Promoting Differentiation

At the onset of therapy, Isabel's discourse could be summarized as: "I suffer because my husband makes me feel inadequate". Her narrative was disorganized (Dimaggio & Semerari, 2001) and vague, and the only clear emotion was anger. Consequently, at the early stage of therapy, it was impossible to encourage her to consider that her schemas were not incontrovertible facts but instead were simply perspectives she firmly believed. With time, her narratives become more organized and metacognition grew, giving therapy more material for the schema-level formulation as well as forming an initial step towards Isabel recognizing her ideas were subjective. Isabel started to understand that the core of her distress was the conflict between her wish for appreciation and attention from her husband and the reality that this rarely occurred. She considered herself as inferior and a victim and him as superior, but she showed no ability to see this as a subjective view of her relationships and the world.

A crucial element of therapy revolved around a painful autobiographical memory. Isabel had been at a spring lunch in the countryside with friends. After lunch, her husband was sitting in the garden, chatting with a female colleague he had met there. She asked her husband something, but he responded without even looking at her, remaining focused on his other conversation. Isabel sudden felt inferior and thought: "Here they are, they talk about things that interest them while I have nothing to say". At that point the thought intruded that she thinks she is "just a cleaning lady", and so she went to help the hosts tidy up. She felt sad, dejected, and deprived of agency. She then sat on a chair, alone, and felt like crying but unable to do so.

The therapist helped Isabel notice that her social rank schema was active – she felt inferior vis-à-vis someone she perceived as a rival for her husband's affections. The therapist proposed Isabel role-played the scene. The story began with Isabel facing her husband, enacted by her therapist, whilst he was going away to his female colleague. At that moment Isabel felt empty, deprived of energy, and abandoned. The therapist used body work to regulate this state: she asked Isabel to breath mindfully, open up her shoulders, and stand up fiercely (a power pose) until she no longer felt empty and instead felt empowered. Then, the therapist asked her to contact with a healthy self-aspect of self-esteem and dignity, which Isabel felt she could do. The therapist asked Isabel to focus on the broom for cleaning, experiencing the urge to take it, and clean the garden, but not to do so. After successfully resisting the urge, the therapist invites Isabel to pay attention to herself as the husband. Isabel said: "Are you going to chat with your colleague? I'll join you, would you introduce me to her?". After saying this, she had a different wish – to go to a seat in the shadow of a tree and relax, which she eventually did. Isabel said, that once she is on the seat, some other people seek her out for conversation, which she felt happy about. Having connected with the associated positive feelings, the exercise ended.

Isabel now understands that her behaviour changes according to the part of the self that is determining her actions. If she lets healthy self-aspects take control, she has different aims and desires, and she experiences different, more positive feelings. Overall, she acquired greater agency over her mental states, instead of remaining vulnerable to passivity, control, revenge, and rumination.

This exercise was also important as she first embodied the self-image of the "cleaner with a broom" vis-à-vis her husband, embodied by her therapist, but then she let it go, realizing that was just a mental representation. Instead, she could relate to her husband whilst she embodied a position of herself as worthy and filled with dignity. Through this insight, she also changed her attitude in real life, becoming able to act as equal to her husband in several situations.

10.6.5 Module 5: Promoting the Healthy Self

Isabel engaged well with her therapist and developed a good therapeutic rapport. In contrast to her pleasant demeanour in therapy sessions, she described herself as "coy" and "a loner", having few friends and preferring to spend her time alone at home. She did not report any interests or hobbies, and when not working, she stated that she "just rests". This was, however, belied by some of the experiences she recounted. During one session, 6 months into therapy, she described going for a walk by a local lake, to pick rocks for her collection. The therapist encouraged Isabel to hold in mind the positive sensations as she described them, at which point she relaxed and looked revitalized. The therapist asked her if this is a new experience or whether she had other, similar memories. She recalled that as a teenager, she used to walk around the city for hours, feeling fine. Once she focused on these memories, she looked even more relaxed. The therapist reflected with Isabel on how she retains the capacity to experience pleasure when alone, which she agreed with. A further developmental memory then spontaneously emerged. In the memory, Isabel was 5 years old. It was a rainy afternoon, and she was in her mother's kitchen together with her two older sisters, who were baking sweets. Isabel said that according to her mother, she was too little to cook like her sisters were, so her mother had sent her to play in her own room. She remembers sitting alone in the room, twiddling with some things, bored. She became sad when recalling the episode, thinking that she is inferior to her sisters and that her mother prefers them. The therapist then asked Isabel to try a guided imagery and rescripting exercise. The goal was to build positive experiences and support positive self-related cognitions in her mind, weakening the established negative schema response pattern.

Once back in the room, she states that she has been left alone because "I'm inferior, and my sisters are better"; this heightens her affect and she reports a mixture of loneliness and dejection. Her body seems "like an empty bag". She experiences a sense that she is spending hours alone and "no one even knows I exist". At this point, the therapist pauses the imagery and suggests adopting a bioenergetic exercise, with the goal of reexperiencing vitality (Lowen, 1971). The exercise requires her to move, shaking her legs and arms as if dancing. Isabel notes that her body is coming back to life. With this new internal state, Isabel closes her eyes and they restart the imagery. The therapist suggests that Isabel can do something she enjoys rather than remaining in the room as instructed. Isabel states that her 5-year-old self would like to walk in the rain – "I'd like that. I don't like baking!". The therapist licences this, and Isabel imagines getting dressed in her rain jacket dressing, walking out and feeling the rain, and experiencing happiness and a sense of energy. Her therapist invites her to label this state, which Isabel calls "joy in the puddles". The exercise ends with Isabel feeling content.

To consolidate healthy self-aspects, over the previous maladaptive patterns, a series of behavioural experiments and behavioural activation interventions were used. The goal here was to help Isabel identify positive experiences that would help her feel validated and empowered, strengthening a representation of self as adequate. Together Isabel and her therapist identified a series of pleasurable activities from previous dialogue, such as painting stones, walking, and floristry. In addition, they identified a number of activities that Isabel was interested in but found difficult, such as learning English and playing racquet sports. Initially, Isabel had approached behavioural exercises with diffidence: she did not believe she was capable of achieving these goals and the tendency towards passivity took over. At the first few attempts at each activity, Isabel quickly abandoned them – her negative cognitions of "not being good enough" led to a sense of resignation. During therapy, the therapist discussed with Isabel how pervasive this negative schema was; however, as therapy progressed, Isabel became increasingly adept at using counteractive coping strategies, with the outcome that she was gradually able to undertake the activities they had identified.

10.6.6 Therapy Outcome

The therapy lasted for 2 years. At the end point, Isabel no longer experienced depressive episodes, and her paranoid presentation had remitted. Although she still experienced a negative schema of "unworthiness", a parallel set of positive and benevolent self-images had appeared. She reported that others also appear less "threatening", and she tried to challenge her perception that others are critical and contemptuous.

After her husband confessed this infidelity, she reported feeling angry for some time, but she decided to stay in the marriage, stating that he had said he still loved her. Importantly, Isabel stated that she felt no longer dependent on him, and she recognized this contrasted with her past beliefs of idealizing him whilst considering herself to be unworthy. She now reported feeling strong and empowered. When he criticizes her, she is able to swiftly retort, and she considers she is in a relationship of equals. Isabel stated that now realizes her husband is arrogant rather than superior, but that façade hides the underlying fragility. With this formulation, she no longer fears him. She also acknowledged that she still loves him and they have shared interests, such as traveling. At 6-month follow up, her gains remained stable. Isabel recognized that she continues to have developmental goals in her interpersonal domain, such as smiling and laughing more, but she feels empowered to work on these herself.

10.7 Conclusions

In this chapter, we make the case that working on complex depression comorbid with PD requires a modular approach – tackling the breadth of psychopathology implicated in the maintenance of depression in this group. We targeted a number of different domains of psychopathology. First, we address metacognition – increasing patients' awareness of psychological and relational functioning as a technique to enable them to discover that distress mostly comes from maladaptive schemas activated in interpersonal relationships. We then we help the patient to contrast cognitive and behavioural coping strategies – particularly worry, rumination, social avoidance, and overchecking. Through enhancing differentiation, we also generate a parallel work on developing healthy self-aspects, aiding the patient to give space to his desires and increase pleasurable activities.

We underscore that modular treatment is not synonymous with sequential treatment. Modules can be delivered in parallel, very often inside the same session, with the clinician guided by an ongoing, evolving case formulation and in-session negotiation of goals and tasks. We also note how many experiential techniques, such as role-playing and imagery with rescripting, are powerful tools in deconstructing crystalized elements of psychopathology, which left unaddressed increase the risk of recurrence of depression.

We acknowledge that we have illustrated this modular approach via a single, successful case example, with no formally assessed outcomes. Future studies could focus on replicating results, assessing therapeutic outcomes and understanding the conditions in which this approach may be useful to individuals with depression and comorbid different underlying personality disorders.

References

Bamelis, L. L., Evers, S. M., Spinhoven, P., & Arntz, A. (2014). Results of a multicenter randomized controlled trial of the clinical effectiveness of schema therapy for personality disorders. *American Journal of Psychiatry, 171*(3), 305–322. https://doi.org/10.1176/appi.ajp.2013.12040518

Bateman, A., & Fonagy, P. (2015). Borderline personality disorder and mood disorders: Mentalizing as a framework for integrated treatment. *Journal of Clinical Psychology, 71*(8), 792–804. https://doi.org/10.1002/jclp.22206

Baumeister, R. F., & Leary, M. R. (1995). The need to belong: Desire for interpersonal attachments as a fundamental human motivation. *Psychological Bulletin, 117*(3), 497. https://doi.org/10.1037/0033-2909.117.3.497

Bordin, E. (1979). The generalizability of the psychoanalytic concept of the working alliance. *Psychotherapy: Theory, Research, and Practice, 16*, 252–260.

Bowlby, J. (1969). *Attachment and loss* (Attachment) (Vol. 1). New York, NY: Basic Books.

Carcione, A., Semerari, A., Nicolò, G., Pedone, R., Popolo, R., Conti, L., … Dimaggio, G. (2011). Metacognitive mastery dysfunctions in personality disorder psychotherapy. *Psychiatry Research, 190*, 60–71. https://doi.org/10.1016/j.psychres.2010.12.032

Carter, J. D., McIntosh, V. V., Jordan, J., Porter, R. J., Frampton, C. M., & Joyce, P. R. (2013). Psychotherapy for depression: A randomized clinical trial comparing schema therapy and cognitive behavior therapy. *Journal of Affective Disorders, 151*(2), 500–505. https://doi.org/10.1016/j.jad.2013.06.034

Centonze, A., Inchausti, F., MacBeth, A., & Dimaggio, G. (2020). Changing embodied dialogical patterns in metacognitive interpersonal therapy. *Journal of Constructivist Psychology*, 1–15. https://doi.org/10.1080/10720537.2020.1717117

Cesario, J., Jonas, K. J., & Carney, D. R. (2017). CRSP special issue on power poses: What was the point and what did we learn? *Comprehensive Results in Social Psychology, 2*(1), 1–5. https://doi.org/10.1080/23743603.2017.1309876
Dimaggio, G., & Lysaker, P. H. (2015). Metacognition and mentalizing in the psychotherapy of patients with psychosis and personality disorders. *Journal of Clinical Psychology, 71*(2), 117–124. https://doi.org/10.1002/jclp.22147
Dimaggio, G., Montano, A., Popolo, R., & Salvatore, G. (2015). *Metacognitive interpersonal therapy for personality disorders: A treatment manual*. London, UK: Routledge. https://doi.org/10.4324/9781315744124
Dimaggio, G., Ottavi, P., Popolo, R., & Salvatore, G. (2020). *Metacognitive interpersonal therapy: Body, imagery and change*. London, UK: Routledge.
Dimaggio, G., & Semerari, A. (2001). Psychopathological narrative forms. *Journal of Constructivist Psychology, 14*(1), 1–23. https://doi.org/10.1080/10720530125913
Fosha, D. (2000). *The transforming power of affect: A model for accelerated change*. New York, NY: Basic Books.
Gazzillo, F., Genova, F., Fedeli, F., Curtis, J. T., Silberschatz, G., Bush, M., & Dazzi, N. (2019). Patients' unconscious testing activity in psychotherapy: A theoretical and empirical overview. *Psychoanalytic Psychology, 36*(2), 173–183. https://doi.org/10.1037/pap0000227
Gendlin, E. (1981). *Focusing* (2nd ed.). New York, NY: Bantam Books.
Gilbert, P. (1989). *Human nature and suffering*. London, UK: Psychology Press.
Gonçalves, M. M., Ribeiro, A. P., Mendes, I. S., Alves, D. E., Silva, J., Rosa, C., … Oliveira, J. T. (2017). Three narrative-based coding systems: Innovative moments, ambivalence and ambivalence resolution. *Psychotherapy Research, 27*(3), 270–282. https://doi.org/10.1080/10503307.2016.1247216
Gordon-King, K., Schweitzer, R. D., & Dimaggio, G. (2018). Metacognitive interpersonal therapy for personality disorders featuring emotional inhibition: A multiple baseline case series. *The Journal of Nervous and Mental Disease, 206*(4), 263–269. https://doi.org/10.1097/NMD.0000000000000789
Greenberg, L. S. (2002). *Emotion focused-therapy. Coaching clients to work with their feelings*. Washington, DC: American Psychological Association.
Hackmann, A., Bennett-Levy, J., & Holmes, E. A. (2011). *Oxford guide to imagery in cognitive therapy*. Oxford, UK: Oxford University Press.
Jørgensen, C. R., Freund, C., Bøye, R., Jordet, H., Andersen, D., & Kjølbye, M. (2013). Outcome of mentalization based and supportive psychotherapy in patients with borderline personality disorder: A randomized trial. *Acta Psychiatrica Scandinavica, 127*(4), 305–317. https://doi.org/10.1111/j.1600-0447.2012.01923.x
Klerman, G., Weissman, M., Rounsaville, B., & Chevron, E. (1984). *Interpersonal psychotherapy of depression* (pp. 7–42). New York, NY: Basic Books. Kupfer, D.
Körük, S., & Özabacı, N. (2018). Şema terapinin depresif bozuklukların tedavisindeki etkililiği: Bir meta-analiz. *Psikiyatride Güncel Yaklaşımlar, 10*(4), 470–480. https://doi.org/10.18863/pgy.361790
Leeds, A. M. (2009). Resources in EMDR and other trauma-focused psychotherapy: A review. *Journal of EMDR Practice and Research, 3*(3), 152–160. https://doi.org/10.1891/1933-3196.3.3.152
Lewinsohn, P. M. (1974). A behavioral approach to depression. In R. J. F. M. M. Katz (Ed.), *The psychology of depression: Contemporary theory and research* (pp. 157–187). Washington, DC: Winston-Wiley.
Lichtenberg, J. D. (1989). *Psychoanalysis and motivation*. Hillsdale, NJ: The Analytic Press Inc.
Liotti, G., & Gilbert, P. (2011). Mentalizing, motivation, and social mentalities: Theoretical considerations and implications for psychotherapy. *Psychology and Psychotherapy: Theory, Research and Practice, 84*(1), 9–25. https://doi.org/10.1348/147608310X520094
Livesley, J. W., Dimaggio, G., & Clarkin, J. F. (Eds.). (2016). *Integrated treatment for personality disorders: A modular approach*. New York, NY: Guilford.
Lowen, A. (1971). *The language of the body*. New York, NY: Macmillan General Reference.

Luborsky, L., & Crits-Christoph, P. (1998). *Understanding transference: The core conflictual relationship theme method* (2nd ed.). New York, NY: Basic Books.
Lynch, T. R., Cheavens, J. S., Cukrowicz, K. C., Thorp, S. R., Bronner, L., & Beyer, J. (2007). Treatment of older adults with comorbid personality disorder and depression: A dialectical behavior therapy approach. *International Journal of Geriatric Psychiatry: A Journal of the Psychiatry of Late Life and Allied Sciences, 22*(2), 131–143. https://doi.org/10.1002/gps.1703
Martin, L. L., & Tesser, A. (1989). Toward a motivational and structural theory of ruminative thought. In J. S. Uleman & J. A. Bargh (Eds.), *Unintended thought*. New York, NY: Guilford.
Matos, M., & Steidl, S. (2020). "You are already all you need to be": A case illustration of compassion focused therapy for shame and perfectionism. *Journal of Clinical Psychology: In Session, 76*(11), 1–18.
McLaughlin, K. A., Borkovec, T. D., & Sibrava, N. J. (2007). The effects of worry and rumination on affect states and cognitive activity. *Behavior Therapy, 38*, 23–38.
Moreno, J. L. (1975). *Psychodrama: Action therapy and principles of practice* (Vol. 3). New York, NY: Beacon House.
Morey, L. C., Shea, M. T., Markowitz, J. C., Stout, R. L., Hopwood, C. J., Gunderson, J. G., … Skodol, A. E. (2010). State effects of major depression on the assessment of personality and personality disorder. *American Journal of Psychiatry, 167*(5), 528–535. https://doi.org/10.1176/appi.ajp.2009.09071023
Newton-Howes, G., Tyrer, P., & Johnson, T. (2006). Personality disorder and the outcome of depression: Meta-analysis of published studies. *The British Journal of Psychiatry, 188*(1), 13–20. https://doi.org/10.1192/bjp.188.1.13
Nolen-Hoeksema, S. (2000). The role of rumination in depressive disorders and mixed anxiety/depressive symptoms. *Journal of Abnormal Psychology, 109*, 504–511. https://doi.org/10.1037/0021-843X.109.3.504
Nolen-Hoeksema, S., Wisco, B. E., & Lyubomirsky, S. (2008). Rethinking rumination. *Perspectives on Psychological Science, 3*(5), 400–424. https://doi.org/10.1111/2Fj.1745-6924.2008.00088.x
Ogden, P., & Fisher, J. (2015). *Sensorimotor psychotherapy*. New York, NY: Norton & Company.
Ottavi, P., Passarella, T., Pasinetti, M., MacBeth, A., Velotti, P., Velotti, A., … Dimaggio, G. (2019). Metacognitive interpersonal mindfulness-based training for worry about interpersonal events: A pilot feasibility and acceptability study. *Journal of Nervous and Mental Disease, 207*(11), 944–950. https://doi.org/10.1097/NMD.0000000000001054
Ottavi, P., Passarella, T., Pasinetti, M., Salvatore, G., & Dimaggio, G. (2015). Adapting mindfulness for treating personality disorders. In W. J. Livesley, G. Dimaggio, & J. F. Clarkin (Eds.), *Integrated treatment for personality disorders*. London, UK: Guilford Press.
Panksepp, J. (1998). The periconscious substrates of consciousness: Affective states and the evolutionary origins of the SELF. *Journal of Consciousness Studies, 5*(5–6), 566–582.
Panksepp, J., & Biven, L. (2012). *The archaeology of mind: Neuroevolutionary origins of human emotions (Norton series on interpersonal neurobiology)*. New York, NY: WW Norton & Company.
Papageorgiou, C., & Wells, A. (2008). *Depressive rumination: Nature, theory and treatment*. Chichester, UK: Wiley.
Perls, F., Hefferline, G., & Goodman, P. (1951). *Gestalt therapy*. New York, NY: Julian Press.
Price, C. J., & Hooven, C. (2018). Interoceptive awareness skills for emotion regulation: Theory and approach of mindful awareness in body-oriented therapy (MABT). *Frontiers in Psychology, 9*, 798. https://doi.org/10.3389/fpsyg.2018.00798
Reich, J. (2003). The effect of Axis II disorders on the outcome of treatment of anxiety and unipolar depressive disorders: A review. *Journal of Personality Disorders, 17*(5), 387–405. https://doi.org/10.1521/pedi.17.5.387.22972
Richman, M., Unoka, Z., Dudas, R., & Demetrovics, Z. (2018). Rumination in borderline personality disorder: Meta-analysis. *PsyArXiv*. https://doi.org/10.31234/osf.io/7twf4

Robichaud, M., & Dugas, M. J. (2006). A cognitive-behavioral treatment targeting intolerance of uncertainty. In A. Wells & G. C. Davey (Eds.), *Worry and its psychological disorders: Theory, assessment and treatment* (pp. 289–304). Chichester, UK: Wiley.

Rossouw, T. I., & Fonagy, P. (2012). Mentalization-based treatment for self-harm in adolescents: A randomized controlled trial. *Journal of the American Academy of Child & Adolescent Psychiatry, 51*(12), 1304–1313. https://doi.org/10.1016/j.jaac.2012.09.018

Safran, J. D., & Muran, J. C. (2000). *Negotiating the therapeutic alliance: A relational treatment guide*. New York, NY: Guilford Press.

Santos, V., Paes, F., Pereira, V., Arias-Carrión, O., Silva, A. C., Carta, M. G., … Machado, S. (2013). The role of positive emotion and contributions of positive psychology in depression treatment: Systematic review. *Clinical Practice and Epidemiology in Mental Health*. https://psycnet.apa.org/doi/10.2174/1745017901309010221

Seligman, M. E., & Csikszentmihalyi, M. (2014). Positive psychology: An introduction. In *Flow and the foundations of positive psychology* (pp. 279–298). Dordrecht, The Netherlands: Springer.

Semerari, A., Carcione, A., Dimaggio, G., Falcone, M., Nicolò, G., Procacci, M., & Alleva, G. (2003). How to evaluate metacognitive functioning in psychotherapy? The metacognition assessment scale and its applications. *Clinical Psychology & Psychotherapy, 10*, 238–261. https://doi.org/10.1002/cpp.362

Semerari, A., Carcione, A., Dimaggio, G., Nicolo, G., Pedone, R., & Procacci, M. (2005). Metarepresentative functions in borderline personality disorder. *Journal of Personality Disorders, 19*(6), 690–710. https://doi.org/10.1521/pedi.2005.19.6.690

Semerari, A., Colle, L., Pellecchia, G., Buccione, I., Carcione, A., Dimaggio, G., … Pedone, R. (2014). Metacognitive dysfunctions in personality disorders: Correlations with disorder severity and personality styles. *Journal of Personality Disorders, 28*(6), 751–766. https://doi.org/10.1521/pedi_2014_28_137

Tomasello, M., Carpenter, M., Call, J., Behne, T., & Moll, H. (2005). Understanding and sharing intentions: The origins of cultural cognition. *Behavioral and Brain Sciences, 28*(5), 675–691. https://doi.org/10.1017/S0140525X05220125

Watkins, E. R., Moberly, N. J., & Moulds, M. L. (2008). Processing mode causally influences emotional reactivity: Distinct effects of abstract versus concrete construal on emotional response. *Emotion, 8*, 364–378. https://doi.org/10.1037/1528-3542.8.3.364

Weiss, J. (1993). *How psychotherapy works: Process and technique*. New York, NY: Guilford Press.

Weissman, M. M., Markowitz, J. C., & Klerman, J. L. (2000). *Comprehensive guide to interpersonal psychotherapy*. New York, NY: Basic Books.

White, M., & Epston, D. (1990). *Narrative means to therapeutic ends*. New York, NY: W. W. Norton.

Zimmerman, M. (1994). Diagnosing personality disorders: A review of issues and research methods. *Archives of General Psychiatry, 51*(3), 225–245. https://doi.org/10.1001/archpsyc.1994.03950030061006

Part III
Concluding Remarks

Chapter 11
Concluding Remarks: Where Do We Come From? Where Are We Moving To? Towards the Development of *Precision Psychotherapy*

Guillermo de la Parra, Alex Behn, and Paula Dagnino

Abstract After our journey through the ongoing paradigm shift from a disorder-centred approach to a person-centred approach and then to a functional domains perspective, we introduce the RDoC framework as a current working model and research agenda to support this paradigm shift. Furthermore, we discuss how it orients the authors of each chapter of this book. After detailing the contents of each chapter, we discuss whether it is possible to define precision psychotherapy and determine its contributions to clinical work.

Keywords Functional domains · Precision medicine · Precision psychotherapy · Personality disorder · Depression

In daily clinical practice, we continue to employ a categorical approach to make mental health diagnoses and plan treatment delivery. For these diagnoses, we resort to the usual DSM/ICD criteria, since they have been used for decades in communications among professionals, at an administrative level, in research, and even to apply for funding, which until recently required DSM/ICD diagnoses to finance

G. de la Parra (✉)
Department of Psychiatry, Pontificia Universidad Católica de Chile, Santiago, Chile

Millennium Institute for Research in Depression and Personality (MIDAP), Santiago, Chile
e-mail: gdelaparra@uc.cl

A. Behn
Millennium Institute for Research in Depression and Personality (MIDAP), Santiago, Chile

School of Psychology, Pontificia Universidad Católica de Chile, Santiago, Chile

P. Dagnino
Millennium Institute for Research in Depression and Personality (MIDAP), Santiago, Chile

Faculty of Psychology, Universidad Alberto Hurtado, Santiago, Chile

G. de la Parra et al. (eds.), *Depression and Personality Dysfunction*, Depression and Personality, https://doi.org/10.1007/978-3-030-70699-9_11

projects. As is well known, this approach derives from the Kraepelinian model, according to which mental disease is a discrete medical condition with clear boundaries between health and disease, and with clear diagnostic boundaries between disorders. In other words, the person either has a disorder – e.g. a personality disorder – or not (Trull & Durrett, 2005). It is further assumed that patients suffering from a disorder require treatment, whereas those not afflicted by one do not (Trull & Durrett, 2005). This approach was once applied to depression, which was largely regarded as a discrete, one-dimensional entity, and to personality disorders. Although this stance was comfortable, especially for clinicians, and even though it was designed to minimize uncertainty and sooth those who felt part of the "non-diseased", categorical diagnoses began to be challenged as early as the 1990s, particularly regarding personality disorders (Arbeitskreis OPD, 1996). Gradually, more and more critical voices echoed these views, drawing attention to the empirical unsustainability of the attempts to differentiate people with and without personality disorders in a categorical manner (Clark, Cuthbert, Lewis-Fernandez, Narrow, & Reed, 2017; Ehrenthal & Benecke, 2019; Haslam, Holland, & Kuppens, 2012; Zimmermann, 2014). Nowadays, authors largely suggest that personality traits are distributed within a continuum allowing for a gradual transition to pathological manifestations, as the evidence supports the existence of a range from normal and abnormal personality (Pukrop, Herpertz, Sass, & Steinmeyer, 1998; Trull & Durrett, 2005; Tyrer, 2020; Widiger, Simonsen, Krueger, Livesley, & Verheul, 2005).

The DSM-5 Alternative Model (American Psychiatric Association, 2013) is informed by these scientific advances; however, it preserves its traditional categories in the rest of its classificatory system. Interestingly, the authors focus on dysfunctions, noting that, in their alternative model, "personality disorders are characterized by impairments in *personality functioning* and pathological personality traits" (p. 761, our emphasis). This concept is also adopted in other classification systems and in the present book, as we will discuss later. Amid this knowledge milieu, the impact caused by the ICD-11 (World Health Organization, 2018) is worth noting. Its presentation and discussion, led by Jeffrey Reed at the 15th International Congress of the International Society for the Study of Personality Disorders (ISSPD) in Heidelberg, Germany, in September 2017, caused great controversy and heated reactions from the audience (Behn A., personal communication, 2017). The ICD-11 abolishes personality disorder categories, but defines a continuum that comprises personality difficulties, mild disorder, moderate disorder, and severe disorder, taking into account a set of dimensional constructs: emotional dysregulation vs stability, extroversion vs introversion, antagonism vs compliance, and impulsiveness vs repression. As we can see, this approach also represents a dimensional perspective informed by the assessment of functionality.

Research Domain Criteria (RDoC; Cuthbert, 2014, 2015), which see pathology "in terms of deviations in fundamental functional systems" (Cuthbert, 2014; p. 31), are the most radical contribution in this regard. RDoC, as described in other chapters of this book, is a "framework that is designed and intended to both foster and accommodate new research findings on a continual basis" (p. 30). It defines five domains of functioning that contain various constructs that can be studied or described and enriched at multiple levels of analysis, ranging from the genetic and the molecular to manifest behaviour and self-reports. These functions are influenced by developmental and environmental factors.

According to RDoC and the accumulated empirical evidence, which increases day by day, human mental/cerebral/behavioural functioning can be evaluated relative to a normal curve: as it deviates from the curve, it becomes dysfunctional and constitutes a pathology. The RDoC is currently the most developed effort within a broader functional domains perspective. An interesting advantage of focusing on functional domains is the chance to develop relevant therapeutic targets within a single traditional diagnostic category. For instance, self-critical dysfunction and behavioural inhibition can be key therapeutic targets for depressive patients. Similarly, one functional domain dysfunction can work as a transdiagnostic therapeutic target so that interventions can have a transdiagnostic utility. For example, interventions to help improve emotional dysregulation can be useful for patients with borderline personality disorder comorbid with depression, or even in patients with anger control issues or mood dysregulation. This can lead to the development of modular treatments that can be eventually tailored to improve affected functional domains. This approach is addressed in the chapters of this book, of which we will highlight some examples below.

Approaching psychopathology and its treatment based on transdiagnostic dysfunctions brings us to the domain of precision medicine (Insel & Cuthbert, 2015). Developed in the oncology field, this concept indicates that, thanks to new insights into the biology and genetics of cancer, it is possible to indicate more effective treatments for specific manifestations of this disease. "In precision medicine, the focus is on identifying which approaches will be effective for which patients based on genetic, environmental, and lifestyle factors" (Genetics Home Reference, 2019). As is well known, mental health treatments are largely based on psychosocial interventions (psychotherapy); psychotherapy influences environmental factors and thus brain functioning across disorders (Barsaglini, Sartori, Benetti, Pettersson-Yeo, & Mechelli, 2014), including personality dysfunction (Gabbard, 2000; Mancke et al., 2018), which can be mediated by epigenetic factors (Jiménez et al., 2018). Therefore, and in line with the aim of this book, namely, to address psychopathology based on a functional domain perspective, we advocate for the application of precision psychotherapy to standard mental health care. In the words of Insel and Cuthbert (2015), "one of the most powerful and precise interventions to alter such (brain) activity may be targeted psychotherapy ... which uses the brain's intrinsic plasticity to alter neural circuits and as a consequence, deleterious thoughts and behavior" (p. 500).

The book's introduction contextualizes the title of our book, "Depression and Personality Dysfunction: An Integrative Functional Domains Perspective" and provides a logic for the delivery of its contents. First, in line with the points made above, the book develops the idea that personality functioning includes relevant domains of functioning to be targeted transdiagnostically, including self and other functioning, self-criticism, affect dysregulation, reflective functioning, social dysfunction, meta-cognitive capacity, and identity regulation. In this context, we express our preference for the term *personality dysfunction* instead of personality disorder. This distinction is quite relevant from a dimensional perspective and also acknowledges a continuum from healthy personality traits to sub-diagnostic threshold dysfunction and into the realm of full-blown personality pathology. In other words, it broadens the scope of clinically relevant deficits in functional domains integrated into the notion of personality functioning. The authors of each chapter work within this contemporary perspective while also incorporating the concept of complex depression, which reflects the multidimensionality of the depression diagnosis and its aetiology – discussed in another volume of this series – as well as the multiple factors that take place in the evolution, prognosis, and therapeutic response of this dysfunction. In the introductory Chap. 1, "Depression and Personality Dysfunction: Towards the Understanding of Complex Depression", the authors adopt the perspective of "functional domains that are differentially affected in depression concurrent with personality dysfunction and on personality styles as well as how the co-occurrence of both impacts on the severity of the condition" (p. 1 of the chapter). Interestingly, the authors stress the relevance of intermediate phenotypes, which underlie complex phenotypes such as depression and its interaction with personality. This approach would allow both understanding of common or differential underlying mechanisms to the respective phenotype and also enabling practitioners to suggest treatments focused on these intermediate phenotypes.

In Chap. 2, "The Functional Domain of Identity", part of Section I, "Domains of Personality Dysfunction Complicating the Presentation and Treatment of Depression", the authors present an in-depth discussion of identity dysfunctions, addressing their role not only in personality disorders but also in depression, with which they have a bidirectional relationship: doubts about one's identity can cause depression and early depression can have an impact on identity development. The authors show how the concept of identity is relevant for understanding the comorbidity between depression and the so-called borderline personality disorder (BPD). They take chronic emptiness to be a manifestation of both depression and BPD and assert that as long as this dysfunction (which could be regarded as an intermediate phenotype) remains untreated, neither depression nor personality dysfunction will show any improvements. Chapter 3, "The Functional Domain of Affect Regulation", presents a detailed exchange and discussion with the RDoC model, understanding affect regulation "as a mechanism that lays at the crossroads of several of the systems proposed by the RDoC" (p. 4 of the chapter). The authors propose a developmental approach based on attachment theory and developmental research in which affect regulation constitutes a fundamental element of self-development, with this function being linked to the RDoC dimensions "social processes" and "arousal/regulatory systems". Chapter 4, "The Functional Domain of Self-Other Regulation", operates as a continuation of the previous chapter: the authors present a model for understanding this functional domain (and its dysfunction) as a result of the interaction of three systems: stress regulation (negative valence system + arousal/modulatory systems), reward (positive valence systems), and mentalizing systems (systems for social processes). These two chapters rise to the challenge of meeting the recommendations of the RDoC initiative in order to understand each functional domain/

dysfunction, including developmental trajectories and environmental effects, especially with respect to the pathogenic role of adversity in childhood. Chapter 5, "The Domain of Social Dysfunction in Complex Depressive Disorders", focuses on the units of analysis of the "behaviour" and "self-report" of the RDoC model and describes how five domains of this dysfunction manifest themselves in various types of complex depression. The authors assert that treatment must address both depressive symptoms and functional improvements, that is, this approach operates at the level of phenotypic expression. In Chap. 6, "Neurobiological Findings Underlying Personality Dysfunction in Depression: From Vulnerability to Differential Susceptibility", after examining the personality-depression link and elaborating on the neurobiology of personality traits in this disorder, the authors address gene-environment correlation and gene-environment interaction. The authors cover a range of topics from RdoC genetic levels of analysis to the phenotypic expression of environment susceptibility. The authors confirm the points made thus far: "there is now increasing consensus that most common psychiatric disorders, such as depression and anxiety, are best explained as complex disorders involving dysfunctions in several biological systems in interaction with environmental factors" (p. 14, Chap. 6). The section concludes with Chap. 7, "The Functional lDomain of Self-Criticism", whose authors conduct a detailed examination of this domain of functioning, described as an aberration in depression and/or personality dysfunctions. This is a good example of how the construct can manifest itself "normally" or reach pathological and self-destructive levels. The situation becomes more complex after interaction with the moderating effect of personality structure, with more vulnerable personality structures exhibiting more pathogenic self-criticism. The authors also show how different therapeutic approaches can deal with the same dysfunction, in this case, one of a self-critical nature.

In Section II: "Integrative Models of Depression and Personality Dysfunction: Implications for Diagnosis and Treatment", the first two chapters address complex depression. In Chap. 8, "Complex Depression and Early Adverse Stress: A Domain-Based Diagnostic Approach", after reviewing the factors that increase depression complexity, the authors discuss the role of childhood adversity in depressive pathology, taking into account its manifestations, complications, prognosis, and treatment. Based on their own research, they propose a model aimed at differentiating complex depression from non-complex depression. Chapter 9, "Complex Depression in High-Pressure Care Settings: Strategies and Therapeutic Competences", addresses complex depression and its underlying dysfunctions, focusing on environmental factors. The authors link complex depression with the concept of *difficult patient*, noting that an adverse environmental context plays a key role regarding not only the patient's dysfunctional manifestations but also the practitioner's therapeutic capabilities and his/her relationship with the patient. The chapter offers multiple therapeutic approaches to specific personality dysfunctions. Chapter 10, "Modular Treatment for Complex Depression According to Metacognitive Interpersonal Therapy", offers a clear example of the therapeutic approach based on tackling specific dysfunctions that underlie the clinical manifestation (intermediate phenotype). The authors detail specific modules aimed at treating specific dysfunctions in order to alleviate depressive symptoms and/or manifestations of personality structure vulnerabilities, representing a clear example of transdiagnostic treatments.

A look at the chapters of this volume reveals certain building blocks of knowledge that, apart from contributing to clinical work, help to ground future research. These building blocks provide several insights: that development results from the interplay of developmental tasks, relatedness, and self-definition; that alterations in this balance lead to different susceptibilities to environmental stressors that generate depression, causing self-critical dysfunction (which can be treated in a number of ways); that there seems to be crossed aetiopathogenesis between personality dysfunctions and depression; that childhood adversity is a critical factor in people's lives that makes them vulnerable to several pathologies (a vulnerability that has been decanted into a single "p" factor) (Caspi et al., 2014); that therapeutic interventions focused on mechanisms (intermediate phenotype) can generate symptomatic responses in depression and personality functioning; and that paradigms in the last few years have shifted from a disorder-centred approach to a person-centred approach and then (nowadays) to a dysfunction-centred approach. The latter approach, based on the insights presented in this book, can be referred to as *precision psychotherapy*. Nevertheless, in the psychotherapy field, the concept of precision medicine can be nuanced: the association between an altered functional domain and the therapeutic approach adopted, as noted above, is not univocal. Many examples can be presented of how a single dysfunction, self-criticism, emotional dysregulation, depressive inhibition, or identity diffusion could be successfully addressed with a variety of approaches. How can we account for this phenomenon? Does each strategy target a variety of unknown, unrecorded intermediate phenotypes that underlie measurable phenotypes, which is where we are recording a change? Future comparative studies might yield more information about intervention accuracy.

The clinical relevance of the RDoC initiative has been disputed in the literature (Carpenter Jr, 2016); however, the approaches presented in this book have all consistently taken into account the clinical perspective. Thus, specific tools such as those discussed here should inform the work of clinicians, who will apply them following the principles of evidence-based practice (American Psychological Association, 2005). As is well known, evidence-based practice rests on three pillars: best available evidence – e.g. some of the guidelines presented in this book – clinician expertise, and patient characteristics, culture, and preferences. In this regard, evidence-based practice presupposes some form of personalization, namely, the balancing of best available evidence with the personal characteristics of the patient, the therapies, and the context in which treatment is delivered. Treatment indication will result from a collaborative decision-making process involving the therapist and the patient (Mulder, Murray, & Rucklidge, 2017), in which the subjectivity of the latter and the possibility of establishing a therapeutic alliance are essential. No specific intervention will have an effect if it is not sown in the fertile ground of a good therapeutic bond, which in all likelihood requires personalization and not the robotic delivery of treatment manuals. In this regard, some problems remain underdeveloped. First, a precision psychotherapy model will heavily rely on the assessment of affected deficits in functional domains. It is yet not clear how to accomplish this, mainly because most evidence-based assessment is geared towards the detection of standard psychopathology and not underlying, transdiagnostic deficits in functional domains. In this regard, the development of broadband measures to capture such deficits is key and can be aided by the use of state-of-the-art adaptive testing technologies. It is clear that even though conceptually sound, the clinical effectiveness of personalized psychotherapy is strongly contingent on the precision and practicality of the initial assessment of functional domains. Following this difficulty, precision psychotherapy requires the development of modularization, that is, the structuring of sets of interventions that target deficits in specific functional domains or intermediate phenotypes. This framework is also conceptually sound, but its implementation poses significant challenges, including the construction of modules, the design of specific delivery algorithms for modules (i.e. what comes first), the specification and creation of sensitive outcome measures to evaluate incremental progress on each functional domain, and, surely, profound changes in clinical training. Furthermore, some questions remain with respect to the role of the relationship in therapeutic change: is it always a moderating factor, or is its mediating effect on change scientifically demonstrable? The practitioner's ability to establish a bond with the patient – whom he/she will try to understand upon the basis of the patient's subjectivity, his/her own expertise, and empirical evidence – will depend on his/her practical wisdom (Jiménez & Botto, 2020). It is our hope that this book will enrich this practical wisdom from a scientific perspective.

Acknowledgements This work was funded by the ANID-Millennium Science Initiative/ Millennium Institute for Research on Depression and Personality-MIDAP.

References

American Psychiatric Association. (2013). *Diagnostic and statistical manual of mental disorders* (5th ed.). Arlington, VA: American Psychiatric Association.

American Psychological Association. (2005). *Policy statement on evidence-based practice in psychology.* https://www.apa.org/practice/guidelines/evidence-based-statement

Arbeitskreis, O. P. D. (1996). *Operationalisierte psychodynamische diagnostik. Grundlagen und Manual.* Bern, Switzerland: Huber.

Barsaglini, A., Sartori, G., Benetti, S., Pettersson-Yeo, W., & Mechelli, A. (2014). The effects of psychotherapy on brain function: A systematic and critical review. *Progress in Neurobiology, 114*, 1–14.

Carpenter, W. T., Jr. (2016). The RDoC controversy: Alternate paradigm or dominant paradigm? *The American Journal of Psychiatry, 173*(6), 562–563. https://doi.org/10.1176/appi.ajp.2016.16030347

Caspi, A., Houts, R. M., Belsky, D. W., Goldman-Mellor, S. J., Harrington, H., Israel, S., … Moffitt, T. E. (2014). The p factor: One general psychopathology factor in the structure of psychiatric disorders? *Clinical Psychological Science: A Journal of the Association for Psychological Science, 2*(2), 119–137. https://doi.org/10.1177/2167702613497473

Clark, L. A., Cuthbert, B., Lewis-Fernandez, R., Narrow, W. E., & Reed, G. M. (2017). Three approaches to understanding and classifying mental disorder: ICD-11, DSM-5, and the National

Institute of Mental Health's Research Domain Criteria (RDoC). *Psychological Science in the Public Interest, 18*(2), 72–145. https://doi.org/10.1177/1529100617727266
Cuthbert, B. N. (2014). The RDoC framework: Facilitating transition from ICD/DSM to dimensional approaches that integrate neuroscience and psychopathology. *World Psychiatry: Official Journal of the World Psychiatric Association (WPA), 13*(1), 28–35. https://doi.org/10.1002/wps.20087
Cuthbert, B. N. (2015). Research domain criteria: Toward future psychiatric nosologies. *Dialogues in Clinical Neuroscience, 17*(1), 89–97.
Ehrenthal, J. C., & Benecke, C. (2019). Tailored treatment planning for individuals with personality disorders: The OPD approach. In U. Kramer (Ed.), *Case formulation for personality disorders: Tailoring psychotherapy to the individual client*. Cambridge, MA: Elsevier.
Gabbard, G. O. (2000). A neurobiologically informed perspective on psychotherapy. *The British Journal of Psychiatry: The Journal of Mental Science, 177*, 117–122. https://doi.org/10.1192/bjp.177.2.117
Genetics Home Reference. (2019). *Lister Hill national center for biomedical communications*. Bethesda, MD: U.S. National Library of Medicine National Institutes of Health Department of Health & Human Services.
Haslam, N., Holland, E., & Kuppens, P. (2012). Categories versus dimensions in personality and psychopathology: A quantitative review of taxometric research. *Psychological Medicine, 42*(5), 903–920. https://doi.org/10.1017/S0033291711001966
Insel, T. R., & Cuthbert, B. N. (2015). Brain disorders? Precisely: Precision medicine comes to psychiatry. *Science, 348*(6234), 499–500. https://doi.org/10.1126/science.aab2358
Jiménez, J., & Botto, A. (2020). Models in depression and clinical judgment, or how to use different etiopathogenic models with a particular patient. In J. Jiménez, A. Botto, & P. Fonagy (Eds.), *Etiopathogenic theories and models in Depression*. Springer. in preparation.
Jiménez, J., Botto, A., Herrera, L., Leighton, C., Rossi, J., Quevedo, Y., … Luyten, P. (2018). Psychotherapy and genetic neuroscience: An emerging dialog. *Frontiers in Genetics, 9*(257), 1–19. https://doi.org/10.3389/fgene.2018.00257
Mancke, F., Schmitt, R., Winter, D., Niedtfeld, I., Herpertz, S. C., & Schmahl, C. (2018). Assessing the marks of change: How psychotherapy alters the brain structure in women with borderline personality disorder. *Journal of Psychiatry & Neuroscience: JPN, 43*(3), 171.
Mulder, R., Murray, G., & Rucklidge, J. (2017). Common versus specific factors in psychotherapy: Opening the black box. *The Lancet Psychiatry, 4*(12), 953–962. https://doi.org/10.1016/S2215-0366(17)30100-1
Pukrop, R., Herpertz, S., Sass, H., & Steinmeyer, E. M. (1998). Personality and personality disorders. A facet theoretical analysis of the similarity relationships. *Journal of Personality Disorders, 12*(3), 226–246. https://doi.org/10.1521/pedi.1998.12.3.226
Trull, T., & Durrett, C. (2005). Categorical and dimensional models of personality disorder. *Annual Review of Clinical Psychology, 1*(1), 355–380. https://doi.org/10.1146/annurev.clinpsy.1.102803.144009
Tyrer, P. (2020). Why we need to take personality disorder out of the doghouse. *The British Journal of Psychiatry: The Journal of Mental Science, 216*(2), 65–66. https://doi.org/10.1192/bjp.2019.125
Widiger, T. A., Simonsen, E., Krueger, R., Livesley, W. J., & Verheul, R. (2005). Personality disorder research agenda for the DSM-V. *Journal of Personality Disorders, 19*(3), 315–338. https://doi.org/10.1521/pedi.2005.19.3.315
World Health Organization. (2018). *International classification of diseases for mortality and morbidity statistics* (11th Revision). https://icd.who.int/browse11/l-m/en
Zimmermann, J. (2014). Paradigmenwechsel in der Klassifikation von Persönlichkeitsstörungen. *Psychotherapie im Dialog, 15*(3), 1–10. https://doi.org/10.1055/s-0034-1388629

Index

G. de la Parra et al. (eds.), *Depression and Personality Dysfunction*, Depression and Personality, https://doi.org/10.1007/978-3-030-70699-9

D

N

O

CPSIA information can be obtained
at www.ICGtesting.com
Printed in the USA
LVHW081258101121
702733LV00015B/63